Blackwell's Five-Minute Veterinary Consult
Clinical Companion

Equine Toxicology

Blackwell's Five-Minute Veterinary Consult
Clinical Companion

Equine Toxicology

Edited by

Lynn R. Hovda, RPh, DVM, MS, DACVIM
University of Minnesota
St. Paul, MN, USA

Dionne Benson, DVM, JD
The Stronach Group
Aurora, ON, Canada

Robert H. Poppenga, DVM, PhD, DABVT
California Animal Health and Food Safety
Laboratory System
Davis, CA, USA

WILEY Blackwell

This edition first published 2022
© 2022 John Wiley & Sons, Inc.

All rights reserved. No part of this publication may be reproduced, stored in a retrieval system, or transmitted, in any form or by any means, electronic, mechanical, photocopying, recording or otherwise, except as permitted by law. Advice on how to obtain permission to reuse material from this title is available at http://www.wiley.com/go/permissions.

The right of Lynn R. Hovda, Dionne Benson, and Robert H. Poppenga to be identified as the author of the editorial material in this work has been asserted in accordance with law.

Registered Office
John Wiley & Sons, Inc., 111 River Street, Hoboken, NJ 07030, USA

Editorial Office
111 River Street, Hoboken, NJ 07030, USA

For details of our global editorial offices, customer services, and more information about Wiley products visit us at www.wiley.com.

Wiley also publishes its books in a variety of electronic formats and by print-on-demand. Some content that appears in standard print versions of this book may not be available in other formats.

Limit of Liability/Disclaimer of Warranty
The contents of this work are intended to further general scientific research, understanding, and discussion only and are not intended and should not be relied upon as recommending or promoting scientific method, diagnosis, or treatment by physicians for any particular patient. In view of ongoing research, equipment modifications, changes in governmental regulations, and the constant flow of information relating to the use of medicines, equipment, and devices, the reader is urged to review and evaluate the information provided in the package insert or instructions for each medicine, equipment, or device for, among other things, any changes in the instructions or indication of usage and for added warnings and precautions. While the publisher and authors have used their best efforts in preparing this work, they make no representations or warranties with respect to the accuracy or completeness of the contents of this work and specifically disclaim all warranties, including without limitation any implied warranties of merchantability or fitness for a particular purpose. No warranty may be created or extended by sales representatives, written sales materials or promotional statements for this work. The fact that an organization, website, or product is referred to in this work as a citation and/or potential source of further information does not mean that the publisher and authors endorse the information or services the organization, website, or product may provide or recommendations it may make. This work is sold with the understanding that the publisher is not engaged in rendering professional services. The advice and strategies contained herein may not be suitable for your situation. You should consult with a specialist where appropriate. Further, readers should be aware that websites listed in this work may have changed or disappeared between when this work was written and when it is read. Neither the publisher nor authors shall be liable for any loss of profit or any other commercial damages, including but not limited to special, incidental, consequential, or other damages.

Library of Congress Cataloging-in-Publication Data

Names: Hovda, Lynn R., 1951– editor. | Benson, Dionne, editor. | Poppenga, Robert H., editor.
Title: Blackwell's five-minute veterinary consult clinical companion. Equine toxicology / edited by Lynn R. Hovda, Dionne Benson, Robert H. Poppenga.
Other titles: Equine toxicology | Five minute veterinary consult.
Description: First edition. | Hoboken : Wiley, 2022. | Series: Blackwell's five-minute veterinary consult series | Includes bibliographical references and index.
Identifiers: LCCN 2021027324 (print) | LCCN 2021027325 (ebook) | ISBN 9781119671497 (paperback) | ISBN 9781119671503 (adobe pdf) | ISBN 9781119671534 (epub)
Subjects: MESH: Horses | Poisoning–veterinary | Drug-Related Side Effects and Adverse Reactions–veterinary
Classification: LCC SF959 (print) | LCC SF959 (ebook) | NLM SF 959 | DDC 636.1/0895952–dc23
LC record available at https://lccn.loc.gov/2021027324
LC ebook record available at https://lccn.loc.gov/2021027325

Cover Design: Wiley
Cover Images: © Mahlon Bauman, Shelley Paulson, Lynn Hovda

Set in 10.5/13pt Berkeley by Straive, Pondicherry, India

Printed in Singapore

M105523_300821

Dedications

This textbook in equine toxicology is an extension of *Blackwell's Five Minute Veterinary Consult: Canine and Feline* by Drs. Larry Tilley and Frank Smith. We are thankful for their foresight and wisdom in beginning this series and grateful to be a part of the stream with the first edition of this textbook.

The editors of this textbook would like to thank the authors whose dedication to toxicology and depth of knowledge helped make this book a reality. It would not have been possible without their donation of time and effort. A special thank you as well to the veterinary students who each day challenge us to become better at our respective jobs, whether it is teaching, industry, or private practice.

In fond remembrance of Dr Gary Osweiler, mentor and friend. I miss his wisdom, support and enthusiasm for toxicology. There are not enough words in the English language to adequately express my appreciation for my co-editors, Dr Dionne Benson and Dr Bob Poppenga. Somehow "whew" and "you rock" don't say nearly enough. To my colleagues at Pet Poison Helpline – a heartfelt thank you. Finally, to old friends, many gone but forever in my heart, and to Bob and Tyne, the cornerstones of my world.

Lynn R. Hovda

Thank you to each of my mentors – both human and horse. Especially Dr Lynn Hovda, Dr Rick Arthur, and Dr Mary Scollay. You have taught me and inspired me. To Oliver and Henry who taught me to fly – if only for a moment. And to my family, especially Paul, who singlehandedly makes our crazy life work.

Dionne Benson

I want to thank all of my veterinary toxicology colleagues for their enthusiasm and advocacy for and commitment to the specialty. It is a small but mutually supportive group which embraces a One Health approach to keeping animals, humans, and our environment healthy. A special thanks to those veterinary toxicology trailblazers who, over the years, influenced me and confirmed that I made the right career choice.

Robert H. Poppenga

Contents

Contributor List xi
About the Companion Website xv

SECTION 1 Clinical Toxicology 1

Chapter 1 Forensic Investigation of Equine Intoxications 3
Chapter 2 Necropsy Analysis. 7
Chapter 3 Laboratory Testing Considerations 14
Chapter 4 Treating an Intoxicated Animal: Antidotes and Therapeutic Medications . . . 19
Chapter 5 Compounded Medication 29

SECTION 2 Specific Toxins and Toxicants 33

Drugs: Illicit and Recreational 35

Chapter 6 Cobalt. 37
Chapter 7 Cocaine 41
Chapter 8 Dermorphin 45
Chapter 9 Growth Hormone and Secretagogues 49
Chapter 10 Marijuana. 53
Chapter 11 Methamphetamine/Amphetamine 58
Chapter 12 Opioids 62
Chapter 13 Selective Androgen (SARMS) and Estrogen Receptor (SERMS) Modulators . 67
Chapter 14 Synthetic Cannabinoids 72

Drugs: Prescription 77

Chapter 15 Antipsychotic Agents – Reserpine and Fluphenazine. 79
Chapter 16 Benzodiazepines. 84
Chapter 17 Beta$_2$ Agonists – Clenbuterol and Albuterol 88
Chapter 18 Bisphosphonates 92
Chapter 19 Gabapentin 97
Chapter 20 Iodine. 101
Chapter 21 Medroxyprogesterone Acetate 106
Chapter 22 Methylxanthine: Caffeine, Theobromine, Theophylline 110
Chapter 23 Nonsteroidal Anti-inflammatory Drugs (NSAIDs) 116
Chapter 24 Levothyroxine. 121
Chapter 25 Vitamin D (Calciferol) 125

Insecticides, Herbicides and Farm Chemicals 129

Chapter 26	Amitraz	131
Chapter 27	Cholinesterase-Inhibiting Carbamate Pesticides	137
Chapter 28	Cholinesterase-Inhibiting Organophosphate Pesticides	142
Chapter 29	Fertilizers – Nitrates, Urea, Phosphates, and Others	147
Chapter 30	Herbicides	151
Chapter 31	Paraquat and Diquat	156
Chapter 32	Pentachlorophenol (PCP)	161
Chapter 33	Pyrethrins and Pyrethroid Insecticides	165

Ionophores and Growth Promotants 171

Chapter 34	Ionophores	173
Chapter 35	Ractopamine	178
Chapter 36	Zilpaterol	182

Metals 187

Chapter 37	Arsenic	189
Chapter 38	Fluoride	193
Chapter 39	Iron	197
Chapter 40	Lead	202
Chapter 41	Selenium	207

Mycotoxins / Fungus 213

Chapter 42	Aflatoxins	215
Chapter 43	Fescue (Endophyte-infected Tall Fescue)	220
Chapter 44	Fumonisins	227
Chapter 45	Fusaria	231
Chapter 46	Slaframine	235
Chapter 47	Tremorgenic Mycotoxins	238

Other Toxins 243

Chapter 48	*Clostridium botulinum* Toxin	245
Chapter 49	Cyanide	250
Chapter 50	Sodium Chloride (Salt)	254

Plants and Biotoxins 259

Chapter 51	Alsike Clover (*Trifolium hybridum*)	261
Chapter 52	Blue-green Algae (Cyanobacteria)	265
Chapter 53	Cardiotoxic Plants	271
Chapter 54	Day Blooming Jessamine (*Cestrum diurnum*)	277

Chapter 55	Death Camas (*Zigadenus* spp.)	282
Chapter 56	Hemlock (Poison Hemlock – *Conium maculatum*; Water Hemlock – *Cicuta* spp.)	287
Chapter 57	Hoary Alyssum (*Berteroa incana*)	294
Chapter 58	Jimsonweed (*Datura stramonium*)	300
Chapter 59	Kleingrass (*Panicum coloratum*)	306
Chapter 60	Lantana (*Lantana camara*)	310
Chapter 61	Locoweed (*Astragalus* and *Oxytropis*) Poisoning in Horses	315
Chapter 62	Narrowleaf Milkweed (*Asclepias fascicularis*)	322
Chapter 63	Nightshades (*Solanum* spp.)	326
Chapter 64	Oleander (*Nerium oleander* and *Cascabela thevetia*)	330
Chapter 65	Pyrrolizidine Alkaloids	336
Chapter 66	Rayless Goldenrod (*Isocoma pluriflora*)	344
Chapter 67	*Rhododendron* spp.	350
Chapter 68	Sudangrass (*Sorghum* spp.)	355
Chapter 69	Tansy Ragwort (*Senecio jacobaea*)	359
Chapter 70	White Snakeroot (*Ageratina altissima*)	364
Chapter 71	Yellow Star Thistle (*Centaurea solstitialis*) and Russian Knapweed (*Acroptilon repens*)	369
Chapter 72	Yew (*Taxus* spp.)	374

Rodenticides 381

Chapter 73	Anticoagulants	383
Chapter 74	Bromethalin	388
Chapter 75	Cholecalciferol	393
Chapter 76	Phosphides	398
Chapter 77	Sodium Fluoroacetate (Compound 1080)	403
Chapter 78	Strychnine	408

Toxic Gases 413

| Chapter 79 | Air Contaminants: CO, NH_3, H_2S | 415 |
| Chapter 80 | Smoke | 421 |

Trees 427

Chapter 81	Black Locust (*Robinia pseudoacacia*)	429
Chapter 82	Black Walnut (*Juglans nigra*) Toxicosis	433
Chapter 83	Boxelder (*Acer negundo*)	437
Chapter 84	Oak (*Quercus* spp.)	442
Chapter 85	Red Maple (*Acer rubrum*)	446

Zootoxins **451**

Chapter **86**	Blister Beetles (*Epicauta* spp. and *Pyrota* spp.)	453
Chapter **87**	Snakes – Crotalids (Pit Vipers)	460
Chapter **88**	Snakes – Elapids (Coral Snakes)	467
Chapter **89**	Spiders – Brown Recluse and Black Widow	474

Section 3 — Reference Information — 483

Appendix **1**	Abbreviations	485
Appendix **2**	Herbicides	489
Appendix **3**	Information Resources for Toxicology	496

Index by Toxins and Toxicants **503**
Index by Clinical Signs **511**

Contributor List

Dionne Benson, DVM, JD
Chief Veterinary Officer
The Stronach Group
Aurora, ON, Canada

Laurie Bohannon, DVM, Candidate DACVS
Senior Veterinarian
Santa Anita Park
Arcadia, CA, USA

Casille Batten, DVM
Senior Veterinarian
Golden Gate Fields
Berkeley, CA, USA

Ryan Carpenter, DVM, MS, DACVS
Partner
Equine Medical Center
Cypress, CA, USA

Cynthia Cole, DVM, PhD, DACVCP
Clinical Associate Professor and Director
University of Florida, Racing Laboratory
Gainesville, FL, USA

Jay Deluhery, DVM, MBA, CJF
Veterinarian
Santa Anita Racetrack
Arcadia, CA, USA
&
Veterinarian
Pacific Coast Equine Veterinary Services
Laguna Niguel, CA, USA

Thomas J. Divers, DVM, DACVIM, DACVECC
Steffen Professor of Veterinary Medicine
Cornell University
Ithaca, NY, USA

Steve Ensley, DVM, PhD
Toxicology Section Head
Kansas State University
College of Veterinary Medicine
Manhattan, KS, USA

Tim J. Evans, DVM, MS, PhD, DACT, DABVT
Associate Professor and Toxicology Section Head
Veterinary Medical Diagnostic Laboratory
University of Missouri
Columbia, MO, USA

Langdon Fielding, DVM, MBA, DACVECC, DACVSMR
Loomis Basin Equine Medical Center
2973 Penryn Rd
Penryn, CA, USA

Scott Fritz, DVM
Kansas State Veterinary Diagnostic Laboratory
College of Veterinary Medicine
Kansas State University
Manhattan, KS, USA

Tam Garland, DVM, PhD, DABVT
Garland and Bailey Associates
College Station, TX, USA

Tamara Gull, DVM, PhD, DACVIM (LAIM), DACVPM, DACVM
Veterinary Medical Diagnostic Laboratory
University of Missouri
Columbia, MO, USA

Petra Hartmann-Fischbach, MS, FAORC
Director, DTS
Industrial Laboratories
Wheatridge, CO, USA

Stephen B. Hooser, DVM, PhD, DABVT
Head, Toxicology Section, Animal Disease Diagnostic Laboratory & Professor of Veterinary Toxicology
Purdue University, Department of Comparative Pathobiology
West Lafayette, IN, USA

Lynn R. Hovda, RPh, DVM, MS, DACVIM
Director of Veterinary Medicine
Pet Poison Helpline & Safetycall International, PLLC
Bloomington, MN, USA
&
Adjunct Assistant Professor
Professor College of Veterinary Medicine
University of Minnesota
St. Paul, MN, USA

Tyne K. Hovda, DVM
Anesthesia Resident
College of Veterinary Medicine
North Carolina State University
Raleigh, NC, USA

Emma V. Hummer, DVM
Anesthesiology Resident
College of Veterinary Medicine
Texas A and M University
College Station, TX, USA

Sarah Jarosinski, DVM
Anesthesiology Resident
College of Veterinary Medicine
Texas A and M University
College Station, TX, USA

Dijana Katan, DVM, MPH, DABT
Associate Veterinarian – Clinical Toxicology
Pet Poison Helpline & Safetycall International, PLLC
Bloomington, MN, USA

Daniel E. Keyler, BS, PharmD, FAACT
Consulting Senior Clinical Toxicologist
Pet Poison Helpline and Safetycall International, PLLC
Bloomington, MN, USA
&
Adjunct Professor
Dept Experimental & Clinical Pharmacology
University of Minnesota
Minneapolis, MN, USA

Christy Klatt, DVM
Assistant Commission Veterinarian
Minnesota Racing Commission
Shakopee, MN, USA

Heather K. Knych, DVM, PhD, DACVCP
Professor of Clinical Veterinary Pharmacology
KL Maddy Equine Analytical Pharmacology Lab
School of Veterinary Medicine
University of California – Davis
Davis, CA, USA

Benjamin C. Moeller, PhD, DABT
Assistant Professor
KL Maddy Equine Analytical Chemistry Laboratory
School of Veterinary Medicine
University of California – Davis
Davis, CA, USA

Michelle Mostrom, DVM, MS, PhD, DABVT, DABT (1995-2020)
Veterinary Toxicologist
North Dakota State University – Veterinary Diagnostic Laboratory, Toxicology Secion
Fargo, ND, USA

Robert H. Poppenga, DVM, PhD, DABVT
Head, Toxicology Section
California Animal Health and Food Safety Laboratory System
School of Veterinary Medicine
University of California
Davis, CA, USA

Scott L. Radke, DVM, MS
Head, Analytical Chemistry Services
Veterinary Diagnostic and Production Animal Medicine
Iowa State University Veterinary Diagnostic Laboratory
College of Veterinary Medicine
Ames, IA, USA

Felipe Reggeti, DVM, PhD, DACVP
Toxicology and Clinical Pathology sections
Animal Health Laboratory
Laboratory Services Division
University of Guelph
Guelph, Ontario, Canada

Tabatha Regehr, DVM
Consulting Veterinarian, Clinical Toxicology
Pet Poison Helpline & Safetycall International, PLLC
Bloomington, MN, USA

Sherry Rippel, DVM, DABT, DABVT
Senior Veterinary Toxicologist
Pet Poison Helpline & Safetycall International, PLLC
Bloomington, MN, USA

Megan C. Romano, DVM, DABVT
Head, Toxicology Section
University of Kentucky Veterinary Diagnostic Laboratory
Lexington, KY, USA

Wilson K. Rumbeiha, DVM, PhD, DABT, DABVT, ATS
Professor of One Environmental Health Toxicology
Dept of Molecular Biosciences
School of Veterinary Medicine
University of California
Davis, CA, USA

Renee Schmid, DVM, DABT, DABVT
Senior Veterinary Toxicologist
DVM Supervisor
Pet Poison Helpline & Safetycall International, PLLC
Bloomington, MN, USA

Mary Scollay, DVM
Executive Director
Racing Medication Testing Consortium
Lexington, KY, USA

Arya Sobhakumari, DVM, PhD, ERT, DABT, DABVT
Research Scientist – Quality and Applied Science
Nestle Purina PetCare
1 Checkerboard Square, 3S
St. Louis, MO, USA

Bryan L. Stegelmeier, DVM, PhD, DACVP
Research Medical Officer
USDA Poisonous Plant Research Laboratory
Logan, UT, USA

Ashley Smit, DVM
Consulting Veterinarian, Clinical Toxicology
Pet Poison Helpline & Safetycall International, PLLC
Bloomington, MN, USA

Patricia A. Talcott, MS, DVM, PhD, DABVT
Clinical Professor, Dept. of Integrative Physiology and Neuroscience
Toxicology Section Head, Washington Animal Disease Diagnostic Laboratory
Pullman, WA, USA

Christie Ward, DVM, MVSc, PhD, DACVIM
Assistant Clinical Professor
College of Veterinary Medicine
University of Minnesota
St. Paul, MN, USA

Katherine D. Watson, DVM, PhD, DACVP
Assistant Professor of Anatomic Pathology
California Animal Health and Food Safety Laboratory System
School of Veterinary Medicine
University of California
Davis, CA, USA

About the Companion Website

This book is accompanied by a companion website:

www.wiley.com/go/hovda/equine

The Website includes:
- Figures from the book
- Appendix 3 – Information Resources for Toxicology

Clinical Toxicology

section 1

Forensic Investigation of Equine Intoxications

Chapter 1

DEFINITION/OVERVIEW

- Determining underlying causes for sudden or unexplained equine deaths has significant medicolegal importance. Potentially all horses are at risk, but horses are less commonly intoxicated than other species due to more selective dietary habits, more controlled environments, and more observant owners.
- Clues that might point towards an intoxication include sudden death of one or more otherwise healthy horses, recent feed or environmental changes, easy access to chemical storage areas or trash piles, access to areas with potentially toxic plants, or threats of poisoning.
- Malicious poisoning does occur due to disputes or in situations in which animals are insured or involved in some form of competition.
- Determining the cause and manner of death is critical to substantiating claims and the ultimate liability of insurers.
- A systematic and thorough postmortem examination is essential to confirm death caused by toxicant exposure.
- Documentation (e.g., use of chain-of-custody procedures) of proper sample collection, storage, and laboratory submission is crucial, especially with accidental feed contamination or malicious poisoning suspicions.
- Toxicant testing can be targeted (i.e., testing for specific toxicants) or non-targeted (i.e., looking for unknowns). While non-targeted testing can identify many toxicants, there is no single comprehensive test for unknowns.
- It is important to keep an open mind when investigating the death of any animal and not to be misled by allegations of malicious intent.

SIGNALMENT/HISTORY

- Exclusive of plants for which ingestion is associated with sudden death, potential toxicants include strychnine, phosphides, cholinesterase-inhibiting insecticides (e.g., OPs, carbamates), nicotine, metaldehyde, cyanide, fluoroacetate, illicit drugs (e.g., amphetamines, cocaine, heroin, morphine), metals (e.g., mercury, arsenic, lead, selenium, iron), drugs (e.g., insulin, barbiturates, reserpine, succinylcholine), electrolytes (e.g., potassium, calcium) and vitamins A, D, and E.

Blackwell's Five-Minute Veterinary Consult Clinical Companion: Equine Toxicology,
First Edition. Edited by Lynn R. Hovda, Dionne Benson, and Robert H. Poppenga.
© 2022 John Wiley & Sons, Inc. Published 2022 by John Wiley & Sons, Inc.
Companion website: www.wiley.com/go/hovda/equine

- Ingestion of toxic plants is a less common cause of malicious poisoning but still a possibility. Exposure to extremely toxic plants (e.g., *Taxus* spp. [yew], *Nerium oleander* [oleander], *Conium maculatum* [poison hemlock], *Cicuta* spp. [water hemlock]) should be considered, as should zootoxins (e.g., cantharidin).

CLINICAL FEATURES

- Signs vary considerably depending on the specific toxicant to which a horse is exposed.
- Most malicious intoxications are associated with administration of highly toxic drugs or chemicals intended to kill quickly.
- An ideal toxicant used maliciously would cause rapid death, not result in specific postmortem lesions, and be difficult to detect in postmortem tissue or fluid samples. Fortunately, the list of toxicants meeting all three criteria is rather limited.
- Most toxicants that result in sudden death impair the central or peripheral nervous systems, cardiovascular system, or respiratory system. Thus, if signs are noted before death, they generally relate to failure of one or more of these systems.
- Intoxications can result in more chronic disease and multiple exposures might be required before onset of clinical signs (e.g., ingestion of pyrrolizidine alkaloid-containing plants).
- Depending on the toxicant, there might be evidence of struggle before death, as might occur following central nervous system (CNS) stimulation or respiratory impairment. Alternatively, some toxicant-induced deaths are associated with no struggle before death, as might occur after administration of a barbiturate or other CNS depressant.

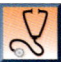

DIFFERENTIAL DIAGNOSIS

- There are many causes of sudden or unexplained death other than toxicants:
  - Physical causes – trauma, electrocution, lightning strike, suffocation, heat stroke, and gunshot.
  - Natural or genetic causes – hyperkalemic periodic paralysis, cardiac conductive disturbances, acute myocardial necrosis, cerebral thromboembolism, aortic aneurysm or other vessel rupture, and neoplasia.
  - Infectious or parasitic causes – acute clostridial diseases, salmonellosis, Tyzzer's disease, anthrax, equine monocytic ehrlichiosis, foal actinobacillosis, babesiosis, and verminous arteritis.
  - Metabolic and nutritional causes – hypoglycemia, hypocalcemia, hypomagnesemia, and selenium or vitamin E deficiencies.

DIAGNOSTICS

CBC/Serum Chemistry/Urinalysis

- When possible, collect whole blood, serum, plasma, and urine before death for routine clinicopathologic tests; this helps to delineate pathophysiologic processes, which aids in refining an initial differential list.

Other Laboratory Tests

- In addition to samples collected for clinicopathologic testing, other samples for toxicologic analysis include stomach contents, urine, liver, kidney, brain, eyeball, and heart blood. Given the delay in the possible incorporation of a chemical into hair, hair samples are not generally useful for testing.
- With any suspicion of an injection site, obtain tissue from around that site.
- Collect representative feed and water samples.
- Submit plants for identification if necessary (submit fresh whole plants, wrap plant [at least the base of the plant] in moistened paper towels, place in a plastic bag and keep chilled; representative samples of hay can also be collected for identification of contamination).
- Because of medicolegal considerations, handle all samples under chain-of-custody procedures. These records specifically identify each specimen, document their condition and container in which they are packaged, time and date of both transfer and receipt of samples, and all individuals involved in their handling, transfer, or receipt.
- Testing can be targeted or non-targeted depending on whether there are known exposures or unknown exposures. Mass spectrometry is a powerful technique for broad-based targeted testing. However, there is no one or two analytical procedures that can rule out all possible chemical exposures.

Pathological Findings

- Conduct a complete and thorough postmortem examination.
- Consider transporting the animal to a veterinary diagnostic facility as soon as possible. If this is not an option, conduct a thorough field postmortem examination, and record any actual or suspected abnormalities.
- If an animal cannot be taken to a veterinary diagnostic facility, consultation with a veterinary pathologist or toxicologist might be warranted to ensure collection and appropriate preservation of useful samples in sufficient quantities.
- Carefully examine stomach and GI tract contents for evidence of toxic plant fragments or unexpected grain or forage ingestion.
- Collect formalin-fixed samples from all major organ systems and any gross lesions, and submit these samples to a veterinary pathologist for histopathologic examination.

THERAPEUTICS

- In many situations, treatment is not possible; however, if the animal is alive, direct treatment toward stabilization of vital organ systems – establish and maintain an open airway, control seizures, correct life-threatening cardiac dysrhythmias, and begin fluid administration.
- Once the animal is stabilized, initiate oral and dermal decontamination.

Detoxification

- AC (1–4 g/kg PO in water slurry [1 g of AC in 5 mL of water]).
- One dose of cathartic PO with AC if no diarrhea or ileus – 70% sorbitol (3 mL/kg) or sodium or magnesium sulfate (250–500 mg/kg).
- Administration of other drugs depending on the individual situation.

Appropriate Health Care

Appropriate monitoring and follow-up depend on the specific toxicant under suspicion or analytically confirmed.

Antidotes

- Antidotes are not available for most toxicants, but fortunately, many animals survive with timely decontamination and appropriate symptomatic and supportive care.
- If an antidote is available, consider giving it first before further treatment.

COMMENTS

Prevention/Avoidance

- Routinely inspect the immediate environment of an animal and note any unusual human activity.
- Routinely inspect feed and water for any foreign material.
- Encourage clients to know sources of feeds and forages.
- To minimize malicious poisoning opportunities, camera surveillance can be considered, particularly for valuable animals.

Possible Complications

- Potential complications depend on the specific toxicant involved.

Expected Course and Prognosis

- Variable depending on the chemical.

See Also

Necropsy Analysis
Other specific toxicant topics

Abbreviations

See Appendix 1 for a complete list.

Suggested Reading

Haliburton JC, Edwards WC. Medicolegal investigation of the sudden or unexpected equine death: toxicologic implications. In: Robinson, NE, ed. Current Therapy in Equine Medicine 4. Philadelphia: WB Saunders, 1997; pp. 657–659.

Johnson BJ. Handling forensic necropsy cases. Vet Clin N Am: Equine Practice 2001; 17(3):411–418.

Poppenga RH. Toxicology. In: Southwood LL, Wilkins PA, eds. Equine Emergency and Critical Care. Boca Raton: CRC Press, 2015.

Author: Robert H. Poppenga DVM, PhD, DABVT
Consulting Editor: Robert H. Poppenga DVM, PhD, DABVT

Chapter 2

Necropsy Analysis

DEFINITION/OVERVIEW

- The key components of a diagnostic toxicology work-up include history, clinical signs, clinical chemistry, analytical toxicology, and, if animals die, a postmortem examination (necropsy).
- The first goal of a postmortem examination is to determine the cause of death, circumstances surrounding the death, and/or the extent of disease.
- Systematic gross and microscopic inspections of all organ systems after death are indispensable diagnostic tools that can help the clinician gain clues about what the physical findings likely represent and are important should litigation become an issue.
- The second goal is to collect appropriate specimens for analytical toxicology testing. Samples typically collected for toxicology testing include stomach contents, liver, kidney, fat and brain.

ETIOLOGY/PATHOPHYSIOLOGY

- See individual topic discussions on absorption, distribution, metabolism, and excretion (ADME), mechanisms of action, systems affected and diagnostic approaches for individual toxicants.

SIGNALMENT/HISTORY

- History and clinical signs should be kept in perspective for determining differential diagnoses while completing the necropsy.
- Poisonings often affect many animals in a very short period of time and thus attract substantial public attention and interest.
- Many clues can increase the suspicion of a toxic etiology. Obvious cases involve sudden onset of disease in a number of animals. Common feed or environmental conditions will further support a suspicion of an intoxication. Intoxication is also suggested in the otherwise healthy animal that is found "suddenly dead".

Blackwell's Five-Minute Veterinary Consult Clinical Companion: Equine Toxicology,
First Edition. Edited by Lynn R. Hovda, Dionne Benson, and Robert H. Poppenga.
© 2022 John Wiley & Sons, Inc. Published 2022 by John Wiley & Sons, Inc.
Companion website: www.wiley.com/go/hovda/equine

- However, chronic and subchronic intoxications also occur and are more challenging to diagnose because they are subtle. Sporadic mortality in a group of animals along with poor animal condition should raise suspicion of a chronic intoxication.
- Other situations suggesting testing from a toxicology laboratory include drug testing in the racehorse industry, testing for nutritional adequacy (especially selenium and vitamin E status), or providing testing in suspect cases of malicious poisoning.
- Reasons to suspect a poisoning:
  - Many animals are sick with no known exposure to infectious disease.
  - Affected individuals have been exposed recently to a new environment.
  - There has been a recent change in feed.
  - Recent construction activity in the environment.
  - Recent pesticide application in the environment.
  - Unusual weather conditions.
  - The animal has limited feed or pasture, resulting in consumption of plants not normally consumed.
  - An uncommon clinical condition exists.
  - There has been a potential threat of malicious poisoning.
  - Unexplained death(s) has/have occurred.
  - Persistent poor health condition.

CLINICAL FEATURES

- Toxicants typically target specific organs or systems (e.g. the cardiovascular, the nervous or the urogenital systems). However, multiple organs can be affected.
- If a toxicant targets a specific organ this can help narrow down the differential list.
- However, many toxicants target the same organ or system, likely causing similar clinical signs. Therefore, one should not rely on clinical signs alone to make a diagnosis.
- Templates can be useful guides for collecting diagnostic information (see Table 2.1), but no template can possibly account for all scenarios. Thus, a thorough, thoughtful and organized investigation is needed without over-reliance on a template.

DIFFERENTIAL DIAGNOSIS

- Establishing an accurate diagnosis depends heavily on a systematic approach because toxicants often have clinical signs that overlap with other non-toxicologic causes and lesions may or may not be present.
- Even if a poisoning is suspected, the practitioner has to be a neutral observer considering toxic as well as non-toxic causes of disease. For example, lead poisoning may cause few or very subtle lesions while oak or monensin intoxications cause consistent lesions helpful for making a diagnosis.
- The absence of lesions is as important as their presence and is helpful in narrowing down a differentials list.
- An accurate diagnosis is central to providing adequate treatment for affected animals and preventing new cases.

TABLE 2.1. Checklist for information collection in a suspected poisoning.

Owner Data:
Date:_____
Owner:_____
Manager:_____
Address:_____
Phone:_____
Fax:_____
E-mail:_____

Patient Data:
Species:_____
Breed:_____
Sex:_____
Pregnancy:_____
Weight:_____
Age:_____

Health History:
- Illness past 6 months
- Exposure to other animals last 30 days
- Vaccination history
- Medications: sprays, dips, hormones, minerals, wormers past 6 months
- Last exam by a veterinarian

Current Clinical History:
- Herd size; housing
- Are other similar groups on the same premises?
- Common feed or water among groups?
- Morbidity_____ Mortality _____
- When first observed sick?
- How long has problem been in the herd?
- If found dead, when last seen alive and healthy?
- Any recent malicious threats?

Environmental Data:
- Location: pasture, woods, dry lot, near river or pond, confined indoors; recent location changes
- Housing: group-housed or individually; type of ventilation; new construction
- Recent changes in weather, transport, shows or competitions; unexplained deaths; access to trash, old construction materials; recent burning of materials
- Pesticide use (i.e. insecticides, rodenticides, herbicides) and specific types or names if available (ask for tags or bags to ID)
- Materials used for construction/renovation
- Services such as lawn care, pasture seeding, tree planting, and fertilization
- Access to old machinery, automotive products, treated lumber, burn piles, flowing water

Dietary Data:
- Nutritionist (contact information)
- Diet components: whole grains or ground; sweet feed; pelleted complete feed; other (list)
- Recent changes in total diet or specific diet component(s)
- Method of feeding (hand feeding, full feed, mechanical delivery)
- Type of hay (e.g. grass, alfalfa, mixed; weed contaminants)
- Presence of molded or spoiled feed or hay
- Pasture: type, scant, abundant, weed contamination; trees or brush present
- Water source (flowing stream, pond, well, county or city water)

Clinical Signs:

Ataxia	Anorexia	Anemia
Salivation	Colic	Hemorrhage
Blindness/vision	Vomiting	Hematuria
Depression	Diarrhea	Icterus
Excitement	Melena	Hemoglobinuria
Seizures	Polyphagia	Methemoglobinemia
Cerebellar signs	Polydipsia	Straining
Dysphonia	Polyuria	Fever
Other (describe)	Dyspnea	Weakness
	Lameness	Alopecia

- A conclusive diagnosis depends heavily on a systematic investigation, appropriate sample choice based on a good knowledge of ADME and appropriate sample handling and storage to preserve specimen integrity.

DIAGNOSTICS

- Discriminating between differential diagnoses may require ancillary diagnostics:
  - Histopathology:
    - Samples for histopathology should be collected in 10% formalin.
    - Bouin's solution can be used for delicate tissues (i.e. ophthalmic, gastrointestinal and reproductive tissues). Bouin's solution is not a good fixative for preserving ultrastructure for electron microscopy.
    - Tissues should not exceed 0.5 cm thickness to permit proper fixation. Bloody tissues (i.e. liver and spleen) should be thinner.
    - A set of samples should minimally include liver, kidney, lungs, GI tract and any tissues with lesions.
    - Brain and/or spinal cord are needed if there are neurologic signs.
    - Do not freeze formalin-preserved tissues.
  - Microbiology:
    - Sterile culture swabs or large sections of any tissues with lesions should be sent fresh (refrigerated, not frozen) for microbial work-up.
  - Serology/immunology:
    - Whole blood
    - Serum
    - Plasma
  - Molecular diagnostics:
    - 1 cm square section of fresh (unfixed) tissue with the lesion in a sterile container refrigerated or frozen depending on transport time.
  - Analytical toxicology:
    - Use laboratories accredited by the American Association of Veterinary Laboratory Diagnosticians (AAVLD). These can be accessed at https://www.aavld.org/accredited-labs
    - Freeze appropriate unfixed tissue specimens for toxicology testing.
    - Use separate containers for each specimen (i.e., do not combine samples into one container). Label each sample.
    - If in doubt, contact the toxicology laboratory for advice on sample types and amounts, including collection and preservation of environmental samples.
- Conduct a detailed field investigation to identify, remove and/or restrict access to source(s) of toxicants.
- Samples for toxicology fall into three general categories (see Table 2.2):
  - Environmental (e.g. pasture samples, weeds, feed and feed supplements, water, soil, pesticide containers).
  - Antemortem (e.g. whole blood, serum, urine, hair).
  - Postmortem (e.g. stomach contents, liver, kidney, perirenal fat, brain).

TABLE 2.2. Samples for toxicology: guide to collection and analysis.

Sample Type	Amount	Condition	Potential Analyses
Environmental			
Hay, grain, concentrate feeds, mineral supplements	500 g to 1 kg composite	In paper or plastic bags, glass jars; avoid spoilage during shipping	Pesticides (insecticides, rodenticides, herbicides), heavy metals, salts, feed additives, antibiotics, ionophores, mycotoxins, nitrates, sulfate, cyanide, plant toxins, cantharidin, botulinum toxin, vitamins
Plants	Entire plant	Press and dry or refrigerate or freeze	Identification, alkaloids, tannins, grayanotoxins (rhododendron), cardiac glycosides (oleander, foxglove, adonis)
Mushroom	Whole	Keep cool and dry in paper bag	Identification; chemical test for amanitins
Water	1 L	Preserving jar	Pesticides, salts, heavy metals, microcystins, anatoxin-a, sulfate, nitrate, pH. For blue green algae identification mix water:10% neutral buffered formalin (50:50) to preserve the cells
Source/bait; soil	500 g to 1 kg	Freeze in bag or glass jar	Include package label; variety of toxicants
Antemortem			
Whole blood*	5–10 mL	EDTA anticoagulant	Cholinesterase activity, lead, selenium, arsenic, mercury, cyanide, some organic chemicals, anticoagulant rodenticides
Serum*	5–10 mL	Spin and remove clot; special tube for zinc	Copper, zinc (no rubber contact if testing for zinc), iron, magnesium, calcium, sodium, potassium, drugs, alkaloids, oleandrin, vitamins, anticoagulant rodenticides
Urine*	50 mL	Send in plastic, screw-cap vial	Illicit drugs, some metals (arsenic, mercury), alkaloids, cantharidin (blister beetle), fluoride, paraquat, oleandrin
Feces (collect at different time points)	100 g plus	Freeze	Plant identification (if not too macerated), seed identification, cardiac glycosides (oleander, foxglove, adonis), grayanotoxins (rhododendron), alkaloids (yews, poison hemlock), tannins, pesticides, illicit drugs, cyanide, ammonia, cantharidin (blister beetle), 4-aminopyridine (Avitrol®), petroleum hydrocarbons, antifreeze, heavy metals, ionophores, algal toxins
Biopsy specimens	E.g., liver, fat	Freeze	Metals, pyrrolizidine alkaloids (histopathology), potentially other toxicants depending on size of the sample

(Continued)

TABLE 2.2. Continued

Sample Type	Amount	Condition	Potential Analyses
Hair	10 g	Tie mane/tail hair so origin and base are evident	Pesticides, some heavy metals
Postmortem			
Ingesta (collect stomach, small intestine and large intestine contents; keep separate)	500 g	Freeze, collect separate samples from stomach, small and large intestine	Plant identification (if not too macerated), seed identification, cardiac glycosides (oleander, foxglove, adonis), grayanotoxins (rhododendron), alkaloids (yews or poison hemlock), tannins, pesticides, drugs, cyanide, ammonia, cantharidin (blister beetle), Avitrol®, petroleum hydrocarbons, antifreeze, heavy metals, ionophores, algal toxins
Liver	100 g	Freeze†	Heavy metals, pesticides, some plant toxins, some pharmaceutical or illicit drugs, vitamins
Kidney (cortex)	100 g	Freeze†	Heavy metals, calcium, some plant toxins, ethylene glycol
Brain	Half of brain	Freeze†; sagittal section (leave midline in formalin for pathologist; unfrozen for AchE)	AchE activity, sodium, organochlorine insecticides; yellow star thistle (histopathology), bromethalin
Fat	100 g	Freeze†; smaller OK for biopsy samples	Organochlorine insecticides, PCBs
Ocular fluid	One eye	Freeze†	Potassium, ammonia, magnesium, nitrate
Injection site	100 g	Freeze†	Injectable drugs; malicious injectable toxicants
Miscellaneous	100 g	Special tests, usually freeze†	Special tests, e.g., spleen (barbiturates), lung (paraquat)

* If possible, whole blood, serum and urine should also be collected during a postmortem examination.
† Frozen is best for toxicology samples, but refrigerated is best for bacterial cultures.

THERAPEUTICS

- See individual toxicant topics.
- There are relatively few toxicants most likely to poison horses for which specific antidotes exist.
- In most suspected intoxications, the best approach to decontamination is administration of an adsorbent such as activated charcoal (AC):
  - Early and appropriate decontamination and vigorous symptomatic and supportive care often result in recovery.
  - Always observe appropriate precautions during decontamination procedures to avoid self-exposure or exposure of others to the toxicant.

- Often, mineral oil is given after suspected exposure to a toxicant. This practice should be discouraged because there is no evidence that mineral oil is an effective adsorbent for most toxicants. Mineral oil should not be administered with AC because of a possible diminution of the adsorptive capacity of the administered AC.
- If the specific toxicant is known, make sure to verify what additional treatment options (antidotes) are available.
- Keep in mind that multiple toxicants might be involved particularly in malicious poisonings.

COMMENTS

- Contact a pathologist at the diagnostic laboratory in your region if you are performing the necropsy. It is preferable to get some of the animals into the diagnostic laboratory for a pathologist to examine, but if this is not possible, then discussing options with a pathologist prior to performing field necropsies is recommended.
- If you suspect intoxication, contact a toxicologist prior to sample collection for guidance on appropriate samples to collect and sample storage and submission guidelines.
- In the event of a reportable disease, contact the state veterinarian in your region to keep them informed and allow for timely intervention if necessary.
- Keep in mind the safety of you and your client, the environment and other animals. Always wear personal protection equipment for your safety.
- Carcass disposal can be an important consideration and your state veterinarian or diagnostic laboratory can provide advice.
- Keep in mind infectious diseases that can mimic an intoxication. A few examples of possible infectious diseases that might cause multiple deaths in a short time-frame are anthrax, emerging diseases to which animals are naïve, and rare bacterial and viral diseases. If anthrax is a possible differential (multiple species or large numbers of animals affected; blood from all orifices – but not always), collect an eyeball and submit to the diagnostic laboratory for stain and culture. Opening the carcass will contaminate the soil with spores that will remain infectious for decades.

See Also

Specific topics

Abbreviations

See Appendix 1 for a complete list.

Suggested Reading

Barr AC, Reagor JC. Toxic plants: what the horse practitioner needs to know. Vet Clin N Am: Equine Practice 2001;17:529–546.

Puschner B, Galey FD. Diagnosis and approach to poisoning in the horse. Vet Clin N Am: Equine Practice 2001; 17:399–409.

Davis GJ, McDonough SP. Writing the necropsy report. In: Brooks JW, ed. Veterinary Forensic Pathology, Volume 2. Springer International Publishing, 2018.

Murphy LA, Kagan R. Poisoning. In: Brooks JW, ed. Veterinary Forensic Pathology, Volume 2. Springer International Publishing, 2018.

Authors: Katherine D. Watson, DVM, PhD, DACVP; Wilson K. Rumbeiha, DVM, PhD, DABT, DABVT, ATS
Consulting Editor: Robert H. Poppenga, DVM, PhD, DABVT

Chapter 3

Laboratory Testing Considerations

Background Information

- The best laboratory testing starts with the collection and handling of the correct sample. Sample collection and handling errors are referred to as "pre-analytical" errors and some studies estimate that these types of errors account for between 40% and 75% of diagnostic errors.
- Drug concentrations in various body fluids are a snapshot in time. Toxicity may precede elevated blood or urine levels.
- Searching for an "unknown" compound is time-, sample-, and labor-intensive and will cost accordingly.
- There are thousands of toxic agents, but organisms have a limited number of clinical/physiological responses. Providing the laboratory with a description of clinical signs may be helpful in determining the best analytical strategy.
- A "tox screen" varies in scope and may include different analytical techniques, but none are 100% encompassing. The most comprehensive screens can identify 95–98% of *common* toxicants.
- A negative screen does not mean a toxicant is not present in the sample. Potential reasons why a toxicant is not identified include:
  - The unknown compound may be present at a level that is too low for the test to detect.
  - The compound was lost during sample preparation.
  - The wrong instrument parameters were used.
  - The compound is not included in the screening panel.
- When it is known that the sample contains certain drugs, such as in blood samples collected immediately following the administration of euthanasia drugs, the laboratory should be alerted to the presence of these compounds. When the laboratory uses highly sensitive instrumentation for testing, the euthanasia medications will be present at levels that can overload detectors and contaminate equipment.

Communication is Key

- Asking the laboratory very specific questions about the scope of testing will improve and speed up results. For example: "Does this screen detect monensin?/metals?/blood doping agents?/pesticides?" etc.

Blackwell's Five-Minute Veterinary Consult Clinical Companion: Equine Toxicology, First Edition. Edited by Lynn R. Hovda, Dionne Benson, and Robert H. Poppenga.
© 2022 John Wiley & Sons, Inc. Published 2022 by John Wiley & Sons, Inc.
Companion website: www.wiley.com/go/hovda/equine

Common Terms and Definitions

- **Detection limits**. The lowest level at which a test can reliably detect the analyte. The more sensitive the test, the lower the detection limit. For drug concentrations, general units range from picograms per milliliter (pg/mL; most sensitive) to micrograms per milliliter (µg/mL; least sensitive).
- **Drug**. A substance that has a physiological effect when introduced into the organism.
- **ELISA** (enzyme linked immunosorbent assay). The assay uses an enzyme linked to either antibody or antigen. When the analyte is present, the coupled enzyme reacts with a substrate, causing a color change.
- **FID** (flame ionization detector). Can be coupled to gas chromatographs for separation of analytes. Toxicology applications include ethanol testing.
- **Forensic testing**. Test results may be used in a legal setting and any sample collected for this purpose will require special handling to document the chain of custody of the sample. Data to support a test result must be scientifically and legally defensible.
- **GC** (gas chromatography). A separation technique that can separate components of a mixture for detection and/or quantification. The sample must be able to be *volatilized* and is generally restricted to lower-molecular-weight compounds (less than 500–600 amu).
- **ECD** (electron capture detector). Used to detect halogenated compounds, i.e., compounds containing bromine, chlorine, fluorine, or iodine. Can be coupled to gas chromatographs for separation of analytes. Toxicology applications include pesticide analysis in body fluids.
- **GC-MS** (gas chromatography–mass spectrometry). A technique used for the separation, detection, and confirmation of volatile, non-polar, and lower-molecular-weight (< 500–600 amu) compounds within a test sample. It is generally not suitable for analysis of larger molecules, such as peptides, proteins, or metals. It is considered a "gold standard" test for positive identification when the right parameters are used. Crucial parameters for successful performance include the ability of the target molecule to be volatilized, choosing the correct extraction, temperature range for separation, column chemistry, carrier gas, and ionization mode. If the identity of the target molecule is not known, the test can yield a false negative. Toxicology applications are numerous in the field of small molecule drug analysis.
- **HS** (headspace). Involves sampling of volatile analytes from a sample. Toxicology analytes include alcohols (ethanol, methanol, isopropanol, etc.) and carbon dioxide/carbon monoxide. Headspace sampling can be coupled to gas chromatography for separation of analytes and FID or MS detection techniques. An example is HS-GC-MS.
- **HPLC** (high performance liquid chromatography). A technique that can separate components of a mixture for detection and/or quantification. Unlike gas chromatography, the sample is in a liquid state and can also test larger-molecular-weight compounds such as peptides and proteins under the correct conditions. Another significant advantage over gas chromatography is that the technique is much faster and offers the user more flexibility with separation of analytes.
- **IA** (immunoassay). Any test using an antigen–antibody interaction. Examples include radioimmunoassay, enzyme immunoassay (EIA or ELISA), fluorescence immunoassay (FIA), or chemiluminescence immunoassays (CLIA). Immunoassays can be fast and economical, if targeting a specific compound, and offer varying degrees of sensitivity. However, immunoassays can also lack specificity and are not available for every type of drug/toxin/toxicant. Quantitation can be unreliable due to cross-reactivity with structurally similar compounds. The test cannot be used for legally defensible test results.

- **ICP-MS** (inductively coupled plasma-mass spectrometry). Uses a plasma state to ionize samples and is used mainly for the detection of elements. It has wide application in the fields of inorganic trace analysis and food testing. Nearly every element in the periodic table can be analyzed by ICP-MS. Toxicology applications include the analysis of metals in body fluids, such as cobalt, arsenic, nickel, etc.
- **LC-MS** (liquid chromatography-mass spectrometry). Like GC-MS, except using a liquid sample state. It is also a gold standard for scientifically and legally defensible testing. It is generally faster than GC-MS and provides more user flexibility to optimize separation, sensitivity, and specificity.
- **MS** (mass spectrometry). After separation of components in a sample using gas or liquid chromatography, the individual compounds are introduced into the mass spectrometer, where molecules are ionized and fragmented. The fragmentation pattern of individual molecules is highly specific under standardized conditions. Each ion fragment can be measured by the instrument and the resulting mass spectrum can be compared with certified reference materials for identification.
- **RIA** (radioimmunoassay). A type of immunoassay using radio-labeled antigens or antibodies. If the target analyte is present, it will bind to the radio-labeled component and the resulting radioactive complex can be very accurately measured. While a very sensitive technique, it has fallen out of favor due to exposure hazards and problems with disposal of used test materials.
- **Toxin**. A toxin is an antigenic poison or venom produced by living cells. Nature provides it as either a weapon for predation or as a defense mechanism:
  - If it bites you and you die, it is venomous. If you bite it and you die, it is poisonous.
  - Examples: botulinum toxin (from *Clostridium botulinum*), muscarine (from mushrooms), tetrodotoxin (puffer fish).
- **Toxicant**. A toxicant is any substance (natural or synthetic) capable of causing ill health.
  - Examples: pesticides, benzene, cyanide.
- **UHPLC** (ultra-high-performance liquid chromatography). As implied by the term "ultra", UHPLC offers higher speed of analysis, and better sensitivity, reproducibility, and specificity over HPLC.

Seeking a Laboratory

- *Define your testing objective first and foremost*. Different laboratories offer different types of tests. A test is a tool. Always use the right tool for the job.
- Toxicology laboratories can be subdivided into different functionalities:
  - Environmental, occupational, experimental, and pharmaceutical toxicology laboratories engage in very specific subsections of toxicology.
  - Veterinary diagnostic laboratories and equine drug testing or doping control laboratories offer many of the tests that can be useful to the practitioner looking to determine a cause of illness or death. If there are legal implications (lawsuits, penalties, etc.), the laboratory should be experienced in forensic sample handling and chain of custody procedures. Contacting the laboratory as soon as possible should allow them to provide information to ensure that proper procedures are performed from collection to shipping as well as for testing. The designated laboratory should be accredited for the testing technology requested and utilized.

- **Veterinary diagnostic laboratories (VDLs).** The focus of a VDL is on the diagnosis and prevention of disease in animals. Individual specialized test offerings may vary from laboratory to laboratory. The VDL should be the first stop when the causative agent is unknown, and a consultation with the chief toxicologist should be conducted prior to collecting/submitting samples, whenever possible.
- **Equine drug testing/doping control laboratory.** These laboratories are specialized in testing methods designed for the detection of prohibited compounds in performance animals. Due to the large number of drug compounds these laboratories routinely test for, and the availability of advanced analytical instrumentation, many laboratories can offer a very broad scope of drug coverage with superior sensitivity. However, the scope of coverage is not always uniform among different laboratories beyond a base panel of commonly regulated medications, and most do not offer testing for pesticides, rodenticides, industrial chemicals, etc. Test results obtained from previous testing at a VDL and clinical history should be shared, when possible, to ensure the best possible test selection and avoid analyte overlap.
- **Private analytical laboratories.** These laboratories perform a variety of testing on food, water, dietary supplements, industrial chemicals, pharmaceuticals, etc. Larger facilities can offer state-of-the-art equipment and scientific staff and may be able to test for exotic analytes.

Samples

- High-quality samples are essential for optimizing the laboratory testing to be performed. The best sample should be chosen based on the suspected compound/analyte. Communication with the laboratory about specific samples to obtain and submit often improves the outcome.
    - Blood (whole blood – not clotted) (serum/plasma). Avoid hemolysis. Some compounds may require specific collection tubes (check with laboratory).
    - Saliva.
    - Ocular fluid.
    - Urine.
    - Hair.
    - Bile/stomach contents.
    - Liver/kidney/spleen.
    - Injection site/muscle.
    - Materials found in the animal's environment (syringes, unlabeled pharmaceuticals, tongue ties, feed remnants, dietary supplements/botanicals, etc.).
- The minimum volume for collection will depend on the number of tests to be performed on the sample(s). Check with the laboratory before collection, whenever possible.
- Store samples under appropriate conditions for the analyte.

Potential Analytical Targets

Rodenticides, insecticides, herbicides, fertilizers, feed additives, drugs (human/veterinary, OTC/prescription/compounded products), research chemicals, paint components, household products, poisonous plants, microbial toxins, animal venoms, heavy metals, ionophores, fumonisin, taxine, cardiac glycosides, and others.

Abbreviations

See Appendix 1 for a complete list.

Suggested Reading

Ghaedi M, El-Khoury JM. Pre-analytical variation: the leading cause of error in laboratory medicine. Clinical Laboratory News 2016. Available at: https://www.aacc.org/cln/articles/2016/july/preanalytical-variation-the-leading-cause-of-error-in-laboratory-medicine (accessed April 3, 2021).

https://www.vet.cornell.edu/animal-health-diagnostic-center/laboratories/toxicology
http://www.vdl.uky.edu/LaboratoryServices/Sections/Toxicology.aspx
https://cahfs.vetmed.ucdavis.edu/tests-and-fees/diagnostic-services/toxicology
https://vet.purdue.edu/addl/Toxicology-Analytical-Chemistry.php

Author: Petra Hartmann-Fischbach, MS, FAORC Director, DTS
Consulting Editors: Dionne Benson, DVM, JD; Lynn R. Hovda, RPh, DVM, MS, DACVIM

Treating an Intoxicated Animal: Antidotes and Therapeutic Medications

Chapter 4

DEFINITION/OVERVIEW

- The incidence, prevalence, case fatality rate, and mortality rate vary with each specific toxicant, dose, animal factors such as age, nutritional status, or concurrent disease, or exposure to other toxicants.
- If information is available, determine how and when the animal was exposed to the toxicant.
- Clinical signs vary with the different toxicants. Not all potential signs are seen in each affected animal. Signs can vary with disease progression. The current clinical observation is just a snapshot of the toxicosis.
- There is limited availability of FDA-approved drugs to treat animals. The majority are used in an extra-label or unapproved manner.
- Currently, only seven FDA-approved "antidotes" are used to treat animal toxicoses. Of these, only two are used in horses (pralidoxime hydrochloride and tolazoline hydrochloride).
- Some antivenoms and antitoxins are approved by the USDA for equine use.

ETIOLOGY/PATHOPHYSIOLOGY

Mechanism of Action

- Mechanisms of action vary with different toxicants and are discussed in the specific chapters dealing with those toxicants.
- Briefly, toxicants can cause local or general systemic effects. Injury to one organ could potentially negatively impact other body systems.

Systems Affected

- All systems have the potential to be affected by toxicants. The GI system, including the liver, is the primary system, with the nervous, renal, and cardiovascular systems also affected. Many toxicants cause clinical signs in more than one system.
- Different systems are targeted depending on the inherent toxicity of the specific toxicant. A toxic outcome, however, can be modulated by animal factors (e.g., genetics) or by the dose or the route of exposure, or by environmental conditions such as season, among others.
- The effects can occur concurrently, sequentially, or independently of each other.

Blackwell's Five-Minute Veterinary Consult Clinical Companion: Equine Toxicology, First Edition. Edited by Lynn R. Hovda, Dionne Benson, and Robert H. Poppenga.
© 2022 John Wiley & Sons, Inc. Published 2022 by John Wiley & Sons, Inc.
Companion website: www.wiley.com/go/hovda/equine

SIGNALMENT/HISTORY

- Some toxicants can have an age predilection, most often related to eating habits (and, therefore, dose ingestion) or to management practices.
- Some toxicants have breed or gender predispositions, e.g., reproductive toxicants.
- Current or past health problems and treatments may reveal factors that can affect toxicity and influence therapeutic outcomes.

Risk Factors

- Risk factors can be due to the toxicant, the individual, or the environment.
- Toxicant-related risk factors include the toxicity of the substance, physical nature (e.g., solid, powdered, nanoparticle), dose, and exposure route (e.g., dermal, oral, inhaled, injected).
- Individual risk factors may include age, breed, sex, reproductive status, nutrition, weight, previous health status, and current treatments.
- Environmental factors include specific season, drought, floods, ambient temperatures, etc.

CLINICAL FEATURES

- Clients may not be forthcoming with complete information if they feel guilty because poisoning resulted from their own mistakes. Conversely, clients may give biased information if they believe poisoning resulted from a faulty product, the negligence of others, or suspected malicious intent.
- The clinician should determine how many animals are affected or at risk of poisoning and collect detailed information regarding the current poisoning situation, including clinical signs, date of onset, time of onset, treatment given by the owner, and number of ill and dead animals.

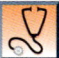

DIFFERENTIAL DIAGNOSIS

- Establishing a conclusive diagnosis of poisoning is like assembling multiple pieces of a giant puzzle. The importance of a complete history, physical examination, and complementary diagnostic tests cannot be overstated.
- Steps in diagnosis and formulating a treatment plan are:
  - Determine if signs are a result of an actual poisoning rather than of an infectious, metabolic, or nutritional disease.
  - Determine if signs or lesions are compatible with a toxic exposure. This requires appropriate selection and testing of specimens.
  - Determine if it is an acute or chronic exposure and establish a timeline as treatment will vary.
  - Utilize services available, including an animal poison control center or diagnostic laboratory, to narrow diagnosis (see Appendix 3).

CBC/Serum Chemistry/Urinalysis

- These tests are often more helpful in determining the course of treatment, but not in making a diagnosis.

Other Diagnostic Tests

- Laboratory confirmation can be made for many toxicants via sample submission to diagnostic laboratories
- At a minimum, whole blood, serum, and urine from live animals or liver, kidney, brain, fat, urine, and GI contents from dead animals should also be submitted. Hair, feces, and bone, may be helpful in some cases.

Imaging

- Radiographs, ultrasonography, and other modern imaging techniques may help identify foreign objects and/or assess the severity of toxicosis.

THERAPEUTICS

Goals

- Remove animal from source.
- Determine if acute or chronic condition and decontaminate as appropriate.
- If it is a life-threatening situation, immediately provide life support by maintaining respiratory and cardiac function.
- Control seizures and tremors as needed.
- Provide antidote or antitoxin if available. Most toxicants lack specific antidotes.
- The type, duration, and intensity of supportive care coupled with an ideal environment to heal will, on most occasions, determine whether the animal lives or dies.
- Supportive and symptomatic care.

Appropriate Health Care

- Maintain adequate hydration and control acid–base imbalances if present.
- Maintain proper body temperature. Seizures or tremors can result in elevated temperatures. Conversely, severely depressed or comatose animals may have low body temperatures.
- Dermal – with a dermal route of exposure, bathe the animal with mild dishwashing detergent. Use personal protective equipment (wearing gloves etc.) to prevent self-exposure.
- Ocular – with an ocular route of exposure, lavage the eye with copious amounts of water or normal saline.
- Inhalation – with an inhalation exposure, provide fresh air or humidified oxygen. Be careful to ensure the safety of human workers, especially with smoke, gas, and phosphide intoxications.
- Provide sufficient rest to the animal as necessary to allow healing to occur.
- Dietary restrictions or additions vary with each toxic incident. Parenteral alimentation may be required in some cases.

Antidotes

- Relevant antidotes are discussed in those sections dealing with the specific toxicants, but several important ones are reviewed here.
- Very few antidotes exist in medicine, and those that do are generally not approved for veterinary use. Any use associated with non-veterinary-approved antidotes is considered extra-label. The dosages used are often extrapolated from the human literature with very little scientific animal data available. Veterinarians are allowed to legally use medications in an extra-label manner, but when doing so assume all the responsibility associated with their use.
- Little effort has been made by manufacturers to produce antidotes approved for use in veterinary medicine. There is little financial incentive for them to do this as the use of antidotes is limited, making research and manufacturing cost-prohibitive.

Antivenom

- Intravenous antivenom can be used in horses to prevent paralysis, coagulopathies, and thrombocytopenia from snake and black widow spider bites. They have little to no effect on tissue necrosis. Early administration is preferred as it not only lessens the severity of signs but attenuates the need for a large number of doses at a later date.
- Anaphylactoid, anaphylactic, and serum sickness reactions can occur, especially if the animal has received antivenom at a prior time.
- Sensitivity testing for antivenom reactions is frequently unreliable with false-positive and -negative results.
- Elapid antivenin (coral snakes):
  - North American Coral Snake Antivenin (LLC [subsidiary of Pfizer Inc.] has a new product, Lot Y 03625 [3-year shelf life]) available. Product is prescription only. Contact for new in-date antivenin: +1 (844) 646-4398. However, cost is considerable, and as such veterinary use may be difficult.
  - Mexican, Costa Rican, and Australian antivenoms have been shown to be effective in neutralizing North American coral snake venoms (Coralmyn™, Instituto Bioclon, Mexico; Anticoral antivenom, Instituto Clodomiro Picado, Costa Rica; Australian ANG Polyvalent Snake Antivenom, CSL Limited, Australia). These antivenoms may be available through some zoos or by contacting a regional poison center with Antivenom Index access.
  - Neostigmine (AChE inhibitor) has been used in animals and humans to successfully reverse *Micrurus* venom-induced cholinesterase actions (Vital Brazil, 1996). In the absence of antivenom this may be considered for rescue and short-term use.
- Crotalid antivenin (pit vipers; rattlesnakes, copperheads, and cottonmouths):
  - Antivenin (Crotalidae) polyvalent (equine origin) (ACP); lyophilized IgG preparation; (Antivenin™; Boehringer Ingelheim Vetmedica, Inc., St Joseph, MO – +1 866-638-2226); canine indication. Administration of one vial (reconstituted in 10–50 mL normal saline) diluted to 100–250 mL (volume depends on animal size) administered IV may be adequate for many cases, but three or more vials may be required in more severe envenomations.
  - Antivenin Crotalidae polyvalent equine origin; liquid plasma preparation (Rattler Antivenin™; Mg Biologics, Ames, IA – +1 877-769-2340); canine and equine indication. Product is a whole IgG preparation. The product comes in 50 mL bags for

use with an IV filtration administration set. A unique feature is that it contains all the clotting factors in addition to venom antigen antibodies. Typically, one or two 50 mL doses are adequate.
- Antivenin polyvalent Crotalidae (F(ab')$_2$ equine origin; liquid injectable preparation; (VenomVet™; MT Venom, LLC, Canoga Park, CA – +1 800-385-6914). Product is an F(ab')$_2$ preparation (two-thirds molecular size of whole IgG). Slow IV administration over first 10 minutes. If no adverse effects entire dose should be given with 60 minutes.
- Additionally, there are two human FDA-approved antivenin products for treating North American pit viper envenomation; however, implementation of use must be carefully considered as they may be difficult to obtain and are significantly more costly:
    □ Antivenin (Crotalidae) Polyvalent Immune Fab (ovine origin); lyophilized preparation; (CroFab®; BTG International, West Conshohocken, PA).
    □ Crotalidae Immune F(ab')$_2$ (equine); lyophilized preparation; (Anavip®; Rare Disease Therapeutics, Inc., Franklin, TN).
- Black widow (*Latrodectus* spp.) spider:
  - Antivenin (*Latrodectus mactans*) (Black Widow Spider Antivenin, Equine Origin) (Merck & Co., Inc., Whitehouse Station, NJ 08889 – +1 800-444-2080) – this is a biologic drug, whole IgG antibodies, for use in humans; there is no scientific information on the use in horses. A single 2.5-mL vial diluted to 100 mL administered IV may be successful in reversing signs (in humans, signs begin to subside in 1–2 h).

Chelating agents
- These antidotes are generally used to remove heavy metals from the body. The chelating agent combines with a metal ion to form a complex that is then excreted.
- Calcium disodium ethylenediaminetetraacetic acid or CaNa2EDTA (Calcium Disodium Versenate, Medicis):
  - Labeled for use in pediatric and adult humans with acute and chronic lead poisoning. The use has declined over the years due to side-effects and the decreased incidence of lead toxicosis in human beings.
  - Still widely used in veterinary medicine to chelate lead, zinc, inorganic mercury, and perhaps cadmium, particularly in birds.
  - Calcium disodium EDTA and *not* disodium EDTA must be used. These two should not be confused.
  - Should not be used while lead remains in the GI tract as it may enhance the systemic absorption of lead.
  - Use may result in GI signs.
  - Nephrotoxic, so caution needs to be taken to ensure hydration; should not be used in animals with chronic renal failure.
  - Dose: 73 mg/kg/day divided into two or three doses. Dilute product in 5% dextrose or 0.9% sodium chloride and give by slow IV over the course of the day. Administer for 3–5 days. Rest for 2 days. Repeat as needed.
  - Alternate dose: 110 mg/kg IV BID × 2 days. Rest 2 days. Repeat as needed.
  - IM injection is painful and not recommended.

- Deferoxamine (Desferal, Novartis Pharmaceutical Corporation):
    - Labeled in human beings for the treatment of acute iron intoxication and chronic iron overload due to transfusion-dependent anemia. Veterinary experience is limited.
    - Deferoxamine is most effective if used within the first 24 hours while iron is still in circulation and has not been distributed to tissues.
    - Contraindicated in patients with severe renal disease or anuria and those with high circulating levels of aluminum.
    - Complexes with iron; deferoxamine chelated complex is water-soluble and excreted primarily in urine.
    - A recommended dose of deferoxamine is 40 mg/kg IM every 4–8 h; can be given as a continuous infusion at the rate of 15 mg/kg/h. Chelation should continue until serum iron concentrations fall below 300 μg/dL (3 ppm) or below the TIBC.
    - The excreted complex turns the urine pink or salmon-colored and is sometimes referred to as the "vin rose" of iron poisoning. Continue treatment until the urine is clear or serum iron levels are within normal limits.
- Dimercaprol (BAL in oil, Taylor):
    - Labeled in human beings for use in the treatment of arsenic, gold, and mercury poisoning. Can also be used in acute lead poisoning concomitantly with $CaNa_2EDTA$.
    - Dimercaprol (British anti-lewisite) is the classic arsenic chelator.
    - Complex is water-soluble and excreted in urine.
    - A loading dose of 4–5 mg/kg is given by deep muscular injection, followed by 2–3 mg/kg q4h for 24 hours and then 1 mg/kg q4h for 2 days.
    - IM injections are painful (peanut oil carrier) and should only be given deep IM.
    - Adverse reactions include tremors, convulsions, and coma.
    - Dimercaprol is nephrotoxic so limit use and monitor BUN and creatinine. Be sure that patients are adequately hydrated while product is used.
- Dimercaptosuccinic acid (also referred to as DMSA or Succimer; Chemet, Schwartz):
    - Labeled for use in pediatric human beings for lead poisoning when the blood levels are > 45 μg/mL. Unlabeled use includes mercury and arsenic toxicosis.
    - Used in equines for arsenic toxicosis.
    - DMSA is a less toxic chelator (equine dose not established, but 10 mg/kg PO q8h is suggested).
    - Advantages over other chelators:
        - Can be given PO or rectally if GI signs are severe.
        - Incidence of adverse GI signs is much lower.
        - Can be used while lead is still present in the GI tract.
    - Disadvantages:
        - Cost – expensive.
        - Availability – often difficult to find.
        - May have a transient increase in AST and ALT.
- Digoxin immune Fab fragments – ovine (Digibind, Glaxo Smith Kline; Digifab, BTG Specialty Solutions):
    - Specific antidote used for digoxin toxicosis. It may also be useful for cardiac glycoside containing plant intoxications.

- Fab fragments should be reserved for the treatment of life-threatening cardiac arrhythmias that do not respond to conventional antiarrhythmic therapy.
- Expensive and will likely have to be obtained from a human hospital.
- Unknown equine dose; start with one or two vials and adjust up from there.
■ Pralidoxime hydrochloride (2-PAM – Protopam Chloride, Wyeth):
  - Pralidoxime is used in organophosphate (OP) toxicosis to reactivate cholinesterase enzymes inactivated by the insecticide. It binds to the enzyme attached to the OP and forms a pralidoxime–OP complex that detaches (reactivating the enzyme) and is excreted.
  - Helps to prevent nicotinic signs and should be used in conjunction with atropine (see medications below).
  - Limited benefits with carbamate toxicosis.
  - Generally, pralidoxime should be used within 24 hours of exposure, but may still be effective when given at 36–48 h. These is some evidence that it is also effective when used for treatment of the intermediate syndrome of OP toxicosis.
  - Dose: 20 mg/kg slow IV q 4–6 hours. May have to increase dose to 35 mg/kg.
  - Rapid IV administration has resulted in tachycardia, neuromuscular blockade, laryngospasm, muscle rigidity and death.

Drug(s) of Choice

■ Relevant medications and dosages are provided in the chapters for specific toxicants, but several are reviewed here.

Detoxification

■ Activated charcoal (AC):
  - Many toxicants are adsorbed by AC, thereby reducing the amount of toxicant absorbed from the GI tract.
  - Mix the AC (1–4 g/kg) with warm water to form a slurry.
  - AC binds many organic compounds but is relatively ineffective against inorganic compounds (e.g., heavy metals), mineral acids, and alkali.
  - Follow the AC with a laxative (cathartic) to hasten removal of the toxicant from the intestinal tract.
■ Cathartics can result in significant diarrhea; therefore, ensure the horse is adequately hydrated:
  - Magnesium sulfate (Epsom salts) is an osmotic laxative that draws water into the intestines. The recommended dose is 250–500 mg/kg mixed in several liters of water.
  - Sorbitol 70% (3 mL/kg) or sodium sulfate (250–500 mg/kg mixed in several liters of water) are alternative cathartics.
  - The efficacy of mineral oil for treating intoxicated patients has not been established and its use is discouraged for routine GI decontamination.
■ Cholestyramine (cholestyramine) is useful in some intoxications.
  - Some toxicants are eliminated primarily by the fecal route or undergo enterohepatic recirculation. AC/cholestyramine followed by a laxative is the most effective means for increasing elimination of these toxicants.
■ Many toxicants are eliminated by the kidneys, and, in some cases, renal excretion can be enhanced by increasing urine output via fluid administration. Diuretics can be used

to increase urine flow – furosemide (1 mg/kg IV); mannitol (0.25–1.0 g/kg as 20% solution by slow IV infusion).
- Manipulating the urine pH can increase the excretion of some toxicants in the urine via ion trapping. Weak acids are ionized in alkaline urine, whereas weak bases are ionized in acidic urine. The normal range of pH for urine in adult herbivores is alkaline (pH 7–9).

Medications
- Toxicants typically are metabolized and/or excreted by the liver, GI tract, and/or kidneys. Select medications that will minimally affect these systems.
- Before administering oral products, determine that the horse is not exhibiting gastric reflux.

Alpha$_2$-adrenergic antagonists
- Atipamezole (Antisedan):
    - Used off-label for reversal of xylazine, other alpha$_2$-adrenergic antagonists, and potentially amitraz.
    - Dose: 0.1 mg/kg slow IV.
- Tolazoline (Tolazine):
    - Used primarily to reverse xylazine. The effects may be partial and transient.
    - Dose: 0.5–2 mg/kg IM or very slow IV; labeled dose is 4 mg/kg slow IV.
- Yohimbine (Yoban):
    - Used off-label to reverse the effects of xylazine, other alpha$_2$-adrenergic agonists, and potentially amitraz.
    - The half-life is short (1.5–2 h) and the drug will likely need to be repeated if used to reverse longer-acting agonists. Yohimbine has more side-effects including CNS excitation, tremors, and hypersalivation.
    - Dose: 0.05–0.2 mg/kg IM or very slow IV.

Atropine (generic)
- Antimuscarinic agent used for treatment of SLUDGE (salivation, lacrimation, urination, defecation, and gastroenteritis) that accompanies OP and carbamate insecticide toxicity.
- Competes with acetylcholine at the postganglionic parasympathetic sites.
- Dose 0.2–2 mg/kg. One-quarter of the dose should be given IV and the remainder IM or SC. The dose will likely need to be repeated; heart rate and secretions should be used to guide redosing.
- It is important that enough atropine be provided, especially in large overdoses of OP or carbamates. Atropine should be given despite initial tachycardia, in order to adequately compete with acetylcholine. Without adequate therapy for OP toxicosis, patients may drown in their own secretions.

Skeletal muscle relaxants
- Methocarbamol (Robaxin, Generic):
    - Used for the treatment of tremors associated with pyrethrins and pyrethroids, tremorgenic mycotoxins, strychnine, and CNS stimulant toxicosis.
    - Centrally acting skeletal muscle relaxant.
    - Dose: 4.4–22 mg/kg IV to effect (moderate conditions); 22–55 mg/kg IV (severe conditions). Do not exceed 330mg/kg/day.

- Dantrolene (Dantrium):
  - Used for the treatment of malignant hyperthermia reactions, acute rhabdomyolysis, or as an adjunct therapy for black widow spider bites.
  - Direct-acting skeletal muscle relaxant.
  - Dose: 2–4 mg/kg PO q 24 hours × 3–5 days
  - Hepatotoxic so limit use in horses ingesting known hepatotoxins or those with preexisting liver disease.

Others
- Intravenous fat emulsion/intravenous lipid emulsion (Intralipid, others):
  - Used in human and small animal medicine to reverse the signs associated with several toxins such as lidocaine, mepivacaine, ivermectin, moxidectin, beta blockers, calcium channel blockers and others.
  - Has been used successfully in a miniature horse and foals with ivermectin toxicosis.
  - There is no equine dose available. Information and dosage have been extrapolated from small animal and human data.
  - Dosage: using a 20% solution, inject 1.5 mL/kg through a jugular catheter over 5–15 minutes; follow with a CRI of 0.25 mL/kg/min over 1–2 h. Repeat in several hours if signs of toxicosis return. Check serum for lipemia prior to giving additional doses and do not administer if lipemia is present.
- Methylene blue (generic, various):
  - Infrequently used to treat methemoglobinemia formed secondary to oxidative agents such as hydroxyurea, nitrates, and phenols.
  - Dose: 1% solution, 4.4 mg/kg IV; repeat dose in 15–30 minutes if no response.
- Neostigmine:
  - Neostigmine (AChE inhibitor) has been used in animals and humans to successfully reverse *Micrurus* venom-induced cholinesterase actions.
  - Dose: 0.02 mg/kg SC or IV.

COMMENTS

Client Education
- This is an important component of management of intoxications. Client education is essential to prevent recurrent exposure, prevent new exposures, and affect the outcome of case management.

Prevention/Avoidance
- Minimize the risk of intoxication by using medications and pesticides according to the label directions, storing all chemicals safely, and identifying and removing all potentially toxic plants in the animal's environment.

Possible Complications
- The type and severity of complications as well as potential sequelae will vary with each toxic incident.

- Laminitis is a possible secondary condition to any severe disease in horses.
- Abortion or teratogenic disease may be a concern in pregnant mares depending on the toxicant and stage of pregnancy at the time of exposure
- Some poisons can affect the fertility of mares or stallions.

Abbreviations

See Appendix 1 for a complete list.

Suggested Reading

Bright SJ, Murphy MJ, Steinscheider JC, et al. Treatment of animal toxicosis: a regulatory perspective. Vet Clin NA: Food Anim Pract 2011; 27(2):481–512.

Bruenisholz H, Kupper J, Muentener CR, et. al. Treatment of ivermectin overdose in a miniature Shetland pony using intravenous administration of a lipid emulsion. J Vet Int Med 2012; 26(2):407–411.

Landolt GA. Management of equine poisoning and envenomation. Vet Clin NA: Eq Pract 2007; 23(1):31–34.

Poppenga RH. Treatment. In: Plumlee KH, ed. Clinical Veterinary Toxicology. St Louis, MO: Mosby, 2004; pp. 13–21.

Smollin CG. Toxicology: pearls and pitfalls in the use of antidotes. Emergency Medicine Clinics. 2010 Feb 1; 28(1):149–161.

Acknowledgement: The author acknowledges the prior contribution of Wilson K. Rumbeiha.
Author: Lynn R. Hovda, RPH, DVM, MS, DACVIM
Consulting Editor: Lynn R. Hovda, RPH, DVM, MS, DACVIM

Chapter 5

Compounded Medication

The use of compounded medication is an area of much confusion in veterinary medicine. The law in this area is ever-changing and subject to discretionary enforcement. Legitimate veterinary compounding is an important part of an equine practitioner's arsenal to treat horses.

What is Compounding?

There are four types of substances that must be discussed to understand compounding:
- **Brand name medication**. These are medications developed by pharmaceutical companies and approved through the FDA drug process. Ketofen® and GastroGard® are examples of brand name medications. These medications need to successfully complete safety and efficacy trials and then each batch is regulated to ensure purity.
- **Generic medication**. These are developed by pharmaceutical copies as mimics of previously approved brand name medications. These are developed when the patent on a brand name medication expires. These medications still must satisfy FDA regulations and are subject to FDA testing. These are not considered to be compounded medications.
- **Compounded medication**. These are created when an approved (generic or brand name) medication is customized to meet the needs of a specific patient for a specific diagnosis. The following are examples of legal compounding:
  - Adding flavoring and creating a paste from FDA-approved products such as phenylbutazone pills, etc.
  - Combining FDA-approved version of hyaluronic acid and corticosteroids prior to intra-articular administration.
  - Mixing FDA-approved versions of butorphanol and detomidine prior to intravenous administration.
- **Illegal new medication**. Mixing of multiple substances and marketing it as a new product to treat or prevent disease is considered the creation of an illegal new medication. This type of activity lacks research regarding the efficacy and effects of mixing two products together. They could potentially inactivate one another, increase the reaction when mixed, or, in the cases of some combinations, create a toxic product. One example of an illegal new medication is misoprostol mixed with bulk omeprazole. These types of products have been marketed by companies directly to trainers for gastric ulcers.

Blackwell's Five-Minute Veterinary Consult Clinical Companion: Equine Toxicology,
First Edition. Edited by Lynn R. Hovda, Dionne Benson, and Robert H. Poppenga.
© 2022 John Wiley & Sons, Inc. Published 2022 by John Wiley & Sons, Inc.
Companion website: www.wiley.com/go/hovda/equine

Toxicity and Compounding (see Figs 5.1–5.3)

Legal and illegal instances of compounding as well as the use of illegal new medications do not come without significant risk to the horse. In several instances, administration of improperly compounded medication has been associated with death. For example:
- Compounded clenbuterol linked to three horse deaths in Louisiana.
- Compounded pyrimethamine and toltrazuril sold in Pennsylvania and Kentucky associated with at least seven horse deaths.
- Compounded selenium administered to 21 polo ponies that died in Florida.
- Thirty-two human deaths associated with methylprednisolone acetate that was compounded in non-sterile conditions.

These are just examples of fatalities that have occurred after the administration of a compounded medication.

Why Extra Caution is Needed for Compounded Products

When compared to FDA-approved generic or brand name medications, compounded medications inherently have higher risk. FDA-approved medications (including generic medications) are required to prove:
- Purity.
- Efficacy.
- Consistent concentration.
- Stability.

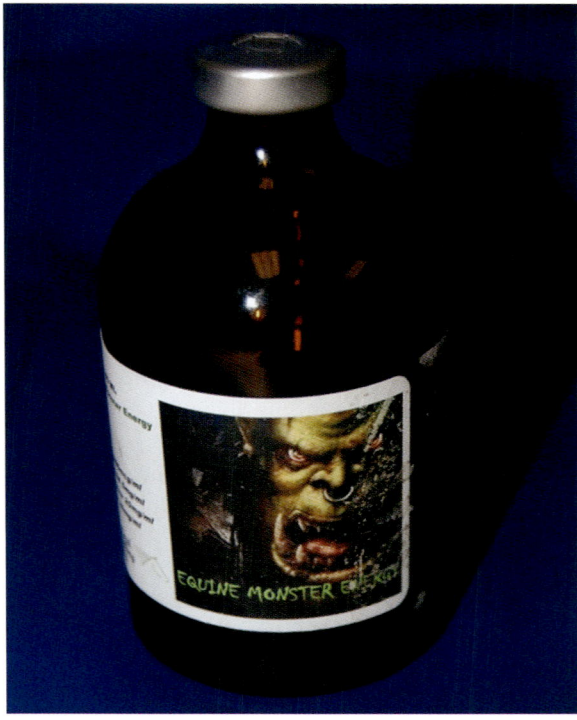

■ **Fig. 5.1.** Compounded substance labeled Equine Monster Energy. Interestingly, this product also violates copyright law due to the image on the bottle. *Source*: Photo courtesy of Dionne Benson.

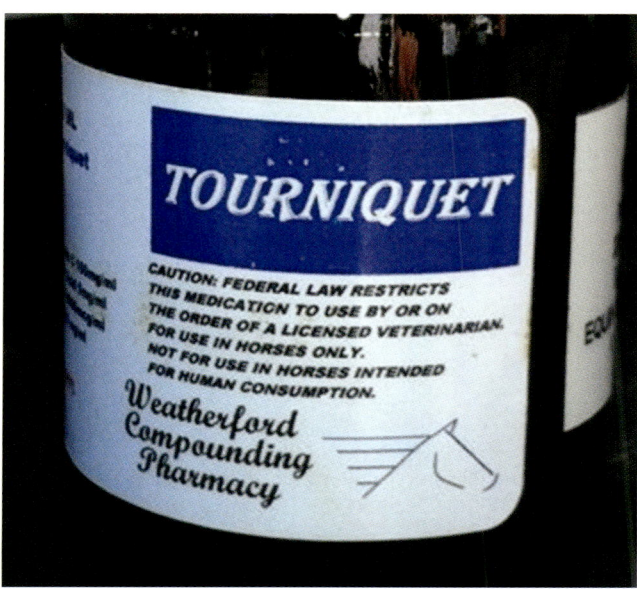

■ **Fig. 5.2.** Compounded substance labeled Tourniquet. *Source*: Photo courtesy of Dionne Benson.

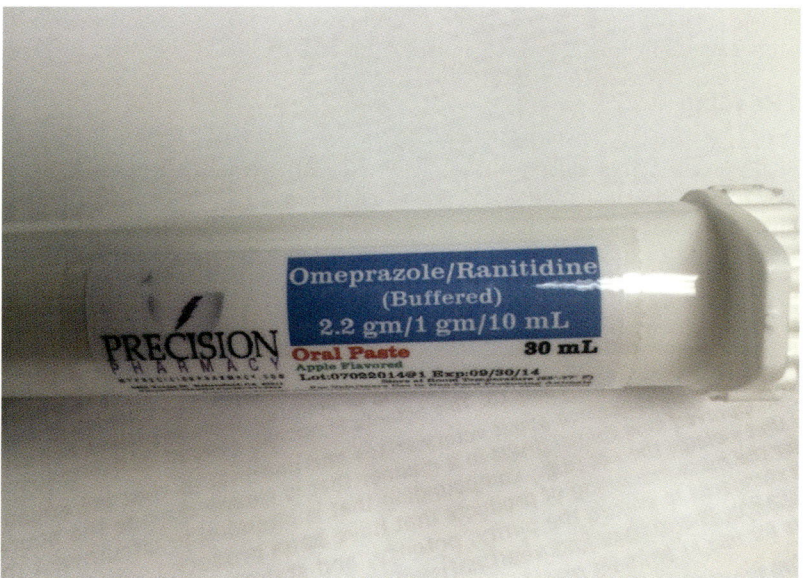

■ **Fig. 5.3.** Compounded substance labeled omeprazole/ranitidine. *Source*: Photo courtesy of Dionne Benson.

These requirements are not imposed for compounded medications. In fact, the FDA involvement in compounded medications is often limited to investigation after incidents occur such as those listed above.

Additionally, it is important to consider that the use of compounded medications for cost-saving purposes is prohibited under FDA regulation. For example, purchasing compounded ketoprofen to avoid paying for brand name Ketofen® is illegal.

Finally, practitioners should know that the use of compounded medication is often specifically excluded on professional liability insurance. In other words, if you are treating a horse and prescribe a compounded medication and something goes wrong, your insurance company may not have to defend you from or indemnify you for any liability.

The safest course of action is to avoid the use of compounded medication altogether whenever possible and find a reputable compounder to use in those instances where it is the only alternative.

Abbreviations

See Appendix 1 for a complete list.

Internet Resources

American Association of Veterinary Medicine, Veterinary Compounding, undated. Available at https://www.avma.org/resources-tools/avma-policies/veterinary-compounding (accessed February 8, 2021).

Thomas K. Polo ponies were given incorrect medication. The New York Times, April 23, 2009. Available at: https://www.nytimes.com/2009/04/24/sports/othersports/24polo.html (accessed February 5, 2021).

United States Food and Drug Administration. Compounded Unapproved Animal Drugs from Rapid Equine Solutions Linked to Three Horse Deaths, July 23, 2019. Available at: https://www.fda.gov/animal-veterinary/cvm-updates/compounded-unapproved-animal-drugs-rapid-equine-solutions-linked-three-horse-deaths (accessed February 5, 2021).

United States Food and Drug Administration. FDA Alerts Horse Owners and Veterinarians About Adverse Events Associated with Certain Unapproved Compounded Drugs in Horses, May 15, 2014. Available at: https://wayback.archive-it.org/7993/20170406075905/https:/www.fda.gov/AnimalVeterinary/NewsEvents/CVMUpdates/ucm397345.htm (accessed February 5, 2021).

Suggested Reading

Thompson J, Mirza M, Barker S, et al. Clenbuterol toxicosis in three quarter horse racehorses after administration of a compounded product. J Am Vet Med Assoc 2011; 239:842–849.

Barlas S. Deaths from contaminated methylprednisolone highlight failures of compounding pharmacies: Less hospital access to outside vendors and more visits from state pharmacy boards. P T. 2013; 38(1):27–57.

Author: Dionne Benson, DVM, JD
Consulting Editor: Dionne Benson, DVM, JD

Specific Toxins and Toxicants

section

Drugs: Illicit and Recreational

Drugs: Prescription

Insecticides, Herbicides and Farm Chemicals

Ionophores and Growth Promotants

Metals

Mycotoxins/Fungus

Other Toxins

Plants and Biotoxins

Rodenticides

Toxic Gases

Trees

Zootoxins

Drugs: Illicit and Recreational

Chapter 6

Cobalt

DEFINITION/OVERVIEW

- Cobalt is a trace element that is a necessary part of the equine diet.
- There are no reported cobalt deficiencies in horses.
- Cobalt is present in feed, supplements, and injectables that are marketed for equine use.
- Cobalt is also purchased from compounding pharmacies.
- Cobalt is used in the equine hindgut to make vitamin B_{12}.
- In humans, cobalt has been used to mimic hypoxia, stimulating RBC production.
- In horses, no RBC production has been observed with IV administration of varying doses.
- Intentional administration of excessive amounts of cobalt have led to toxicosis.
- Controlled substance under ARCI rules.

ETIOLOGY/PATHOPHYSIOLOGY

Mechanism of Action

- Unknown – in humans cobalt stabilizes HIF factors, causing increased erythropoiesis. Although studied, the same effects have not been observed in horses.

Toxicokinetics

- Onset is rapid with effects occurring within minutes of IV administration.
- Duration of action is minutes to hours for a single exposure. Repeated exposure effects have not been studied.
- Absorption through the GI tract – in studies in sheep bioavailability varied by preparation. In horses, they are most often administered IV.
- Hepatic metabolism: horses administered cobalt often have elevated concentrations in liver tissue.
- Excretion – urinary excretion.

Toxicity

- Highly toxic – clinical signs observed at doses as low as 0.25 mg/kg.
- Toxic effects may vary by dose with some clinical signs observed more often at higher doses.

Blackwell's Five-Minute Veterinary Consult Clinical Companion: Equine Toxicology,
First Edition. Edited by Lynn R. Hovda, Dionne Benson, and Robert H. Poppenga.
© 2022 John Wiley & Sons, Inc. Published 2022 by John Wiley & Sons, Inc.
Companion website: www.wiley.com/go/hovda/equine

Systems Affected

- Neurological – anxiety, ataxia, tremors, muscle fasciculations.
- Cardiovascular – tachycardia, arrhythmias (including VT), increases in MAP, SAP, DAP.
- Gastrointestinal – colic.
- Renal – hematuria.

SIGNALMENT/HISTORY

Risk Factors

- Iatrogenic administration.
- Exposure to cobalt salts intended for other species (e.g., goats).

Historical Findings

- Iatrogenic administration.
- Owners or trainers may be reluctant to admit administration due to regulations.
- Incidental exposure to cobalt salt intended for another animal.

Location and Circumstances of Poisoning

- Worldwide problem, especially in racehorses.
- Often intentional exposure in horse racing due to perceived increased erythropoietic effects.
- Unintentional exposure by placement of cobalt salts, especially when co-mingling of horses in pasture with animals requiring cobalt supplementation.

CLINICAL FEATURES

- Variable by dose received.
- Common signs include agitation, ataxia, muscle fasciculations, tachycardia, arrhythmias, hematuria, colic.

DIFFERENTIAL DIAGNOSIS

- Colic of other etiology.
- UTI or bladder stone for hematuria
- Rhabdomyolysis.
- HYPP.
- WNV.
- WEE, VEE, EEE.
- Rabies.

DIAGNOSTICS

CBC/Serum Chemistry/Urinalysis

- Routine laboratory work including serum chemistry and urinalysis.
- Transient increase RBC for 1 hour post-administration.
- Mild increase in lactate and glucose within 1 hour of administration.
- RBCs and urinary epithelial cells in urine.
- ± hypocalcemia.
- Specialized testing for elevated cTnI within 24–48 hours of administration.

Other Diagnostic Tests

- ECG as needed for tachycardia and cardiac effects.
- Presence in serum and urine:
  - No rapid, commercially available urine tests.
  - ICP-MS useful for diagnosis, but the time delay would hinder therapeutics.

Pathological Findings

- No specific lesions reported in horses.

THERAPEUTICS

- The goal of therapy is to provide supportive care.

Detoxification

- Large ingestions – gastric lavage or reflux with large-bore tube.
- Supportive care if symptomatic.

Appropriate Health Care

- Most can be treated in the field.
- Most clinical parameters return to baseline within 2 hours.

Antidote

- No specific antidote.

Drugs of Choice

- IV fluids as needed for dehydration and volume expansion; may be helpful to increase elimination.
- Agitation:
  - Acepromazine 0.01–0.05 mg/kg IV, IM, SC prn.
  - Adrenergic agonist: detomidine 10–40 μg/kg IM, IV or xylazine 0.5–1 mg/kg IV.
- GI protectants:
  - Omeprazole 2–4 mg/kg PO q24h.

- Tremors, twitching:
  - Acepromazine 0.01–0.05 mg/kg IV, IM, SC prn/
  - Methocarbamol 4.4–22.2 mg/kg IV to effect. Administer half estimated dose and pause until the horse has relaxed. Administer the remainder of the dose to effect. Repeat as needed but do not exceed 330 mg/kg/day.

Precautions/Interactions

Protection to the head and limbs may be necessary in severely agitated horses.

COMMENTS

Client Education

- There is no purpose for cobalt supplementation in horses.
- ICP-MS may be useful in legal cases.

Prevention/Avoidance

- Educate trainers and owners about the adverse effects in horses.

Possible Complications

- Acute kidney injury.
- Cardiac damage.
- Injury due to ataxia/colic.
- Long-term potential to cause arrhythmias resulting in sudden death.

Expected Course and Prognosis

- Toxicity – for experimentally induced cases, prognosis is good with effects generally subsiding after 2 hours.
- Fatality – prevalence of fatality in clinical cases is unknown as reports are limited.

Abbreviations

See Appendix 1 for a complete list.

Internet Resources

Racing Medication and Testing Consortium, Cobalt. Available at: https://rmtcnet.com/wp-content/uploads/2015-10-Cobalt-Brochure.pdf (accessed January 15, 2021).

European Food Safety Authority, Scientific Opinion on Safety and Efficacy of Cobalt Carbonate as Feed Additive for Ruminants, Horses and Rabbits. Available at: https://efsa.onlinelibrary.wiley.com/doi/pdf/10.2903/j.efsa.2012.2727 (accessed January 15, 2021).

Suggested Reading

Burns TA, Dembek KA, Kamr A, et al. Effect of intravenous administration of cobalt chloride to horses on clinical and hemodynamic variables. J Vet Intern Med 2018; 32:441–449.

Knych, HK, Arthur, RM, Mitchell MM, et al. Pharmacokinetics and selected pharmacodynamics of cobalt following a single intravenous administration to horses. Drug Test Anal 2015; 7:619–625.

Author: Dionne Benson, DVM, JD
Consulting Editor: Dionne Benson, DVM, JD

Chapter 7

Cocaine

DEFINITION/OVERVIEW

- A white pearlescent powder in its purest form, usually present as a hydrochloride salt. The street drug typically looks like a fine, white, crystalline powder and often contains substances such as cornstarch, talcum powder, or flour as extenders. Occasionally other drugs such as caffeine, levamisole, fentanyl, aminorex, or amphetamines are mixed with the cocaine.
- "Crack" cocaine is the freebase form that has been precipitated into rocks that can be smoked.
- Schedule II drug used for local anesthesia, where vasoconstriction may be advantageous.
- Cocaine is a tropane alkaloid obtained from leaves of shrubs in the genus *Erythroxylaceae*, which are domesticated tropical plants native to the Amazon and the eastern slope of the Andes in Bolivia and Peru.
- Although the active ingredient, cocaine, was only isolated in 1859 by German chemist Albert Niemann, the coca leaves have been used for both medicinal and recreational purposes by the native populations in South American for thousands of years.
- Cocaine is the only naturally occurring local anesthetic. It is also one of the most abused drugs in the world.
- Because of its use as a recreational drug and its powder formulation, residues of cocaine are occasionally found in blood and urine samples collected from horses in drug and medication control programs.
- Prohibited substance under USEF, FEI, AQHA, and ARCI regulations.

ETIOLOGY/PATHOPHYSIOLOGY

Mechanism of Action

- The pharmacodynamics of cocaine involve the complex relationships of multiple neurotransmitters.
- It directly prevents the re-uptake of dopamine, serotonin, and norepinephrine into presynaptic neurons.
- Like other local anesthetics, it produces direct effects on cell membranes – cocaine blocks sodium channel activity and thus prevents the generation and conduction of nerve impulses in electrically active cells, such as myocardial and nerve cells.

Blackwell's Five-Minute Veterinary Consult Clinical Companion: Equine Toxicology,
First Edition. Edited by Lynn R. Hovda, Dionne Benson, and Robert H. Poppenga.
© 2022 John Wiley & Sons, Inc. Published 2022 by John Wiley & Sons, Inc.
Companion website: www.wiley.com/go/hovda/equine

Toxicokinetics

- Cocaine has not been well studied in the horse. Based on the scientific literature examining the effects of cocaine in other species, however, in the horse one would expect it to be well absorbed when administered via mucous membranes (e.g. intranasally) or the GI tract.
- In humans, peak concentrations occur within 5–10 minutes of smoking and within 60 minutes of intranasal administration.
- Some cocaine is excreted unchanged in the urine, but the vast majority is metabolized to benzoylecgonine, ecgonine methyl ester, norcocaine and other metabolites.
- Although cocaine has a short elimination half-life, the half-lives of cocaine metabolites are substantially longer.

Toxicity

- The lethal dose for cocaine in horses has not been determined and there are no reports of acute toxicity in the scientific literature.
- In mice the LD_{50} is reported to be 96 mg/kg following oral administration.
- In humans, recreational cocaine abusers typically have peak serum concentrations between 0.5 and 5 µM, but lethal toxicity has been observed with serum concentrations of cocaine of 10 µM.

Systems Affected

- Neurological – ataxia, disorientation, euphoria, agitation, anxiety, seizures.
- Cardiovascular – tachydysrhythmia, severe hypertension, acute coronary syndrome in humans, stroke.
- Musculoskeletal – hyperthermia, cocaine-induced rhabdomyolysis.

SIGNALMENT/HISTORY

Risk Factors

- Accidental ingestion is unlikely.
- Illicit administration for performance-enhancing effects in racehorses could occur.
- Inadvertent exposure from by a human abuser or from a contaminated environment is theoretically possible.

Historical Findings

- Owners and trainers may be reluctant to admit possession and use.
- In many cases, the source may not be identified.

Location and Circumstances of Poisoning

- Worldwide problem, not just limited to the United States.
- Intentional exposure by direct administration to horse.
- Unintentional exposure by careless placement of product or inadvertent transfer from personnel could theoretically cause detectable concentrations of cocaine or its metabolites to be present in blood and urine samples, but toxic concentrations are unlikely.

CLINICAL FEATURES

- With pharmacologically significant doses:
  - CNS stimulation.
  - Tachycardia.
  - Arrhythmias.
  - Bilateral mydriasis.
  - Increased locomotor activity.
- Many exposures are not pharmacologically significant, although they produce detectable concentrations of cocaine metabolites in urine and blood samples.

DIFFERENTIAL DIAGNOSIS

- CNS stimulants (amphetamines, methamphetamine).
- High doses of beta$_2$-adrenergic agonists.
- High doses of caffeine or other methylxanthines.

DIAGNOSTICS

CBC/Serum Chemistry/Urinalysis

- BUN, creatinine, and creatine kinase for evidence of rhabdomyolysis

Serum Samples/Urine Samples

- Immunoassay screening.
- LC-MS.

Other Diagnostic Tests

- ECG as needed for tachydysrhythmia and cardiac effects.

Pathological Findings

- None reported in the horses, but from other species, if dose was high enough one would predict:
  - Myocardial necrosis and hemorrhage.
  - Pulmonary hemorrhage.

THERAPEUTICS

Appropriate Health Care

- Monitor ECG and treat arrhythmias.
- Maintain blood volume, pH, and electrolyte balance.
- Monitor for hyperthermia.
- Avoid CNS stimulation; dark quiet stall if possible.

Antidotes

No specific antidote.

Drugs of Choice

- IV fluids as needed.
- For excitation:
    - Detomdine 20–40 µg/kg IV.
    - Romifidine 40–120 µg/kg IV.
- Control life-threatening cardiac arrhythmias:
    - Propranolol 0.02 mg/kg IV slowly, maximum of 1 mg/kg.
    - Esmolol CRI 25–75 µg/kg/min.

Precautions/Interactions

- Ethanol potentiates the effects and may increase the risk of toxicity.
- Protection of the head and limbs may be necessary with excitation.

COMMENTS

Client Education

- LC-MS may be useful in legal cases.

Prevention/Avoidance

- Prevent exposure to illegal drugs.
- Keep animals away from illegal drugs.
- Educate trainers/riders/grooms of the risk of low-level contamination.
- Avoid access to illegal drugs.

Expected Course and Prognosis

- Acute fatal toxicity has not been reported. Toxic effects would likely reside within hours.

Abbreviations

See Appendix 1 for a complete list.

Suggested Reading

Kollias-Baker C, Maxwell L, Stanley S, Boone T. Detection and quantification of cocaine metabolites in urine samples from horses administered cocaine. J Vet Pharmacol Ther. 2003; 26(6):429–434.

Richards JR, Hollander JE, Ramoska EA, et al. β-Blockers, cocaine, and the unopposed α-stimulation phenomenon. J Cardiovasc Pharmacol Ther 2017; 22(3):239–249.

Zimmerman JL. Cocaine intoxication. Crit Care Clin 2012; 28(4):517–526.

Author: Cynthia Cole, DVM, PhD, DACVCP
Consulting Editor: Dionne Benson, DVM, JD

Chapter 8

Dermorphin

DEFINITION/OVERVIEW

- Dermorphin ("derm" = skin, and "morphin" = morphine) is just one compound in a family of peptides secreted by the skin of South American hylid frogs, genus *Phyllomedusa*.
- Most commonly found as a synthesized series of amino acids.
- Dermorphin is a hepta-peptide known to have exceptionally long-lasting and potent opioid activity.
- Potency is about 30–40 times greater than that of morphine, and less likely to cause a drug tolerance effect and addiction in humans.
- In humans it has been shown to block pain effectively.
- First detected in post-race testing in Quarter Horse racing in the southwestern United States in 30 horses in 2011–2012.
- Dermorphin stimulates locomotor activity and purportedly improves focus and determination in equines.
- The D-isomer is biologically active, but the L-isomer is not.
- Prohibited under ARCI and AQHA rules.

ETIOLOGY/PATHOPHYSIOLOGY

Mechanism of Action

- Dermorphin is a mu-opioid receptor-binding peptide that causes central and peripheral effects after intravenous administration to rats, dogs, and humans.
- In addition to dermorphin, the family of mu-opioid agonists include seven naturally occurring dermorphin analogs, and at least 30 known synthetic analogs. The inactive L-isomer of dermorphin is also known as "pseudomorphin". Another close relative is HYP^6-dermorphin, which contains hydroxyproline instead of proline in the otherwise same amino acid sequence.
- Some members of the dermorphin peptide family can cross the blood–brain barrier (BBB) and produce central antinociception after peripheral administration, but dermorphin itself is not able to cross the BBB.

Toxicokinetics

- Onset of action is rapid with clinical signs appearing in minutes.

Blackwell's Five-Minute Veterinary Consult Clinical Companion: Equine Toxicology,
First Edition. Edited by Lynn R. Hovda, Dionne Benson, and Robert H. Poppenga.
© 2022 John Wiley & Sons, Inc. Published 2022 by John Wiley & Sons, Inc.
Companion website: www.wiley.com/go/hovda/equine

- Duration of action is short, with most clinical signs subsiding within hours.
- Hepatic and renal metabolism was observed in rats.
- Urinary excretion primarily.

Toxicity

- Toxicity observed in horses in doses of 5 mg.
- Compounded versions may have variable toxicity.
- Dermorphin is unstable at room temp, with some studies showing > 50% degradation after 4 hours at room temperature which may contribute to toxicity. The L-isomer (inactive stereoisomer) is more labile than the D-isomer (active form).

Systems Affected

- Neurological – head shaking, sedation, sweating, increased locomotion, catalepsy.
- Gastrointestinal – colic, decreased borborygmi.
- Cardiovascular – tachypnea.
- Musculoskeletal – antinociception.

SIGNALMENT

Risk Factors

- Iatrogenic.

Historical Findings

- Owners and trainers may be reluctant to admit possession or use.

Location and Circumstances of Poisoning

- Likely in competitive equine sports environment (e.g., racing, barrel racing, etc.).

CLINICAL FEATURES

- Clinical signs begin less than a minute after administration.
- Common signs include head shaking, sedation, sweating, trance-like state, colic, tachypnea, and antinociception.

DIFFERENTIAL DIAGNOSIS

- CNS depressants (benzodiazepine, opioids).
- Hallucinogenic plants and mushrooms.
- Ethanol.
- Rabies.
- Colic of other etiology.

DIAGNOSTICS

CBC/Serum Chemistry/Urinalysis

- Routine bloodwork:
  - Hyponatremia/hypokalemia reported in humans but may be attributable to other causes.
- Presence in serum and urine:
  - Detection times of 12 hours in plasma and approximately 48–72 hours in urine using LC-MS detection which is useful for diagnosis.

Pathological Findings

- None reported in horses.

Therapeutics

- The goal of therapy is to provide supportive care.

Detoxification

- None.

Appropriate Health Care

- Field treatment.

Antidotes

- None.

Drugs of Choice

- None.

Precautions/Interactions

- Protection for the head and limbs may be necessary due to headshaking, increased locomotion, and anti-nociception.

COMMENTS

Client Education

- LC-MS/MS may be useful in legal cases.

Prevention/Avoidance

- Education trainers and owners about potential issues.

Possible Complications

- Musculoskeletal injury due to antinociception.
- Sudden death reported in humans.

Expected Course and Prognosis

- No reported fatal toxicosis in horses. Effects generally subside after 1 hour.

Abbreviations

See Appendix 1 for a complete list.

Suggested Reading

Melchiorri P, Negri L. The dermorphin peptide family. Gen Pharm 1996; 27(7):1099–1107.

Negri L, Espamer GF, Severini C, et al. Dermorphin-related peptides from the skin of *Phyllomedusa bicolor* and their amidated analogs activate two μ opioid receptor subtypes that modulate antinociception and catalepsy in the rat. Proc Natl Acad Sci 1992; 89: 7203–7207.

Negri L, Improta G. Distribution and metabolism of dermorphin in rats. Pharmacol Res Commun 1984; 16(12):1183–1191.

Robinson MA, Guan F, McDonnell S., et al., Pharmacokinetics and pharmacodynamics of dermorphin in the horse. J Vet Pharmacol Ther 2015; 38(4):321–329.

Author: Petra Hartmann-Fischbach, MS, FAORC
Consulting Editor: Dionne Benson, DVM, JD

Growth Hormone and Secretagogues

Chapter 9

 DEFINITION/OVERVIEW

- Growth hormone (GH) is a protein hormone that is produced in the pituitary gland and is essential to normal growth, development, and overall health of animals.
- Recombinant GH, growth hormone-releasing peptides, or small molecule drugs capable of stimulating the release of GH have been developed or approved as pharmaceutical agents.
- Cases may be a result of accidental or illicit use in performance horses.

 ETIOLOGY/PATHOPHYSIOLOGY

- There are no FDA-approved GH formulations approved for use in the horse. There are no peptide or small molecule mimetics of GH approved by the FDA for use in the horse.
- There are many compounds that are currently undergoing pre-clinical development or clinical trials.
- Illicit formulations of GH and its mimetics are readily available on the internet, primarily directed towards body builders and other performance athletes.
- The prevalence of use is unknown, and administrations may be unreported to practitioners due to illicit use.

Mechanism of Action

- Natural production:
  - Hormone produced in the anterior pituitary gland which is under the control of either GH stimulatory hormone (+) or somatostatin (−) produced in the hypothalamus.
  - Following release into systemic circulation, GH binds to GH receptors found on target cells.
  - GH has several effects, both directly acting on target tissues and via downstream mediators such as insulin-like growth factor 1 (IGF-1).
  - GH increases muscle, bone, and organ growth and increased cellular protein synthesis and intracellular lipolysis.
- Recombinant GH:
  - Synthetically produced to mimic the effects of naturally produced GH.
  - FDA has approved recombinant GHs for both human and bovine versions.
  - Equine recombinant GH was developed in the late 1990s and marketed in Australia.

Blackwell's Five-Minute Veterinary Consult Clinical Companion: Equine Toxicology,
First Edition. Edited by Lynn R. Hovda, Dionne Benson, and Robert H. Poppenga.
© 2022 John Wiley & Sons, Inc. Published 2022 by John Wiley & Sons, Inc.
Companion website: www.wiley.com/go/hovda/equine

- GH-releasing peptides:
  - Synthetically produced to mimic the effects of GH-releasing hormone binding to either the GH-releasing hormone receptor or the GH secretagogue receptor.
  - These may also act as mimetics to the natural hormone ghrelin.
  - Examples include hexarelin, sermorelin, hexarelin, tesamorelin, GHRP 2, GHRP 6, CJC-1295, CJC-1295-DAC.
- Small molecule mimetics:
  - Small molecule drugs synthesized to mimic the effects of GH-releasing peptides.
  - Examples include Ibutamorelin and Anamorelin.

Toxicokinetics

- Little is known about onset of action or duration of toxicity for GH.
- Recombinant GH:
  - Typical routes of administration are SC or IM injection (8 µg/kg daily) as oral bioavailability is minimal.
  - Variable pharmacokinetics depending on dose/route with Cmax ~ 4 hours post-dose, ~2 hours terminal half-life. Cleared by proteolytic digestion and urinary excretion.
- GH-releasing peptides – limited pharmacokinetic information in the horse:
  - Typically dosed via SC or IM administration as oral bioavailability is < 1% for most compounds.
  - Rapid half-lives < 1 hour except for CJC-1295-DAC due to the presence of the drug affinity complex which increases binding to free thiols in blood.
  - Cleared by proteolytic digestion and urinary excretion.
- Small molecule mimetics – limited pharmacokinetic information in the horse:
  - Oral bioavailability is good (> 50%), distribution, metabolism and excretion are not well characterized.

Toxicity

- Acute – injection site reaction and muscle stiffness. Potential pyrexia. Overdose can result in hypoglycemia followed by hyperglycemia and fluid retention. Acute effects are not fully understood in the horse.
- Chronic – acromegaly and gigantism noted in humans and other species. Chronic effects are unknown in the horse.

Systems Affected

- Cardiovascular – cardiomegaly, hypo/hypertension.
- Endocrine/metabolic – hypopituitarism, hypothyroidism, disturbances in maintenance of blood glucose levels.
- Gastrointestinal – potential for increased feed and fluid intake.
- Hemic/lymphatic/immune – injection site reactions, potential neutralizing antibody formation.
- Musculoskeletal – potential for increased muscle mass and weight gain, stimulation of skeletal growth. Potential for increased osteoarthritis.
- Renal/urologic – fluid retention.
- Reproductive – potential for mammary stimulation at high doses.
- Skin/exocrine – injection site reactions, excessive sweating.

SIGNALMENT/HISTORY

Potential for increased illicit use in performance horses.

Risk Factors

- Higher potential for use in performance horses
- Incomplete medical records and failure to disclose administrations by owners/trainers.

Historical Findings

- History of use of GH substances. Owner or trainer may be reluctant to disclose.
- History of use of other performance-enhancing drugs with similar desired effects such as anabolic steroids, selective androgen receptor modulators and beta-agonists.
- Performance supplement use.

CLINICAL FEATURES

- Clinical exam may not suggest exposure.

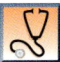
DIFFERENTIAL DIAGNOSIS

- Administration of other pharmaceutical agents such as anabolic steroids.
- Stimulation of hypothalamic–pituitary axis by other environmental or pharmaceutical agents.
- Evaluate for pituitary gland disorders or neoplasms.
- Administration of IGF-1.

DIAGNOSTICS

- IGF1 levels can be determined from blood samples.
- Hyperglycemia or hypoglycemia depending upon time course.
- Detection of parent compounds (GH or its secretagogues) is not a routine clinical diagnostic test.
- Potential to send samples to specialized laboratories for LC-MS testing.

THERAPEUTICS

- Objectives of treatment are to prevent further exposure to compounds and provide symptomatic treatments.

Detoxification

- No well-characterized treatment strategies. Detoxification strategy based upon reducing potential for exposure.

Antidotes

- Somatostatin analogs (octreotide and lareotide) have strong suppression on GH production.

Appropriate Health Care

- Monitor blood glucose levels.
- CBC and biochemistry panel to evaluate hydration status and overall health.
- Evaluate thyroid and parathyroid levels.
- Potential for increased urinary excretion of inorganic phosphorus and calcium.
- Hepatic function panel to evaluate abnormal alkaline phosphatase.
- Evaluate for elevated IGF-1 in blood sample.

Precautions/Interactions

- Decreased insulin sensitivity and glucose intolerance.
- Avoid co-administration with CYP450 substrates.
- Decreased efficacy of corticosteroids.

COMMENTS

Client Education

- Educate client on the potential for exposure from performance-enhancing supplements marketed on the internet.

Prevention/Avoidance

- Remove compounds from the environment.

Possible Complications

- Contaminants or adulterants found in supplements.
- Unknown exposure to other related compounds.

Expected Course and Prognosis

- Compounds are relatively quickly eliminated following administration.
- Effects are time- and dose-dependent, with lower dosages and duration of exposure having better prognosis.

Abbreviations

See Appendix 1 for a complete list.

Suggested Reading

Sigalos JT, Patuszak AW. The safety and efficacy of growth hormone secretagogues. Sex Med Rev 2018; 6:45–53.

Anderson LJ, Tamayose JM, Garcia JM. Use of growth hormone, IGF-I, and insulin for anabolic purpose: pharmacological basis, methods of detection, and adverse effects. Mol Cell Endocrinol 2018; 464:65–74.

Bailly-Chouriberry L, Pinel G, Garcia P, et al. Identification of recombinant equine growth hormone in horse plasma by LC-MS/MS: A confirmatory analysis in doping control. Anal Chem 2008; 80(21):8340–8347.

Author: Benjamin C. Moeller, PhD, DABT
Consulting Editor: Dionne Benson, DVM, JD

Chapter 10

Marijuana

DEFINITION/OVERVIEW

- Marijuana comes from the *Cannabis sativa* plant.
- The plant has a long history of use by humans for recreational, medicinal, religious, and industrial purposes.
- Marijuana is also known as pot, weed, grass, hemp, hashish, and many other names.
- *Cannabis sativa* has very distinctive leaves, with five to seven long leaflets on each stem.
- The plant also produces small green flowers, also called buds, and fruit that is oval and flat (see Fig. 10.1).
- The two major active compounds contained in the marijuana plant are CBD and THC.
- CBD products are widely available in many states as oils, creams, serums, and other products and may contain THC.
- THC is the compound responsible for producing psychoactive effects.
- The concentration of THC is variable, depending upon growing conditions, plant genetics, which parts of the plant were ingested, whether the plant was fresh or dried, processing after harvest, and time between harvesting of the plant and use (see Fig. 10.2)
- Exposure by ingestion of plant material or inhalation of smoke produced by burning the plant may be harmful to equines.
- The systems most affected by exposure to marijuana in horses are the neurological and GI systems.
- Prohibited substance under USEF, FEI, AQHA, and ARCI regulations.

ETIOLOGY/PATHOPHYSIOLOGY

Mechanism of Action

- Not specifically known in horses.
- In dogs, THC is a CB1 and CB2 receptor antagonist.
- The receptors for CB1 are located in the CNS and, when exposed to THC, may cause adverse effects on the mind and body.
- Colic may result due to irritation of the lining of the GI tract after ingestion of marijuana.

Blackwell's Five-Minute Veterinary Consult Clinical Companion: Equine Toxicology,
First Edition. Edited by Lynn R. Hovda, Dionne Benson, and Robert H. Poppenga.
© 2022 John Wiley & Sons, Inc. Published 2022 by John Wiley & Sons, Inc.
Companion website: www.wiley.com/go/hovda/equine

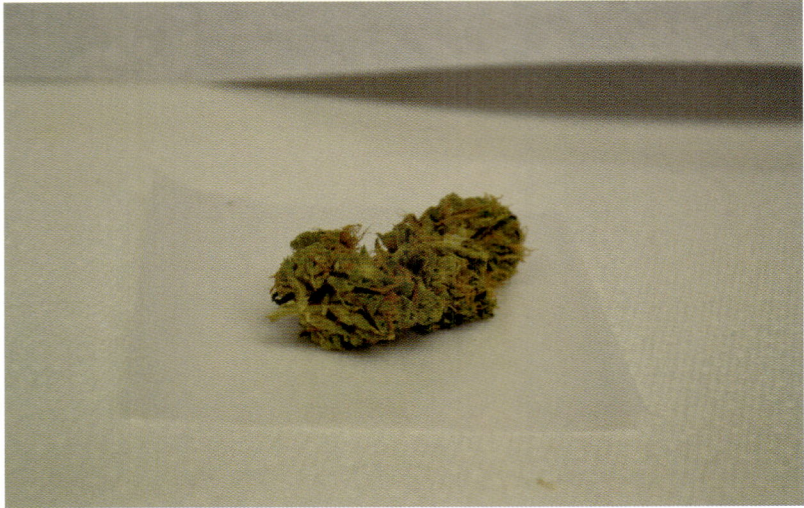

■ **Fig. 10.1.** Marijuana bud (*Cannabis sativa*). *Source*: Photo courtesy of Seth Wong, Industrial Laboratories, Wheat Ridge, CO.

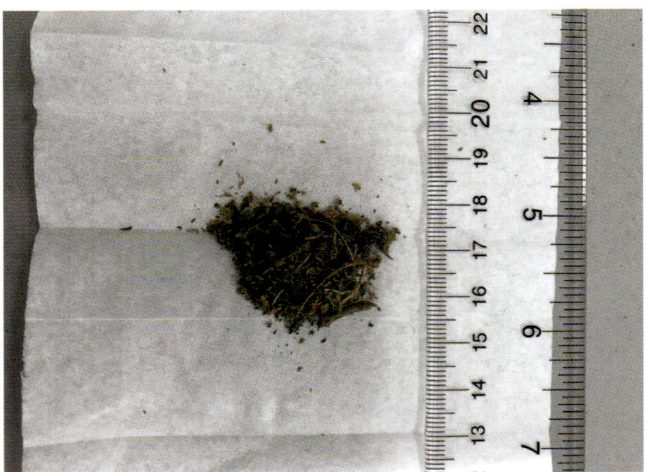

■ **Fig. 10.2.** Ground marijuana plant material. *Source*: Photo courtesy of Seth Wong, Industrial Laboratories, Wheat Ridge, CO.

Toxicokinetics

- Marijuana is absorbed through the GI tract after ingestion or absorbed through the respiratory system after inhalation of marijuana smoke.
- Distribution is not specifically known in equines but in dogs, marijuana is highly distributed to liver, kidney, brain and fat.
- Metabolism is not specifically known in equines but in dogs it occurs primarily in the liver. Metabolites of marijuana do cross the blood–brain barrier.
- Elimination is not specifically known in equines but is through the urine and feces (through bile) in small animals.

Toxicity

- Not specifically known in equines.
- Toxic dose depends on many variables, including amount and route of exposure as well as potency of the marijuana ingested or inhaled.

Systems Affected

- Nervous system – CNS depression or other abnormal behavior in horses. In dogs may include ataxia, disorientation, and coma. CNS stimulation occurs in some dogs.
- GI system – colic.

SIGNALMENT/HISTORY

Risk Factors

- Marijuana use by an owner/trainer/handler may expose an animal to it.
- Consumption of marijuana plant parts (either deliberately or accidentally) or inhalation of second-hand smoke.

Historical Findings

- Some horses may be deliberately exposed to marijuana.
- Owners may not admit possible exposure to an animal as they may be hesitant to disclose marijuana possession or use.
- Some animals may experience exposure in pastures or in baled hay or other feeds or supplements.

Location and Circumstances of Poisoning

- Marijuana use by humans is widespread, and therefore cases can occur anywhere in the country.
- Many states have legalized recreational use of marijuana, making exposure to animals more likely.

CLINICAL FEATURES

- Onset of clinical signs is not specifically known in horses, but in humans the onset of effect of THC occurs in 30–60 minutes post ingestion and 6–12 minutes post-inhalation.
- In dogs, clinical signs are typically seen within 30–60 minutes of exposure but may be as soon as 5 minutes or as long as 12 hours post-exposure.
- In humans, depending on the potency and amount of marijuana used, the half-life can range from about 20 hours to 10 days.
- Systems most commonly affected include:
  - Nervous system – depression, ataxia or other abnormal behavior. Signs of CNS stimulation sometimes occur in dogs and may possibly occur in horses.
  - GI – signs of colic may occur.

DIFFERENTIAL DIAGNOSIS

- Synthetic cannabinoids.
- Substances with CNS depressant effects (opioids, benzodiazepines or others).
- Amphetamines or other substances with CNS stimulant effects.

DIAGNOSTICS

- Careful questioning of the client may reveal exposure to marijuana.
- Inspection of pastures or feed material may reveal an exposure source.
- THC is detectable by LC-MS.
- In humans, metabolites of THC may be detectable in urine for approximately 3–15 days after using marijuana.

THERAPEUTICS

- Treatment objectives are to provide supportive care for affected animals and prevent absorption of marijuana. Removing the source of the marijuana is also important.

Detoxification

- The main goal of therapy would be to remove the marijuana source from the environment.
- Gastric lavage for any horse that has recently ingested a large quantity of marijuana.
- Activated charcoal.

Appropriate Health Care

- Monitor for CNS signs.
- Most common sign is depression which generally is not treated.
- Sedation may be required if hazardous behavior occurs due to CNS stimulation.

Antidotes

- None.

Drugs of Choice

- IV fluids for depressed and/or dehydrated horses.
- Di-Tri-Octahedral (DTO) smectite (Bio-Sponge®)
- Sedation if needed for animals with CNS stimulation:
    - Xylazine 1.1 mg/kg IV or 2.2 mg/kg IM prn.
    - Detomidine 0.02–0.04 mg/kg IV or IM prn.

Precautions/Interactions

- Marijuana compounds can interact with other medications although specifics in horses are not known.

Surgical Considerations

- Not known specifically but if the horse is exhibiting neurologic effects, especially depression, it may be wise to delay procedures requiring anesthesia.

 COMMENTS

Client Education

- Clients should be educated on the need to remove marijuana from the horse's environment.
- A specific withdrawal time for marijuana is not known in horses and so clients should be made aware that marijuana may be detected in drug testing of horses used for racing or showing.

Prevention/Avoidance

- Eliminate marijuana from the environment.

Expected Course and Prognosis

- Marijuana toxicity is rarely fatal in animals.
- Time to recovery will depend on type of exposure (ingested or inhaled) as well as quantity and potency of toxin.
- Marijuana may possibly be detected in drug tests on horses used for racing or showing after clinical signs have resolved.

See Also

Synthetic Cannabinoids

Abbreviations

See Appendix 1 for a complete list.

Suggested Reading

Donaldson CW. Marijuana exposure in animals. Vet Med 2002; 97:437–441.
Hovda L, Brutlag A, Poppenga R, Peterson K. Small Animal Toxicology, 2nd edn. John Wiley & Sons, Inc., 2016.
Stillabower, A. Marijuana Toxicity in Pets. Available at: https://www.petpoisonhelpline.com/pet-safety-tips/marijuana-toxicity-pets/ (accessed April 3, 2021).
Ujvary I, Hanus L. Human metabolites of cannabidiol: A review on their formation, biological activity, and relevance in therapy. Cannabis Cannabinoid Res 2016; 1: 90–101.

Author: Christy Klatt, DVM
Consulting Editor: Dionne Benson, DVM, JD

Chapter 11

Methamphetamine/Amphetamine

DEFINITION/OVERVIEW

- There is no label indication for these compounds in veterinary medicine and exposure is most commonly due to inadvertent exposure.
- Neuroexcitation, agitation, tachycardia, hypertension, and tachypnea are the most common clinical signs noted in the case of toxicity.

ETIOLOGY/PATHOPHYSIOLOGY

Mechanism of Action

- Stimulates the release of monoamine neurotransmitters (dopamine, serotonin, and norepinephrine) from nerve endings.
- Inhibits reuptake and metabolism of catecholamines, increasing amount at nerve endings.

Toxicokinetics

- Pharmacokinetics of methamphetamine have been described in horses.
- Absorption, T_{max}: 15–30 minutes following transmucosal exposure.
- Distribution, V_{ss}: 4.44 ± 0.648 L/kg
- Metabolism: amphetamine is a minor metabolite of methamphetamine.
- Both methamphetamine and amphetamine (at lesser concentrations) are found in urine.
- Terminal half-life: 0.5–1.7 hours
- Urinary alkalization in humans prolongs drug elimination. In horses, urine pH does not appear to affect elimination (10 mg methamphetamine exposure).

Toxicity

- Amphetamine:
  - LD_{50} in rats and mice is 10–30 mg/kg.
- Methamphetamine:
  - LD_{50} (oral) in dogs is 9–11 mg/kg.
  - Ingestion of 1.3 mg/kg in humans – death.

Blackwell's Five-Minute Veterinary Consult Clinical Companion: Equine Toxicology,
First Edition. Edited by Lynn R. Hovda, Dionne Benson, and Robert H. Poppenga.
© 2022 John Wiley & Sons, Inc. Published 2022 by John Wiley & Sons, Inc.
Companion website: www.wiley.com/go/hovda/equine

Systems Affected

- Nervous – agitation, ataxia.
- Cardiovascular – tachycardia, hypertension.
- Respiratory – tachypnea.

SIGNALMENT/HISTORY

Historical Findings
- History of exposure and clinical signs.

Location and Circumstances of Poisoning
- Most likely exposure is from environment including inadvertent by animal handler.

CLINICAL FEATURES

- Clinical signs include hyperactivity, tremors, ataxia, tachycardia, hypertension, hyperthermia, bilaterally dilated pupils, aggression, and circling.
- Severe abdominal pain, bloody diarrhea, and gut ischemia have been reported in humans following ingestion.

DIFFERENTIAL DIAGNOSIS

- CNS stimulants – cocaine, ephedrine, pseudoephedrine, methylxanthines, strychnine.

DIAGNOSTICS

- History of exposure and clinical signs.
- Thrombocytopenia, prolonged PT and activated PTT (consistent with disseminated intravascular coagulation) reported in dogs and humans.
- Quantitation of methamphetamine or amphetamine in urine.
- Drug screening kits available, however, not currently validated for horses.
- LC-MS can assist with diagnostics but may not be timely for therapy.

THERAPEUTICS

- The overall goal is to provide supportive care and allow the animal to clear the drug.

Detoxification
- Urinary acidification with ammonium chloride or ascorbic acid has been suggested to increase the rate of elimination in some species. If this is attempted, acid–base status

should be monitored. In horses, urinary acidification did not enhance elimination following transdermal administration of 10 mg.

Appropriate Health Care

- Monitor closely to ensure animal does not injure itself due to neuroexcitation.
- Monitor blood pressure, heart rate and rhythm and respiration.
- Monitor temperature.

Antidotes

- None available.

Drugs of Choice

- Phenothiazines tranquilizers to control CNS signs:
  - Animal should be monitored as seizure threshold may be lowered.
  - Acepromazine (0.05–1 mg/kg IV).
- Diazepam and other barbiturates – for seizure activity.
- Propranolol for tachycardia (0.02–0.06 mg/kg IV).

COMMENTS

Client Education

- Ensure animal will not be exposed in the future.
- Contact veterinarian if clinical signs return or worsen.

Patient Monitoring

- Behavioral monitoring.
- Monitor heart rate and blood pressure.
- ECG as needed.
- Monitor electrolytes.

Prevention/Avoidance

- Prevent inadvertent exposure by handlers.

Possible Complications

- Self-injury due to excitation/ataxia.
- Death.

Expected Course and Prognosis

- Time to development of clinical signs likely within 15–30 minutes but will vary with degree of exposure and amount exposed to.
- Prognosis depends on severity of poisoning.

Abbreviations

See Appendix 1 for a complete list.

Suggested Reading

Knych HK, Arthur RM, Kanarr KL, et al. Detection, pharmacokinetics and selected pharmacodynamic effects of methamphetamine following a single transmucosal and intravenous administration to exercised thoroughbred horses. Drug Test Anal 2019; 11:1431.

Zengyang P, Zhang X. Methamphetamine intoxication in a dog: case report. BMC Veterinary Research 2014; 10:139.

Author(s): Heather K. Knych DVM, PhD, DACVCP
Consulting Editor: Dionne Benson, DVM, JD

Chapter 12

Opioids

 DEFINITION/OVERVIEW

- Natural opioids are found in the seeds of the opium poppy (*Papaver somniferum*). Opium powder is about 10% morphine and 0.5% codeine. Oxymorphone, codeine, hydromorphone, and heroin are derived from morphine.
- There are numerous synthetic opioids on the market manufactured primarily for human and animal pain relief and tranquilization. Most are not FDA-approved for horses.
- The exact mode of action varies slightly by drug due to different receptor activity and affinity.
- The primary effects are seen in the CNS; however, there are opioid receptors throughout the body.
- Most pain relief is via agonists binding to mu receptors in the CNS and periphery. Mu receptors vary in location and density for horses compared with other species.
- Opioids licensed for equine patients:
    - Butorphanol (kappa agonist and mu antagonist) – schedule IV, pain management (good for equine GI pain).
    - Pethidine (Meperidine) – schedule II, pain management, labeled for spasmodic colic.
    - Buprenorphine (partial mu agonist) – pain management.
- Other opioids used in equine health care, but not licensed specifically for equine patients:
    - Fentanyl (pure mu agonist).
    - Tramadol.
    - Morphine (pure mu agonist).
    - Nalbuphine (partial agonist/antagonist similar to butorphanol) – not DEA.
    - Remifentanil.
    - Methadone (pure mu agonist).
    - Hydromorphone.
- Opioids easily cross the blood–brain barrier allowing for receptors causing cough reflex suppression, respiratory depression, and a depressed CNS.
- Clinical findings include decreased in gut motility and increased water absorption, causing constipation and impaction. Clinically, this is usually observed at high doses.
- Existing toxicology research is in humans, dogs, and cats with variations in the lethal doses in each species.

Blackwell's Five-Minute Veterinary Consult Clinical Companion: Equine Toxicology,
First Edition. Edited by Lynn R. Hovda, Dionne Benson, and Robert H. Poppenga.
© 2022 John Wiley & Sons, Inc. Published 2022 by John Wiley & Sons, Inc.
Companion website: www.wiley.com/go/hovda/equine

- Use of opioids (particularly mu agonists), historically, has been limited in the horse due to adverse side effects. In horses, clinical signs of toxicosis include excitation, agitation, increased locomotor activity and decreased gut motility. Side effects are likely due to the receptors' affinity for the medications and how densely the receptors are in their specific locations in the equine brain.

 ETIOLOGY/PATHOPHYSIOLOGY

Mechanism of Action

- The major opioid receptors are mu (μ), delta (δ), and kappa (κ). Opioid receptors are found in many locations such as the CNS, autonomic nervous system, GI tract, heart, kidney, pancreas, adipocytes, and on the surface of lymphocytes.
- When the body senses pain or stress, opioid receptors are stimulated by endogenous endorphins and enkephalins.
- Similarly, opiates have various affinity and, when administered, they function as agonists, antagonists, or as both at their unique opioid-binding site. When activated, the following specific actions occur:
  - μ 1 – supraspinal analgesia.
  - μ 2 – spinal analgesia, respiratory suppression, decreased gut motility.
  - δ – higher affinity for enkephalins, spinal analgesia.
  - κ – spinal and supraspinal analgesia, sedation, dysphoria.
- Each opiate has a unique half-life and level of toxicity.

Toxicokinetics (based upon morphine – others may vary)

- Onset is 5–10 minutes after IV administration.
- Duration of action is 2–6 hours, which may be prolonged if in the extradural space.
- Poor lipid solubility.
- Hepatic metabolism.
- Renal excretion.

Toxicity

- Toxicity is dose-dependent. Clinical signs, especially respiratory, are observed at therapeutic doses. Severe adverse effects and death can occur at high concentrations.

Systems Affected

- Neurological – decreased CNS activity, initial excitation leading to depression, hypothermia, seizures, coma, death.
- Respiratory – depression.
- Gastrointestinal – decreased motility, increased water absorption.
- Cardiovascular – bradycardia, possible vasodilation, hypotension.

SIGNALMENT/HISTORY

Risk Factors
- Neonates have undeveloped blood–brain barrier, making them more susceptible.
- Opioid toxicosis in the horse is usually iatrogenic.

Historical Findings
- Iatrogenic.
- Inadvertent exposure via ingestion of fentanyl patches.

CLINICAL FEATURES

- Because toxicity would likely result from iatrogenic administration in the horse, it is imperative that the clinician is cognizant of clinical signs associated with CNS excitation then depression, GI stasis causing episodes of colic, and decreased pulmonary/cardiovascular activity.

DIFFERENTIAL DIAGNOSIS

- Dermorphin administration.
- Electrolyte imbalance.
- CNS Stimulants (amphetamine, methamphetamine).
- CNS depressants (benzodiazepine).
- Colic of other etiology.
- Ethanol.
- Ethylene glycol.
- Ivermectin.
- Marijuana toxicosis.

DIAGNOSTICS

CBC/Serum Chemistry
- Hypoglycemia.
- Elevated BUN.

Other Diagnostic Tests
- Arterial blood gas.
- LC-MS.

THERAPEUTICS

Detoxification

- Remove the source of the toxicosis.
- Provide supportive care as needed.
- If suspected, oral overdoses could be evacuated via nasogastric intubation. Once evacuated, administer activated charcoal at 1 g/kg with mineral oil and water to help decrease absorption of the medication, and assist with the potential GI stasis/impaction.

Appropriate Health Care

- Monitor cardiovascular and respiratory activity. Assisted ventilation may be essential if severely overdosed.
- Gastrointestinal activity may be greatly compromised and monitoring for possible GI stasis should be considered.

Antidotes

- Naloxone 0.01–0.02 mg/kg up to 0.05 mg/kg IV bolus. Note: the half life is 1–1.5 hours and may have to be repeated because its half-life is shorter than morphine.
- Butorphanol (for pure mu agonist) – 0.01–0.1 mg/kg IV, IM.

Drugs of Choice

- IV fluids as needed for volume expansion and dehydration.
- Cardiovascular:
  - Atropine (anticholinergic, but will decrease gut motility) – 0.02 mg/kg IV.
  - Glycopyrrolate (anticholinergic, but will decrease gut motility) – 0.005 mg/kg IV.
- GI Protectants:
  - Omeprazole 2–4 mg/kg PO q24h.
  - N-methylnaltrexone (research only) – does not cross blood–brain barrier and may reduce negative GI effects when a mu agonist such as morphine has been given.
- CNS signs:
  - Detomidine 0.02-0.04 mg/kg IV or IM.
  - Xylazine 1.1 mg/kg IV; 2.2 mg/kg IM.

Precautions/Interactions

- Pethidine (Meperidine) is short-acting. Can cause seizures if administered IV. Diazepam or pentobarbitone would help control these clinical signs.
- Avoid use in horses with renal insufficiency.
- Fentanyl has been noted to be a heavy respiratory depressant, and mechanical ventilation should be used with gas anesthesia.
- Caution should be used if administering other depressants with opioids as the negative side effects could increase. Benzodiazepines should be avoided.

- Ethanol is contraindicated.
- Respiratory depression in neonates has been described when morphine has been administered to mares prior to birth.

COMMENTS

Prevention/Avoidance
- Limit opioid use and monitor closely when used.
- Educate clients regarding adverse effects in horses.

Possible Complications
- Seizures.
- Hyperthermia.

Expected Course and Prognosis
- Prognosis for recovery is good if respiratory and cardiovascular functions are maintained.

Abbreviations
See Appendix 1 for a complete list.

Suggested Reading
Boscan P, Van Hoogmoed LM, Farver TB, et al. Evaluation of the effects of the opioid agonist morphine on gastrointestinal tract function in horses. Am J Vet Res 2006; 67:992–997

Boscan P, Van Hoogmoed LM, Pypendop BH, et al. Pharmacokinetics of the opioid antagonist N-methylnaltrexone and its effects on gastrointestinal tract function in horses treated or not treated with morphine. Am J Vet Res. 2006; 67:998–1004

Combie JD, Nugent TE, Tobin T, Pharmacokinetics and protein binding of morphine in horses. Am J Vet Res 1983; 44(5): 870–874.

Gupta GC. Veterinary Toxicology, 2nd edn. San Diego: Elsevier, 2012.

Matthews NS, Carroll GL, Review of equine analgesics and pain management. AAEP Proc 2007; 53:240–244.

Reed SM, Bayly WM. Sellon DC, ed. Equine Internal Medicine, 4th edn. St Louis: Elsevier., 2018.

Roger T, Bardon T, Ruckebusch Y. Colonic motor responses in the pony: relevance of colonic stimulation by opiate antagonists. Am J Vet Res 1985; 46:31–35.

Van Hoogmoed LM, Boscan PL. In vitro evaluation of the effect of the opioid antagonist N-methylnaltrexone on motility of the equine jejunum and pelvic flexure. Equine Vet J 2005; 37:325–328.

Author: Jay Deluhery, DVM, MBA, CJF
Consulting Editor: Dionne Benson, DVM, JD

Selective Androgen (SARMS) and Estrogen Receptor (SERMS) Modulators

Chapter 13

DEFINITION/OVERVIEW

- SARMs and SERMs are non-steroidal small molecule drugs that function on either the androgen or estrogen receptor as agonists or antagonists.
- Cases may be a result of accidental or illicit use in performance horses.
- There are no FDA-approved SARMs for human or veterinary use, although there are many compounds in pre-clinical and clinical development for a variety of conditions, including hypogonadism, muscle wasting, cachexia, benign prostate hyperplasia, osteopenia/osteoporosis, amd cancer (prostate and breast).
  - Endosarm also known as GTX-024, Ostarine, S-22, or MK-2866.
  - LGD-4033 also known as Ligandrol.
  - Testolone also known as RAD-140.
  - Andarine also known as GTx-007 or S-4.
- Illicit formulations of SARMs are readily available on the internet primarily directed towards body builders and other performance athletes.
- There are three FDA-approved SERMs for human use and none approved for any veterinary species:
  - Tamoxifen citrate – approved for treatment of estrogen sensitive breast cancer.
  - Raloxifene hydrochloride – approved for treatment of postmenopausal osteoporosis.
  - Toremifene – approved for treatment of estrogen-sensitive breast cancer.
- The prevalence of use is unknown, and administrations may be unreported to practitioners due to potential illicit use.
- Prohibited by ARCI and FEI.

ETIOLOGY/PATHOPHYSIOLOGY

Mechanism of Action

- Selective binding to the target receptor (androgen/estrogen) and recruitment/repression of specific co-regulators (activators/repressors) depending upon specific chemical structure of compound:
  - SERMs – bind to estrogen receptor.
  - SARMs – bind to androgen receptor.

Blackwell's Five-Minute Veterinary Consult Clinical Companion: Equine Toxicology, First Edition. Edited by Lynn R. Hovda, Dionne Benson, and Robert H. Poppenga.
© 2022 John Wiley & Sons, Inc. Published 2022 by John Wiley & Sons, Inc.
Companion website: www.wiley.com/go/hovda/equine

- Variable activity in specific tissues/cell types due to differences in expression of co-regulators and expression of target receptors.
- Potential species-dependent effects at different tissues/cell types due to differential co-regulatory activity and expression of target receptors.

Toxicokinetics

SARMs
- Orally bioavailable, widely distributed, most are extensively metabolized via phase I and II (glucuronidation) reactions and eliminated via fecal/urinary routes.
- Available data in the horse:
  - Endosarm – extensively metabolized following IV administration, metabolite with largest signal was sulfate conjugate following amide cleavage.
  - LGD-4033 – extensively metabolized to mono-/di-hydroxylated products following PO/IV administrations.
  - Testolone – no data in the horse available. In humans, primarily excreted in urine as glucuronide conjugate.
  - Andarine – extensively metabolized following IV administration with combinations of amide cleavage, hydroxylation, and sulfate conjugation.

SERMs
- Orally bioavailable (~2–13%), widely distributed and highly protein-bound, long terminal half-life, potential for enterohepatic recirculation and fecal/urinary elimination.
- Available data in the horse:
  - Tamoxifen – 3-hour peak plasma concentration after PO dose, metabolites identified include 4-hydroxytamoxifen (active metabolite), N-desmethyltamoxifen and 4-hydroxy-N-desmethtyl-tamoxifen (endoxifen).
  - Raloxifene and toremifene – no data in the horse available.

Toxicity

SARMs
- There is limited information on dosages that result in adverse events:
  - Common dosing in humans at ~ 0.005–0.2 mg/kg SID PO depending on compound.
  - In the horse, Andarine 41.1 mg IV, Ostarine 33.3 mg IV, LGD-4033, 50 mg PO have been reported for investigatory purposes for doping control.

SERMs
- Common dosing in humans 20–60 mg SID PO:
  - Tamoxifen:
    - 4100 mg/kg LD_{50} rats, clinical dose of 20–40 mg/day in humans (0.25 mg/kg in horse).
    - Known human and animal carcinogen following chronic administration
  - Toremifene:
    - 3000 mg/kg LD_{50} in rats, clinical dose of 60 mg in humans.
  - Raloxifene:
    - No lethality noted at 5000 mg/kg in rats, clinical dose of 60 mg in humans.

Systems Affected

- Musculoskeletal – treatment of osteoporosis (Raloxifene), increase in muscle mass (SARMs).
- Hepatobiliary – potential for liver damage with elevated ALT/AST (SARMs).
- Endocrine/metabolic – decreases in HDL (SARMs).
- Reproductive – potential to affect reproductive tissues (SARMs/SERMs).
- Neurological – potential behavioral changes, aggression, depression (SARMs/SERMs).
- Ophthalmic – crystalline retinal deposits, macular edema, corneal changes for SERMs (Tamoxifen).
- Cardiovascular –thromboembolic events noted for SERMS (Tamoxifen).

SIGNALMENT/HISTORY

- Potential for increased illicit use in performance horses.
- SERMs may be used after SARM use as a "post-cycle recovery therapy".

Risk Factors

- Higher potential for use in performance horses.
- Incomplete medical records and failure to disclose administrations by owners/trainers.

Historical Findings

- History of use of other performance-enhancing drugs with similar effects such as anabolic steroids, beta-agonists, growth hormone, growth hormone-releasing peptides.
- Performance supplement use from online vendors.

CLINICAL FEATURES

- Physical exam may not suggest exposure.
- Potential for behavior changes.

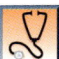
DIFFERENTIAL DIAGNOSIS

- Administration of other pharmaceutical agents:
  - Anabolic steroids such as trenbolone, nandrolone, testosterone and boldenone (esterified or free).
  - Estrogenic steroids such as estradiol, estrone, zeranol, ethinylestradiol (free, conjugated or esterified).
  - Aromatase inhibitors such as anastrozole, testolactone, aminoglutethimide, letrozole, and formestane.
- Stimulation/suppression of hypothalamic–pituitary–gonadal axis by other pharmaceutical or environmental agents.
- Ovarian tumors in female horses.

DIAGNOSTICS

CBC/Serum Chemistry/Urinalysis

- Elevated ALT and AST on serum chemistry.

Other Diagnostic Tests

- Urine or blood samples may be sent to specialized laboratories for testing.
- SARMs/SERMS are not commonly monitored in routine diagnostic testing.
- Reproductive steroid panel to evaluate testosterone and estrogen concentrations.

THERAPEUTICS

- Objectives of treatment are to prevent further exposure to the compounds and provide symptomatic treatment.

Detoxification

- Reduce exposure potential and eliminate repeated administrations.

Antidotes

- No specific antidote is available.

Appropriate Health Care

- Monitor/treat for behavioral changes.
- CBC and biochemistry profile to evaluate hydration status and overall health.
- Hepatic function panel to evaluate ALT and AST elevation.
- Reproductive evaluation and steroid panel to evaluate testosterone and estrogen levels after cessation of exposure.

Precautions/Interactions

- Avoid co-administration with other highly protein-bound drugs.
- SARMs – limited clinical co-administration safety data available.
- SERMs:
    - Toremifene:
        - Avoid co-administration of agents that demonstrate QT prolongation on EKG.
        - Avoid co-administration of CYP3A4 inducers (dexamethasone, carbamazepine, rifampin, phenobarbital) or inhibitors (ketoconazole, itraconazole, clarithromycin, atazanavir, indinavir, nefazodone, nelfinavir, ritonavir, saquinavir, telithromycin, and voriconazole) – may increase or decrease toremifene exposure, respectively.
    - Tamoxifen:
        - Avoid aromatase inhibitors (anatrozole and letrozole).

COMMENTS

Client Education
- Educate client about the potential for exposure from performance supplements marketed on the internet.

Prevention/Avoidance
- Remove compounds from the environment or restrict horse access to them.

Possible Complications
- Contaminants or adulterants found in supplements.
- Unknown exposure to other related compounds.

Expected Course and Prognosis
- Effects are time- and dose-dependent.
- Lower doses and duration – good prognosis.

Abbreviations
See Appendix 1 for a complete list.

Suggested Reading
Gajardo G, López-Muñoz R, Plaza A, et al. Tamoxifen in horses: pharmacokinetics and safety study. Irish Veterinary Journal 2019; 72:5–5.

Hansson, A, Knych H, Stanley S, Thevis M, Bondesson U, Hedeland M. Characterization of equine urinary metabolites of selective androgen receptor modulators (SARMs) S1, S4 and S22 for doping control purposes. Drug Testing Analysis 2015; 7:673–683.

Martinkovich S, Shah D, Planey SL, Arnott JA. Selective estrogen receptor modulators: tissue specificity and clinical utility. Clinical Interventions in Aging 2014; 9:1437–1452.

Solomon ZJ, Mirabal JR, Mazur DJ, et al. Selective androgen receptor modulators: current knowledge and clinical applications. Sexual Medicine Reviews 2019; 7(1):84–94.

Author: Benjamin C. Moeller, PhD, DABT
Consulting Editor: Dionne Benson, DVM, JD

Chapter 14

Synthetic Cannabinoids

DEFINITION/OVERVIEW

- Laboratory-manufactured chemicals that bind to the same receptors as delta-9-tetrahydrocannabinol (THC) and CBD (cannabidiol).
- Chemicals are dissolved in a solvent, sprayed on dried plant or "herbal" plant material until saturated, and allowed to dry; once the solvent has evaporated the plant material is crushed and sold to be smoked or ingested as a recreational drug.
- Some newer ones are sold as liquids to be used in e-cigarettes.
- More potent and toxic than THC or CBD.
- Purchased on the internet and head shops as "Spice", "K2", "Herbal Incense", "Mojo", "Cloud Nine", "Crazy Monkey", "Happy Shaman", "Liquid Incense", and many others.
- Generally labelled "not for human consumption".
- There are currently over 160 synthetic cannabinoids worldwide with a variety of older names such as JWH-018, JWH-081, JWH-250, JWH-073, CP-47, HU-210, and PB-22.
- Fifteen known synthetic cannabinoids are DEA Schedule 1-regulated, but newer compounds are manufactured as rapidly as others are added to the list.
- Many are contaminated with fatty acids, additives, and preservatives and some with fentanyl, kratom, salvia (*Salvia divinorum*), or other street drugs which may increase toxicity.
- Prohibited substance under USEF, AQHA, and ARCI rules.
- Little information on clinical effects in horses; anecdotal reports only.

ETIOLOGY/PATHOPHYSIOLOGY

Mechanism of Action

- Full CB1 and CB2 receptor agonists as opposed to THC which is a partial agonist.
- Greater binding affinity than THC.
- Bind to cannabinoid receptors in the brain and spinal cord (CB1) and periphery (CB2).

Blackwell's Five-Minute Veterinary Consult Clinical Companion: Equine Toxicology, First Edition. Edited by Lynn R. Hovda, Dionne Benson, and Robert H. Poppenga.
© 2022 John Wiley & Sons, Inc. Published 2022 by John Wiley & Sons, Inc.
Companion website: www.wiley.com/go/hovda/equine

Toxicokinetics

- Onset of action varies with each compound and may be minutes to hours.
- Duration of action also variable, but generally 12–24 hours; agitation in humans has lasted for days.
- Hepatic metabolism; some synthetic cannabinoids have metabolites which may be more active than the parent compound.
- Excretion – most of the older products are eliminated in the urine; unknown in newer products.

Toxicity

- Highly toxic.
- Older compounds up to 10 times as toxic as THC; newer ones are up to 100 times as toxic.

Systems Affected

- Neurological – psychotic reactions, agitation (rarely sedation), irritability, ataxia, tremors, nystagmus, hyperflexion, hyperextension, seizures or seizure-like activity.
- Cardiovascular – hypertension, tachycardia (rarely bradycardia).
- Gastrointestinal – retching, colic.
- Renal – acute kidney injury.
- Other – mydriasis or miosis, cough, hyperthermia, rhabdomyolysis.

SIGNALMENT/HISTORY

Risk Factors

- Presence in environment.
- Typically abused by older teenagers and younger adults.

Historical Findings

- Owners and trainers may be reluctant to admit possession and use.
- Difficult to find on routine drug screen as there are so many of them.

Location and Circumstances of Poisoning

- Worldwide problem, not just limited to the United States.
- Intentional exposure by blowing smoke into horse's face or adding to feed.
- Unintentional exposure by careless placement of product; may be "stashed" or hidden in a horse's stall at a show, racetrack, or training center.

CLINICAL FEATURES

- Variability in signs due to large number of compounds and contaminants.
- Common signs include agitation or drowsiness, ataxia, twitching, tremors, tachycardia, and hyperesthesia.

DIFFERENTIAL DIAGNOSIS

- CNS stimulants (amphetamine, methamphetamine).
- CNS depressants (benzodiazepine, opioids).
- Ethanol.
- Hallucinogenic plants and mushrooms.
- Other recreational drugs.
- Rabies.

DIAGNOSTICS

CBC/Serum Chemistry/Urinalysis

- Routine laboratory work including serum chemistry and urinalysis.
- ± Hypokalemia
- BUN, creatinine and creatine kinase for evidence of acute kidney injury or rhabdomyolysis.
- RBCs, casts, excessive protein in urine.

Other Diagnostic Tests

- ECG as needed for tachycardia and cardiac effects.
- Presence in serum and urine:
  - No rapid, commercially available urine tests.
  - LC-MS/MS is useful for diagnosis, but the time delay would hinder therapeutics.

Pathological Findings

- None reported in horses.

THERAPEUTICS

- The goal of therapy is to limit toxin absorption and provide supportive care.

Detoxification

- No emesis.
- Large ingestions – gastric lavage or reflux with large bore tube.
- Activated charcoal 1–3 g/kg BW PO in watery slurry if ingested; follow with a cathartic (magnesium sulfate 250–500 mg/kg) in 2–4 L of water.
- Supportive care if inhaled and symptomatic.

Appropriate Health Care

- Most can be treated in the field.
- Hospitalization for severe cases.

Antidotes

- No specific antidote.

Drugs of Choice

- Intravenous fluids as needed for dehydration and volume expansion; may be helpful to increase elimination.
- Agitation:
    - Acepromazine 0.01–0.05 mg/kg IV, IM, SC prn.
    - Adrenergic agonist: Detomidine 0.02–0.04 mg/kg IM, IV, or Xylazine 1.1 mg/kg IV.
- Seizures:
    - Diazepam 0.02–0.4 mg/kg IV prn (foals); 25–50 mg IV (adult horses).
- GI protectants:
    - Omeprazole 4 mg/kg PO q24h.
- Tremors, twitching:
    - Acepromazine 0.01–0.05 mg/kg IV, IM, SC prn.
    - Methocarbamol 4.4–22.2 mg/kg IV to effect. Administer half estimated dose and pause until animal has relaxed. Administer the remainder of the dose to effect. Repeat as needed but do not exceed 330 mg/kg/day.
- Cardiovascular:
    - Beta-blocker if hospitalized and tachycardia/hypertension non-responsive to IV fluid expansion and sedation.

Precautions/Interactions

- Protection to the head and limbs may be necessary in severely agitated horses.

COMMENTS

Client Education

- There are no commercially available rapid urine tests to detect these substances in horses.
- LC-MS/MS may be useful in legal cases.

Prevention/Avoidance

- Educate young riders about the adverse effects in horses.

Possible Complications

- Acute kidney injury.
- Acute tubular necrosis.
- Cardiac damage secondary to myocardial infarction.
- Rhabdomyolysis.

Expected Course and Prognosis

- Toxicity is rarely fatal, and effects generally reside after 12–24 hours.

Abbreviations

See Appendix 1 for a complete list.

Suggested Reading

Mills B, Yepes A, Nugent K. Synthetic cannabinoids. Am J Med Sci 2015; 350(1):59–62.

Riederer AM, Campleman SL, Carlson RG, et al. Acute poisonings from synthetic cannabinoids. Morb Mortal Wkly Rep 2017; 65(27):692–695.

Tai S. Pharmacological and toxicological effects of synthetic cannabinoids and their metabolites. Curr Top Behav Neurosci 2017; 32:249–262.

Author: Lynn R. Hovda, RPh, DVM, MS, DACVIM

Consulting Editor: Dionne Benson, DVM, JD

Drugs: Prescription

Antipsychotic Agents – Reserpine and Fluphenazine

Chapter 15

DEFINITION/OVERVIEW

- Antipsychotic agents include reserpine and fluphenazine.
- Reserpine is derived from *Rauwolfia serpentina*, a shrub found in India.
- Reserpine is used in humans for hypertension, tardive dyskinesia, and psychiatric disorders.
- Reserpine use in horses is available through compounding pharmacies in an IM version or an oral powder or suspension.
- Fluphenazine is a phenothiazine neuroleptic consisting of a synthetic organofluorine compound.
- Fluphenazine is used in human medicine in the treatment of schizophrenia.
- Human FDA-approved fluphenazine is available for use in horses.
- Fluphenazine and reserpine are used off-label for anxiolytic and long-acting sedative effects – particularly in horses on long-term stall rest.
- Prohibited under ARCI, USEF, FEI, and AQHA rules.

ETIOLOGY/PATHOPHYSIOLOGY

Mechanism of Action

- After administration, reserpine crosses the blood–brain barrier and inhibits the VMAT. This blocks uptake of monoamine neurotransmitters, including dopamine, serotonin, and norepinephrine.
- After administration of fluphenazine decanoate, the drug gradually diffuses into the surrounding lymph nodes and tissues.
- Fluphenazine decanoate is rapidly hydrolyzed by esterases, and the parent compound (fluphenazine) is released.
- Fluphenazine crosses the blood–brain barrier and blocks dopamine receptors – particularly D_2 receptors located in the brain – although in humans, evidence exists that D_2 receptor antagonism is not wholly responsible for antipsychotic effects.

Pharmacokinetics

- Onset of action varies. Reserpine toxicosis has been reported within 5 hours of IM administration. Fluphenazine reactions have been reported within 14–36 hours.

Blackwell's Five-Minute Veterinary Consult Clinical Companion: Equine Toxicology,
First Edition. Edited by Lynn R. Hovda, Dionne Benson, and Robert H. Poppenga.
© 2022 John Wiley & Sons, Inc. Published 2022 by John Wiley & Sons, Inc.
Companion website: www.wiley.com/go/hovda/equine

- Duration of action is also variable, but generally clinical signs resolved within 48 hours for reserpine and 72 hours for fluphenazine toxicosis.
- Fluphenazine primarily undergoes hepatic metabolism, with some renal metabolism. Most excretion occurs via the kidneys with less in feces. Reserpine undergoes hepatic metabolism, but most is excreted unchanged in feces.

Toxicity

- Not well defined. Clinical reports of toxicosis in horses receiving 12.5 mg of reserpine and 25–125 mg of fluphenazine.

Systems Affected

- Neurological – extrapyramidal effects and include agitation, sweating, hypermetria, circling, severe pawing and striking, miosis, ptosis, and swinging of the head and neck.
- Musculoskeletal – skeletal muscle fasciculations.
- Gastrointestinal – colic, diarrhea.
- Reproductive – priapism in male horses.
- Respiratory – nasal congestion, respiratory distress.
- Cardiovascular – bradycardia.

SIGNALMENT/HISTORY

Risk Factors

- Horses prescribed antipsychotics.

Historical Findings

- Horse placed on long-term stall rest and prescribed antipsychotic for management.
- Can also be associated with attempts to calm a show horse prior to competition.

Location and Circumstances of Poisoning

- Horses administered antipsychotics.

CLINICAL FEATURES

- Limited clinical cases reported.
- Common signs include agitation, muscle fasciculations, sweating, intermittent somnolence.
- For male horses, priapism reported with reserpine.

DIFFERENTIAL DIAGNOSIS

- Rabies.
- EHV-1 myeloencephalopathy.

- EPM.
- EEE.
- WEE.
- WNV.
- Toxicosis:
    - Nigropallidal encephalomalacia from the chronic ingestion of yellow star thistle (*Centaurea solstitialis*).
    - Fumonisin.
    - Russian knapweed (*Centaurea repens*) may also be considered as a possible diagnosis.
- Colic of other etiology.
- Trauma.

DIAGNOSTICS

- Blood work – LC-MS screen for antipsychotic.
- Rule out other possible causes, e.g., colic.
- History – re: history of exposure to antipsychotic as well as vaccination history to rule out other causes and potential exposure to other potential toxins

Pathological Findings

- None reported in horses.

THERAPEUTICS

- Supportive care is the goal.

Detoxification

- Supportive care, including quiet stall to limit reactiveness.
- Fluid therapy.

Appropriate Health Care

- Most can be treated in the field.
- Hospitalization for severe cases.

Antidotes

- While not true antidotes, reported effective treatments for fluphenazine intoxication include:
    - Pentobarbital bolus 2 mg/kg IV or 1 mg/kg/hour CRI.
    - Anticholinergics drugs:
        - Benztropine mesylate 0.018 mg/kg IV or 0.035 mg/kg PO q12h
    - Diphenhydramine hydrochloride 0.67–1 mg/kg IV.

Drugs of Choice

- Systemic support: IV fluids as needed for dehydration and volume expansion; may be helpful to increase elimination.
- Agitation:
    - Acepromazine 0.01–0.05 mg/kg IV, IM, SC prn
    - Adrenergic agonist: Detomidine 10–40 µg/kg IM, IV or Xylazine 0.5–1 mg/kg IV
- GI protectants: Omeprazole 2–4 mg/kg PO q24h

Precautions/Interactions

- Protection of the head and limbs may be necessary in severely agitated horses.
- Penile sling for priapism.
- Quiet stall area to decrease agitation.

Alternative Drugs

- No medical alternatives – some practitioners recommend supplements containing magnesium, tryptophan, valerian root, or raspberry leaf extract.

COMMENTS

Client Education

- Important to discuss risks with clients prior to prescribing antipsychotics.

Prevention/Avoidance

- Discontinue use of antipsychotics in patients with toxicosis.

Possible Complications

- Musculoskeletal – injury due to agitation.

Expected Course and Prognosis

- Prognosis is generally good with treatment. Clinical symptoms resolve between 3 and 5 days in reported cases.

See Also

Yellow Star Thistle (*Centaurea solstitialis*) and Russian Knapweed (*Acroptilon repens*)
Fumonisins

Abbreviations

See Appendix 1 for a complete list.

Suggested Reading

Baird JD, Arroyo LG, Vengust M, et al. Adverse extrapyramidal effects in four horse given fluphenazine decanoate. J Am Vet Med Assoc 2006; 229(1):104–110.
Benowitz N. Antihypertensive agents. In: Katzung BG, ed. Basic and Clinical Pharmacology, 10th edn. Connecticut: Appleton & Lange, Norwalk, 2007; pp. 461–467.
Bidwell L, Schott II H, Derksen F. Reserpine toxicosis in an aged gelding. EVE 2007; 19(7):341–343.

Brewer B, Hines M, Stewart J, et al. Fluphenazine induced Parkinson-like syndrome in a horse. Equine Vet J 1990; 22(25):136–137.

Brashier M. Fluphenazine-induced extrapyramidal side effects in a horse. Vet Clin North Am Equine Pract 2006; 22:e37–e45.

Scharman E. Reserpine. In: Wexler P, ed. Encyclopedia of Toxicology, 2nd edn. Elsevier, 2005; pp. 661–662.

Author: Laurie Bohannon, DVM, candidate DACVS
Consulting Editor: Dionne Benson, DVM, JD

Chapter 16

Benzodiazepines

DEFINITION/OVERVIEW

- Laboratory-manufactured medication with an undefined mechanism of action.
- Benzodiazepines are commonly used in equine practice as sedatives, muscle relaxants, anticonvulsants, or as an adjunct to anesthesia.
- Included are diazepam (Valium) and midazolam (Versed).
- Several other benzodiazepines are used in human and small animal medicine.
- Often administered in conjunction with ketamine for induction of general anesthesia.
- The most common clinical signs of benzodiazepine toxicosis are CNS depression, ataxia, muscle fasciculations, and, rarely, coma.
- Overdose is usually a result of iatrogenic administration.
- Benzodiazepines have a wide margin of safety.
- Diazepam is not approved for use in animals by the FDA.
- Regulated in competition in USEF, FEI, AQHA, and ARCI.

ETIOLOGY/PATHOPHYSIOLOGY

Mechanism of Action

- Mechanism of action in veterinary medicine is not well understood. Potential mechanisms include:
  - Serotonin antagonism.
  - Increased GABA concentrations.
  - Increased acetylcholine concentration.
- Primarily affects CNS.

Pharmacokinetics

- Oral absorption is good; however, benzodiazepines undergo rapid hepatic metabolism, thus oral administration is not as effective as IV administration.
- Duration of action up to 2–3 hours. Duration is dose-dependent.
- Onset of action is minutes, with peak plasma concentrations occurring within minutes to hours of dosing.
- Metabolized in liver to several different active metabolites.
- Excretion of metabolites occurs in urine.

Blackwell's Five-Minute Veterinary Consult Clinical Companion: Equine Toxicology,
First Edition. Edited by Lynn R. Hovda, Dionne Benson, and Robert H. Poppenga.
© 2022 John Wiley & Sons, Inc. Published 2022 by John Wiley & Sons, Inc.
Companion website: www.wiley.com/go/hovda/equine

Toxicity

- Benzodiazepines have a wide margin of safety. Signs can be seen at therapeutic doses; however, a single overdose is rarely life-threatening.
- Recumbency seen at doses > 0.2mg/kg. Lower doses commonly cause ataxia.

Systems Affected

- Neurological – sedation, ataxia, occasionally paradoxical stimulation: agitation, anxiety.
- Musculoskeletal – muscle fasciculations, weakness, recumbency (mostly in foals).
- Neuromuscular – muscle relaxation.
- Cardiovascular – respiratory depression.

SIGNALMENT/HISTORY

- All breeds and ages can be affected. Foals more prone to recumbency.
- History of benzodiazepine administration.

Risk Factors

- Iatrogenic.
- Less common – exposure to human prescription medications.

Historical Findings

- History of benzodiazepine administration.
- Signs and observations often reported by the owner.

CLINICAL FEATURES

- The most common signs are CNS depression and recumbency.
- Benzodiazepines are relatively short-acting and the effects in adult horses usually resolve within 10–15 minutes. At higher doses, can last 2–3 hours.
- Occasionally can have paradoxical stimulation causing agitation/anxiety. These effects are usually transient and will resolve within 15 minutes.

DIFFERENTIAL DIAGNOSIS

- Case history will often give definitive diagnosis; however, ataxia/recumbency/sedation can also be attributed to:
    - CNS depressants: phenothiazines, barbiturates, muscle relaxants.
    - Viral encephalitis (WEE, EEE, WNV).
    - EPM.
    - Trauma.
    - Hepatic encephalopathy.
    - Foals:
        - Hypoglycemia.
        - Neonatal maladjustment syndrome in foals.

DIAGNOSTICS

- Patient history and clinical signs should be used for diagnosis
- LC-MS testing for presence of benzodiazepines is useful for diagnostics but not helpful for immediate treatment.

THERAPEUTICS

- The goal of treatment is mainly supportive due to the secondary effects (ataxia, recumbency).

Detoxification

- Focus is on supportive care.

Appropriate Health Care

- Fluid therapy as needed for hypotension.

Antidotes

- Flumazenil: 0.01 mg/kg slowly – only for severe CNS depression.

Drugs of Choice

- IV fluid therapy, if needed, for supportive care.
- Sedation if paradoxical stimulation (however usually transient and will resolve):
  - Detomidine: 0.02–0.04 mg/kg IV.
  - Xylazine: 0.2–1.0 mg/kg IV.
  - Romifidine: 0.04–0.12 mg/kg IV.
  - Acepromazine: 0.02–0.05 mg/kg IM, IV.

Precautions/Interactions

- Protection to head and limbs may be necessary in agitated or severely ataxic horses.
- Drugs that decrease hepatic metabolism can decrease drug clearance.
- Diazepam is not chemically compatible with several drugs, thus mixing drugs in syringes should be avoided. This excludes ketamine.
- Diazepam is not water-soluble and extravenous administration can cause thrombophlebitis/muscle irritation.

Alternative Drugs

- Alternative sedative/anxiolytics:
  - Alpha$_2$-adrenergic agonists: detomidine (Dormosedan), xylazine (Rompun), romifidine.
  - Phenothiazines: acepromazine.
- Muscle relaxant:
  - Methocarbamol (Robaxin).

COMMENTS

Client Education

- Educate client regarding risks of sedation.

Continued Monitoring

- Monitor for any further signs of CNS depression or ataxia.

Expected Course and Prognosis

- A patient with a single overdose has an excellent prognosis for full recovery provided there are no traumatic incidents during the period of CNS depression.

Abbreviations

See Appendix 1 for a complete list.

Suggested Reading

Hovda L, et al., eds. Blackwell's Five-Minute Veterinary Consult Clinical Companion: Small Animal Toxicology. John Wiley & Sons, 2016; pp. 149–156.

Shini S. A review of diazepam and its use in the horse. Journal of Equine Veterinary Science 2000; 20.7:443–449.

Tilley LP, Smith Jr FWK, eds. Blackwell's Five-Minute Veterinary Consult: Canine and Feline. John Wiley & Sons, 2015; p. 172.

Author: Casille Batten, DVM
Consulting Editor: Dionne Benson, DVM, JD

Chapter 17

Beta₂ Agonists – Clenbuterol and Albuterol

DEFINITION/OVERVIEW

- Beta₂ agonists are used therapeutically in horses as bronchodilators.
- Drugs commonly used in horses include clenbuterol (Ventipulmin®) and albuterol (extra-label).
- Tachycardia, muscle tremors or fasciculations, and increased sweating are the most common signs observed with high doses or toxicosis.

ETIOLOGY/PATHOPHYSIOLOGY

Mechanism of Action

- Beta agonists stimulate beta receptors, leading to an increase in adenylate cyclase activity, an increase in intracellular cyclic AMP and relaxation of bronchial smooth muscle.
- Beta agonists decrease the release of inflammatory mediators by binding to beta receptors on mast cells.
- Experimentally there is evidence of an increase in mucociliary clearance.

Pharmacokinetics

- Pharmacokinetics of clenbuterol following oral administration in horses have been well described; albuterol pharmacokinetics in horses have not been described.
- Clenbuterol:
  - Oral bioavailability approximately 84%; peak plasma concentration (C_{max}): 2 hours after oral administration.
  - Extensive tissue distribution (liver, kidney, eyes, fluids, lungs, heart, and spleen) with prolonged tissue clearance relative to serum.
  - Metabolized in liver and excreted in urine.

Toxicity

- Clenbuterol:
  - 1.6–6 4 µg/kg – sweating, muscle tremor and agitation with increasing intensity at higher doses (Ventipulmin® FOI).

Blackwell's Five-Minute Veterinary Consult Clinical Companion: Equine Toxicology,
First Edition. Edited by Lynn R. Hovda, Dionne Benson, and Robert H. Poppenga.
© 2022 John Wiley & Sons, Inc. Published 2022 by John Wiley & Sons, Inc.
Companion website: www.wiley.com/go/hovda/equine

- 100 µg/kg (compounded formulation) – muscle tremors, hyperhidrosis, colic, stiff gait, ataxia, neurologic deficits, tachycardia and prolonged capillary refill time requiring euthanasia reported in one horse.
- 10 µg/kg or greater (compounded formulation) – excitation, hyperhidrosis, muscle tremors, tachycardia, pyrexia, laminitis, acute renal failure, rhabdomyolysis, cardiomyopathy and death reported in two horses.

Systems Affected

- Musculoskeletal/neuromuscular – muscle tremors.
- Skin/exocrine – sweating, urticaria.
- Cardiovascular – tachycardia.
- Nervous – restlessness, ataxia (rare).

SIGNALMENT/HISTORY

Risk Factors

- Do not use in horses suspected of having cardiovascular impairment (per label directions) due to risk of tachycardia.
- Do not use clenbuterol in pregnant mares near full-term as antagonism of prostaglandin F2 alpha and oxytocin can decrease normal uterine contractility.

Location and Circumstances of Poisoning

- Poisonings are most common in cases of overdosing when administering for therapeutic purposes or when administering compounded formulations.

CLINICAL FEATURES

- Most common signs include sweating, muscle fasciculations or tremors, and tachycardia.
- Less common signs that are usually dose-dependent include ataxia, nervousness, restlessness, and cardiac arrhythmias.

DIFFERENTIAL DIAGNOSIS

- CNS stimulants – cocaine, amphetamines.
- Drugs affecting cardiovascular system – alpha$_1$ adrenergic agonists (tricyclic antidepressants), alpha$_2$ adrenergic agonists (xylazine, detomidine).

DIAGNOSTICS

- History of clenbuterol administration, particularly compounded formulations and clinical signs.

CBC/Serum Chemistry/Urinalysis

- Hyponatremia.
- Hypochloremia.
- Hyperglycemia.
- Elevated serum CK and AST.

Other Diagnostics

- ECG-sinus tachycardia.
- LC-MS for presence of clenbuterol in plasma/urine.

Pathological Findings

- Skeletal and cardiac (necrosis) muscle lesions reported at high doses.

THERAPEUTICS

- The overall goal is to provide supportive care and allow the animal to clear the drug.

Appropriate Health Care

- If clinical signs are present, hospitalize.
- Monitor closely to ensure animal does not injure themselves due to ataxia.
- Monitor heart rate and rhythm.

Antidotes

- No specific antidote available.

Drugs of Choice

- Sinus tachycardia:
  - Propranolol (0.01 mg/kg IV); repeated administration may be necessary
  - Potassium chloride (0.08 mEq/kg/hour) IV.
  - IV crystalloid fluids.
- Anxiety and muscle tremors (treatment has had mixed success:
  - Methocarbamol 4.4–22.2 mg/kg IV to effect. Administer half estimated dose and pause until animal has relaxed. Administer remainder of dose to effect. Repeat as needed not to exceed 330 mg/kg/day.
  - Butorphanol tartrate 0.1 mg/kg IV q3–4h for up to 48 hours.
  - Xylazine 1.1 mg/kg IV prn.
  - Phenylbutazone 1–2 g IV per 454 kg q12h.

Precautions/Interactions

A number of potential reported or theoretical drug interactions in humans and animals should be considered:

- Inhalant anesthetics (e.g. isoflurane); may predispose patient to arrhythmias.
- Beta blockers (e.g. propranolol): may antagonize effects of beta agonists.
- Digoxin: may increase risk of cardiac arrhythmias.
- Dinoprost: affects may be antagonized by beta agonists.

COMMENTS

Patient Monitoring

- Electrolytes (sodium and chloride), glucose.
- Heart rate and rhythm.

Prevention/Avoidance

- Don't use compounded formulations.
- Administer according to label doses.

Possible Complications

- Rhabdomyolysis, cardiomyopathy.
- Death.

Expected Course and Prognosis

- Clinical signs may be prolonged due to slow tissue clearance.
- Reports of death at doses of 10 µg/kg.

See Also

Ractopamine.
Zilpaterol.

Abbreviations

See Appendix 1 for a complete list.

Suggested Reading

Thompson JA, Mirza MH, Barker SA, et al. Clenbuterol toxicosis in three quarter horse racehorses after administration of a compounded product. Am J Vet Res 2011; 239:842.

Author: Heather K. Knych, DVM, PhD, DACVCP
Consulting Editor: Dionne Benson, DVM, JD

Chapter 18

Bisphosphonates

DEFINITION/OVERVIEW

- The use of bisphosphonates (BSPs) in equine practice has become very popular with the FDA approval of Tildren® (tiludronate disodium) and Osphos® (Clodronate) for the treatment of navicular disease in horses over 4 years of age.
- Indications for use include: navicular disease with or without osteolytic lesions, chronic back soreness (osteoarthritic lesions of the thoracolumbar vertebral column), and bone spavin (lower hock osteoarthritis).
- Non-nitrogenous BSP, Tildren and Osphos, incorporate into the energy pathways of the osteoclast, resulting in disruption of cellular energy and metabolism leading to cytotoxic effects and osteoclast apoptosis.
- Nitrogenous BSP, zoledronate (Reclast) and pamidronate (Aredia), have been anecdotally reported to have off-label use. Nitrogen-containing BSPs primarily inhibit cholesterol biosynthesis, resulting in the disruption of intracellular signaling and other cellular processes within the osteoclast.
- Nitrogenous BSPs are 100–10,000 fold more potent compared with non-nitrogenous BSPs; therefore, equine-approved products are far less potent than what is currently being used in human medicine.
- Prohibited under ARCI rules

ETIOLOGY/PATHOPHYSIOLOGY

Mechanism of Action

- BSPs are a family of molecules characterized by their ability to bind strongly to bone material; therefore, they accumulate in areas of high calcium deposition, i.e., bone.
- BSPs bind to calcium and other divalent metal ions in circulation and produce inhibitory effects on mature osteoclasts, thus resulting in bone resorption.
- BSPs inhibit osteoclast recruitment, adhesion, differentiation and resorptive activity, and induce cell death.
- BSPs have a strong affinity for bone where it is quickly fixed onto hydroxyapatite crystals; incorporation into bone is higher in bones with high bone turnover such as trabecular bones.

Blackwell's Five-Minute Veterinary Consult Clinical Companion: Equine Toxicology,
First Edition. Edited by Lynn R. Hovda, Dionne Benson, and Robert H. Poppenga.
© 2022 John Wiley & Sons, Inc. Published 2022 by John Wiley & Sons, Inc.
Companion website: www.wiley.com/go/hovda/equine

- BSP release from the hydroxyapatite crystals is very slow as it occurs when a new remodeling cycle is starting; therefore, it is directly linked with the rate of bone remodeling.
- BSPs have strong anti-inflammatory and pain-relieving properties by decreasing the amount of nitric oxide and cytokines released from activation of macrophages, which promote early inflammatory responses.
- Measurable up to 6 months following a single administration.
- BSPs not bound to bone are rapidly cleared from circulation and eliminated in urine.

Pharmacokinetics

- Onset of clinical signs is within minutes of administration but may be intermittent.
- Duration of action is variable, but GI signs resolve within about 90 minutes. Observation is recommended for 4 hours.
- Potential bone fragility can last months if given at high doses or multiple systemic doses.
- IV, IM or RLP administration are recommended routes
- Poor oral absorption from the GI tract (1% in humans).

Toxicity

- Clinical signs occur at therapeutic doses and are more common with systemic administration than RLP.
- Renal toxicity is well identified; therefore, should not be used with impaired renal function.
- Concurrent NSAID administration is not recommended as this may increase the risk of renal toxicity and acute renal failure.
- Use with caution in horse receiving concurrent administration of drugs that reduce serum calcium, such as tetracyclines, or the toxicity of which may exacerbate a reduction in serum calcium, such as aminoglycosides.
- Toxic effects may be minimized with a well-hydrated patient.

Systems Affected

- Musculoskeletal: muscle pain and cramps.
- Renal: increased frequency of urination, renal failure.
- Gastrointestinal: colic is the most common adverse reaction, 10–45% of horses will demonstrate intermittent colic signs that rarely require treatment. Current recommendation is to hand-walk and monitor during the colic episode.
- Neurologic: (rare) depression, lethargy, yawning, headshaking, nodding, or pressing, nystagmus, and paddling.
- Genetic: horses with HYPP, either heterozygous or homozygous, may be at an increased risk of adverse reactions, including colic, hyperkalemic episodes and death.

SIGNALMENT/HISTORY

- Horse treated with BSPs.

Risk Factors

- Prior treatment and reaction to BSPs.
- Patients with impaired renal function.

Historical Findings

- Recent BSP administration for acute clinical signs.
- Special concern if repeated administration within 6 months of previous treatment.

Location and Circumstances of Poisoning

- Iatrogenic administration.

CLINICAL FEATURES

- Common signs include colic, polyuria, muscle pain, and cramps.

DIFFERENTIAL DIAGNOSIS

- Colic of other etiology.
- Rhabdomyolysis.
- For neurologic symptoms: WNV, EEE, WEE, VEE, EHV, rabies.

DIAGNOSTICS

- Routine laboratory work including serum chemistry:
  - ± hypocalcemia and hypophosphatemia
- LC-MS/MS for identification of BSPs is useful for diagnosis but not for treatment due to timing of results.

Pathological Findings

- In horses with fractures that have had been treated with BSP there is a subjective impression that fracture healing is delayed due to the reduction of maturation of woven bone to cancellous bone.

THERAPEUTICS

- The primary objective of treatment is supportive care.

Detoxification

- IV fluid therapy to maintain renal perfusion and minimize the toxic effects.

Appropriate Health Care

- Maintain hydration and monitor renal function.
- Hand-walk as necessary for colic.

Antidotes

- None.

Drugs of Choice

- IV fluids as needed for dehydration and volume expansion.
- GI protectants:
  - 2–4 mg/kg PO q24h
- Colic:
  - Xylazine:
    - 1.1 mg/kg IV.
    - 2.2 mg/kg IM.
  - Detomidine:
    - 0.02–0.04 mg/kg IV.
  - Flunixin meglumine (with caution due to renal effects):
    - 1.1 mg/kg IV.

Precautions/Interactions

- Tildren should not be used with known hypersensitivity to tiludronate disodium or mannitol.
- Surgical considerations:
  - Anti-resorptive agents act to inhibit bone resorption by fewer resorption sites (improves bone microarchitecture), shallower resorption sites (improves bone balance) and slower turnover rate (better mineralization), which results in increased bone mass and improved bone strength and quality.
  - BSPs do not improve bone healing and, in fact, can slow the maturation of woven bone to cancellous bone; therefore, often resulting in delayed fracture healing.

Alternative Drugs

- While nitrogenous-containing BSPs are widely used in human medicine, it is not recommended to use any product that is not approved for use in horses, as potency is greatly different for those products.

COMMENTS

Client Education

- Repeat systemic administration not recommended within 6 months; however, regional administration by RLP can be repeated once a month later.
- Administration to horses below label approval should be discouraged due to potential long-term bone effects.

Prevention/Avoidance

- Educate clients regarding risks of use.

Possible Complications

- Acute kidney injury.
- Pathological fractures.

Expected Course and Prognosis

- Acute toxicity is rarely fatal, and effects usually reside within 4 hours.

Abbreviations

See Appendix 1 for a complete list.

Internet Resources

US Food and Drug Administration, Tildren and Osphos for Navicular Syndrome in Horses – Information for Equine Veterinarians. Available at: https://www.fda.gov/animal-veterinary/resources-you/tildren-and-osphos-navicular-syndrome-horses-information-equine-veterinarians#:~:text=Bisphosphonates%20can%20cause%20signs%20of,associated%20with%20altered%20intestinal%20motility.&text=Bisphosphonates%20have%20been%20shown%20to%20cause%20abnormal%20fetal%20development%20in%20laboratory%20animals (accessed January 26, 2021).

Suggested Reading

Kamm L, McIlwraith WC, Kawcak C. A review of the efficacy of tiludronate in the horse. J Equine Vet Sci 2008; 28:209–214.

Soto SA. Barbara AC. Bisphosphonates: pharmacology and clinical approach to their use in equine osteo-articular diseases. J Equine Vet Sci 2014; 34:727–737.

Author: Ryan Carpenter, DVM, MS, DACVS
Consulting Editor: Dionne Benson, DVM, JD

Chapter 19

Gabapentin

DEFINITION/OVERVIEW

- Gabapentin was created to mimic GABA.
- Human medication used for seizure control and neuralgia.
- Used in horses primarily for neuropathic and laminitis-associated pain.
- Prohibited substance under USEF, AQHA, and ARCI rules.
- Little information on clinical effects in horses; very limited information on toxicology in horses.

ETIOLOGY/PATHOPHYSIOLOGY

Mechanism of Action

- Mechanism of action is poorly understood. Involves control of calcium channels to decrease the release of neurotransmitters.
- Does not affect GABA uptake or release.

Pharmacokinetics

- Side effect of sedation noted 2 hours after administration in a single horse. Sedation resolved without treatment after 1 hour.
- Human reports of nephrotoxicity and hepatotoxicity. Additionally, associated with CNS effects and peripheral edema in humans.
- Sedation and ataxia have occurred in small animals.
- No metabolites identified in plasma.
- Excretion via kidneys.

Toxicity

- Low toxicity – single doses up to 160 mg/kg were associated only with sedation.

Systems Affected

- Neurological – sedation, potentially ataxia at higher doses.
- Hepatic – human reports of hepatotoxicity.
- Renal – human reports of nephrotoxicity.

Blackwell's Five-Minute Veterinary Consult Clinical Companion: Equine Toxicology, First Edition. Edited by Lynn R. Hovda, Dionne Benson, and Robert H. Poppenga.
© 2022 John Wiley & Sons, Inc. Published 2022 by John Wiley & Sons, Inc.
Companion website: www.wiley.com/go/hovda/equine

SIGNALMENT/HISTORY

Risk Factors
- Administration to horse due to laminitis or other neuropathic pain.
- Exposure to human prescription.

Historical Findings
- History of laminitis or other neuropathic pain and associated prescription of gabapentin.

Location and Circumstances of Poisoning
- Any horse prescribed gabapentin.
- Unintentional exposure to human prescription.

CLINICAL FEATURES

- Acute – uncertain but would likely include sedation and ataxia.
- Chronic – nephrotoxicity clinical signs include PU, PD, weight loss with appetite, and anemia.

DIFFERENTIAL DIAGNOSIS

- CNS depressants (benzodiazepine, opioids).
- NSAID toxicosis for nephrotoxicity.
- Rhabdomyolysis for nephrotoxicity.

DIAGNOSTICS

CBC/Serum Chemistry/Urinalysis
- Routine laboratory work including serum chemistry and urinalysis.
- RBC count for CKD.
- BUN and creatinine evidence of kidney injury or rhabdomyolysis.
- Urine concentration.

Other Diagnostic Tests
- Presence in serum:
  - LC-MS/MS useful for diagnosis, especially in unintentional exposure.

Pathological Findings
- None reported in horses.

THERAPEUTICS

- The goal of therapy is to provide supportive care.

Detoxification

- Discontinue use of gabapentin.

Appropriate Health Care

- Most can be treated in the field.
- Hospitalization for severe cases.

Antidotes

No specific antidote.

Drugs of Choice

- Intravenous fluids as needed for dehydration and volume expansion; may be helpful in differential diagnosis of CKD.
- GI protectants:
    - Omeprazole 2–4 mg/kg PO q24h

Precautions/Interactions

- Protection to the head and limbs may be necessary in ataxic horses.

COMMENTS

Client Education

- Acute sedation and potential ataxia present danger to rider.
- Educate clients regarding concerns of long-term gabapentin use.

Prevention/Avoidance

- Routine blood and urine tests to screen for nephrotoxicity when used long term.

Possible Complications

- Chronic kidney injury.
- Ataxia leading to injury.
- Sedation leading to injury.

Expected Course and Prognosis

- No reports of fatal toxicity. Acute toxicity (sedation) resolved 1 hour after onset.

Abbreviations

See Appendix 1 for a complete list.

Internet Resources

Gold JR, Grubb TL, Green S, et al. Plasma disposition of gabapentin after the intragastric administration of escalating doses to adult horses. J Vet Intern Med 2020; 34(2):933–940.

Terry RL, McDonnell SM, Van Eps AW, et al. Pharmacokinetic profile and behavioral effects of gabapentin in the horse. J Vet Pharmacol Ther 2010; 33(5):485–494.

Young JM, Schoonover MJ, Kembel SL, et al. Efficacy of orally administered gabapentin in horses with chronic thoracic limb lameness. Vet Anaesth Analg 2020; 47(2):259–266.

Author: Dionne Benson, DVM, JD
Consulting Editor: Dionne Benson, DVM, JD

Iodine

Chapter 20

 DEFINITION/OVERVIEW

- Iodine is found in the environment, particularly in sea water and organisms nutritionally reliant upon the sea. Generally, there is a decrease in environmental supply of iodine as terrain and land-based organisms exist further from marine life.
- Iodine is the heaviest element required for life, is a halogen in the periodic table, and has been assigned atomic number 53.
- Thyroid hormones circulate within the blood stream. Being key players in metabolic regulation. T3 and T4 maintain fat and carbohydrate usage rates, influence heart rate, regulate protein production, influence proper bone growth and maturation, participate in immune function, and assist in body temperature regulation.
- Iodine is found in mineralized salt blocks, medications, feed additives, supplements, and as an antiseptic in various dilutions. Medical industry uses iodine as a radiocontrast material, and it is also used as a catalyst in the production of acetic acid and some polymers. Sodium and potassium iodide are used in the horse as an antifungal, anti-actinomycetes, and as a selective antibacterial.
- Clinical signs of an iodine deficiency in the horse are goiter (swelling of the thyroid gland), poor hair coats, and contracted tendons and/or angular limb deformity in foals.
- Chronic iodine toxicosis has nearly identical clinical signs as its deficiency, but mild respiratory signs appear in equine iodine toxicity.
- Hypothyroidism can occur because of the Wolff–Chaikoff effect where high concentrations of circulating iodine cause enzyme suppression in the thyroid gland.
- Iodine toxicosis is not commonly reported in the horse. It is usually caused by iatrogenic administration, whether from medication or feed supplementation.
- The organic iodine compound ethylenediamine dihydroiodide is used to treat some conditions and as a feed additive (herbivores and pets) to add iodine to the diet. If suspect iodine toxicosis in an equine patient, consider feed source and possible contamination from mills that manufacture other animal feeds, as iodine is commonly supplemented in food producing animal feeds.

Blackwell's Five-Minute Veterinary Consult Clinical Companion: Equine Toxicology,
First Edition. Edited by Lynn R. Hovda, Dionne Benson, and Robert H. Poppenga.
© 2022 John Wiley & Sons, Inc. Published 2022 by John Wiley & Sons, Inc.
Companion website: www.wiley.com/go/hovda/equine

ETIOLOGY/PATHOPHYSIOLOGY

Mechanism of Action

- Principle dietary iodine is absorbed in the stomach and duodenum and is subsequently absorbed by the thyroid gland. Based on the horse's needs of T3 and T4 in circulation, the hypothalamus releases TSH which signals the thyroid into production.
- Excessive intake of iodine will increase organic iodine production and then sharply decrease production by the thyroid gland. There will also be inhibition of its release into the bloodstream once TSH is released.
- Iodine used as a disinfectant, such as povidone-iodine, is a water-soluble polymer known as polyvinylpyrrolidone. Once free iodine disassociates from its complex, it penetrates microbial cell membranes and interacts with vital cell function, causing rapid bacterial cell death.
- Although low doses of iodine help to make drinking water safe, high doses of iodine in forms commonly used as disinfectants consumed orally can be cytotoxic and will denature proteins if absorbed by cells. Accidental high-dose consumption of these products is likely not to exist in the horse but theoretically would be toxic if consumed in large doses.
- A proposed mechanism of action for the Wolff–Chaikoff effect (which was studied in rats) suggests that during initial high exposures to circulating iodine, the sodium-iodide symporter found on the basolateral membrane of thyroid follicular cells permits an increased amount of iodine into the cells. In turn, there is a transient decrease in thyroid peroxidase and subsequent reduction in thyroid hormone production. Adaptation of the cells occur after approximately 24 hours and cells decrease their expression of sodium-iodide symporter, resulting in less iodine uptake and allowing normal production of thyroid hormone to resume.

Toxicokinetics

- Chronic exposure toxicity is most common.
- Clinical signs for chronic toxicosis resolve in several days.
- High doses of iodine salts will stimulate nerve receptors in the stomach wall, causing vagal stimulation and resulting in upper respiratory tract reflex secretion.
- High bioavailability via GI tract.
- Distributed to entire body via circulatory system, then metabolized in thyroid gland to T3 and T4.
- Primarily urinary excretion, to a lesser degree in feces, sweat, and milk.

Toxicity

- Chronic administration of 50 mg/day can cause toxicosis.

Systems Affected

- Endocrine/metabolic – goiter, hypothyroidism.
- Cardiovascular – pertussis, nasal discharge, tachycardia, tachypnea.
- Neurological – thermoregulation, excessive lacrimation.
- Dermatologic – dermal hypertrophy, lichenification, alopecia, lackluster hair.
- Musculoskeletal – foals: angular limb deformity, abnormal bone development, tendon contracture; adults: cachexia, weight loss.

SIGNALMENT/HISTORY

Risk Factors

- Foals born to mares that have received iodine supplementation during pregnancy.
- Horses fed dietary supplements that are derived from seaweed (which have high iodine concentrations – more specifically, kelp).
- Competition horses that receive significant feed supplementation.
- Iatrogenic.

Historical Findings

- Treatment with IV sodium iodide jugs.
- Feed formulation errors.
- Iodine supplementation.
- Antifungal and antibacterial with iodide at 1–2 mg/kg PO every 12–24 hours for 1 week, then 0.5–1.0 mg/kg PO as needed. As this treatment regimen total dose could exceed 50 mg/horse daily.

Location and Circumstances of Poisoning

- Intentional exposure by iatrogenic administration, supplementation, or feed exposure.

CLINICAL FEATURES

- Not all clinical signs will necessarily be present, but the deficiency and toxicity may or may not have the same clinical signs
- Swelling of the horse's neck next to trachea behind larynx (goiter):
  - The swelling may decrease in 24 hours as the body responds to the high levels of iodine and counters the effect of high plasma concentrations of iodine.
- Chronic clinical signs include generalized poor health, poor hair coat or non-pruritic lesions, alopecia, dermal lesions, poor feed use, lethargy, obesity, and poor metabolic function.
- When exposed to TSH, the thyroid will decrease its release of organic iodine into the bloodstream because of the high amounts of circulating inorganic iodine. The net result is an increased amount of viscosity in the respiratory tract, leading to nasal discharge and non-productive cough.
- Excessive lacrimation.

DIFFERENTIAL DIAGNOSIS

- Hypothyroidism.
- Hyperthyroidism.
- Thyroid adenoma.
- Pituitary pars intermedia dysfunction.
- Other endocrine disorders.

DIAGNOSTICS

- Based on a history of high iodine exposure and clinical signs.

Diagnostic Blood Tests

- High iodine concentrations.
- Lower than normal levels of T3 and T4.

Other Diagnostic Tests

- Collect suspect feed for analysis.

THERAPEUTICS

Detoxification

- Therapy goals are to reduce the exposure to the iodine as soon toxicity is apparent.
- Tissues will rapidly excrete excess iodine and blood levels will be close to normal in a matter of days.

COMMENTS

Client Education

- Inform clients to be cautious when choosing seaweed-based supplements
- Be cognizant when supplementing mares in foal.

Prevention/Avoidance

- Have forage/feeds tested for iodine concentration.
- Avoid supplementation with iodine and iatrogenic administration.

Expected Course and Prognosis

- Prognosis is good if toxicosis is resolved.
- The body will excrete excessive iodine in a matter of days.

Abbreviations

See Appendix 1 for a complete list.

Suggested Reading

Baker, HJ, Lindsey. Equine goiter due to excess dietary iodine. J Am Vet Med Assoc 1968; 153:168.
Drew, B, Barber WP, Williams DG. The effect of excess iodine on pregnant mares and foals. Vet Record 1975; 97:93.
Driscoll, J. et al. Goiter in foals caused by excess iodine. J Am Vet Med Assoc 1978; 173:858.
Fadoc VA, Wild S. Suspected cutaneous iodism in a horse. J Am Vet Med Assoc 1983; 183:1104–1106.
Gupta GC. Veterinary Toxicology, 2nd edn. San Diego; Elsevier; 2012.

National Research Council. Mineral Tolerance of Domestic Animals. Washington DC: National Academy Press, 1980.
Osterc, A, Stibilj V, Raspor P. Iodine in the environment. Encycl Env Health 2011; 280–287.
Reed SM, Bayly WM, Sellon DC, ed. Equine Internal Medicine, 4th edn. St Louis: Elsevier, 2018.
Smith BP, ed. Large Animal Internal Medicine, 4th edn. St Louis: Mosby; 2009.
Stowe CM. Iodine, iodides, and iodism. J Am Vet Med Assoc 1981; 179:334–336.

Author: Jay Deluhery, DVM, MBA, CJF
Consulting Editor: Dionne Benson, DVM, JD

Chapter 21

Medroxyprogesterone Acetate

DEFINITION/OVERVIEW

- Medroxyprogesterone acetate (MPA) is a type of synthetic progesterone.
- In humans it is used for reproductive regulation, reduction in endometrial hyperplasia, and breast and endometrial cancers.
- In the horse, MPA has been used to control estrus in mares and in all sexes for behavior modification.
- MPA use in horses is considered off-label under AMDUCA.
- It is a prohibited substance in competition under USEF and ARCI rules.
- MPA is controlled under the FEI rules.
- Little information exists on clinical toxicity in horses; there are anecdotal reports only.

ETIOLOGY/PATHOPHYSIOLOGY

Mechanism of Action

- The mechanism of action in the horse has not been studied. The sole research study performed in horses showed no efficacy for suppression of estrus.
- In humans, MPA inhibits gonadotropin production. This prevents the maturation of follicles and ovulation. It also downregulates nuclear estrogen receptors and epithelial cell synthesis in the endometrium.

Pharmacokinetics

- Onset of action is immediate to 30 minutes for acute toxicosis.
- Acute toxicosis clinical signs are those of anaphylactic shock and often results in sudden death.
- Toxicosis associated with long-term use has not been studied in the horse but in humans, bone density deficits occurs and lasts more than 24 weeks after the final dose of multiple administrations.
- In humans, metabolism occurs in the intestinal cells and liver and is linked to cytochrome P450 activity.
- Excretion is primarily in the urine.

Blackwell's Five-Minute Veterinary Consult Clinical Companion: Equine Toxicology, First Edition. Edited by Lynn R. Hovda, Dionne Benson, and Robert H. Poppenga.
© 2022 John Wiley & Sons, Inc. Published 2022 by John Wiley & Sons, Inc.
Companion website: www.wiley.com/go/hovda/equine

Toxicity

- Acute toxicity is variable. Acute toxicity has not been reported to have occurred after the first administration of MPA.

Systems Affected

- Multiple organ system – anaphylaxis, collapse, and death.
- Respiratory – apnea interspersed with tachypnea.
- Musculoskeletal – pathologic fractures are unstudied in horses but occur in humans. There is increased risk if a human receives MPA in adolescence.

SIGNALMENT/HISTORY

Risk Factors

- History of MPA administration.

Historical Findings

- Previous administration of MPA.
- Finding of methylprednisolone or MPA in blood.

Location and Circumstances of Poisoning

- Iatrogenic or owner/trainer administration.

CLINICAL FEATURES

- Acute toxicosis associated with unpredictable sudden death.
- Chronic toxicosis unreported but may be associated with pathological fractures.

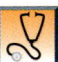
DIFFERENTIAL DIAGNOSIS

- Selenium.
- Aortic rupture.
- Botulism.
- Red oak (*Quercus rubra*).
- Cherry tree (*Prunus spp.*).
- Ionophores.
- Envenomation.
- Aneurysm/embolism.
- Bisphosphonates for pathologic fracture.

DIAGNOSTICS

- History of MPA administration.

CBC/Serum Chemistry

- Routine laboratory work including serum chemistry and urinalysis.
- Anaphylaxis blood work:
  - Polycythemia.
  - Leukopenia.
  - Neutropenia.
  - Hypokalemia.
  - Increase in histamine.

Other Diagnostic Tests

- LC MS/MS useful for diagnosis, but the time delay would hinder therapeutic.

Pathological Findings

- None reported in horses.

THERAPEUTICS

- The goal in acute toxicosis is to treat anaphylaxis.

Appropriate Health Care

- Most treated in the field due to acute nature.

Antidotes

- No specific antidote.

Drugs of Choice

- Fluid therapy – polyionic fluids (e.g., LRS).
- Anaphylaxis:
  - Epinephrine – 3–5 mLs of 1:1,000 per 450 kg of body weight IM or SC.
  - Prednisolone – 50–100 mg IV (slow) or IM q12/24/48h.
  - Dexamethasone – 2.5–5 mg IM or IV.
  - Isoflupredone – 5–20 mg total dose IM prn.

Precautions/Interactions

- MPA in humans may increase blood pressure and risk of clot formation.

COMMENTS

Client Education

- An FDA-approved alternative for estrus control in fillies and mares is available.
- LC-MS may be useful in legal cases.

Prevention/Avoidance

- Recommend use of altrenogest for estrus control in fillies and mares.

Possible Complications
- Pathological fracture.
- Death.

Expected Course and Prognosis
- Toxicity is often fatal.

Abbreviations
See Appendix 1 for a complete list.

Internet Resources
American Association of Equine Practitioners, AAEP Statement on the use of medroxyprogesterone in competition horses, 2019. Available at: https://aaep.org/guidelines/aaep-ethical-and-professional-guidelines/aaep-position-statements/medication#:~:text=Medroxyprogesterone%20acetate%20(MPA)%20is%20a,at%20suppression%20of%20behavioral%20estrus (accessed January 27, 2021).

Bailey M. side effects may include sudden death. Chronicle of the Horse, October 11, 2019, Available at: https://www.chronofhorse.com/article/side-effects-may-include-sudden-death#:~:text=and%20subsequent%20death.-,Dr.,the%20drug%20before%20without%20incident (accessed January 27, 2021).

Abbreviations
See Appendix 1 for a complete list.

Suggested Reading
Gee EK, DeLuca C, Stylski JL, McCue PM. Efficacy of medroxyprogesterone acetate in suppression of estrus in cycling mares. J Equine Vet Sci 2009; 29(3):140–145.

Kobayashi K, Mimura N., Fujii H, et al. Role of human cytochrome P450 3A4 in metabolism of medroxyprogesterone acetate. Clin Cancer Res 2000; 6(8):3297–3303.

Author: Dionne Benson, DVM, JD
Consulting Editor: Dionne Benson, DVM, JD

Chapter 22

Methylxanthine: Caffeine, Theobromine, Theophylline

DEFINITION/OVERVIEW

- Methylxanthine poisoning occurs in horses that ingest toxic amounts of the methylated xanthine compounds, theobromine or caffeine, present in cocoa or coffee products, respectively[1] (Figs 22.1 and 22.2)
- Historically, equids have also been reported to have exhibited theobromine poisoning after being fed chocolate waste.
- Methylxanthines include theobromine and caffeine, which can be found in cocoa and coffee, and theophylline, which is found in smaller amounts in cocoa/chocolate and tea, and is used medicinally as a bronchodilator.
- Theobromine (from cocoa bean hulls) and caffeine from coffee husks have been associated with clinical intoxication in horses.
- Death has been associated with ingestion of theobromine in cocoa bean hulls used as bedding.
- Inappropriate use and detection of methylxanthines in racehorses are of concern.
- They are FEI and USEF controlled substances.
- ARCI has prohibited substance in competition.

ETIOLOGY/PATHOPHYSIOLOGY

Etiology

Cases of methylxanthine poisoning are uncommon. They have been reported related to ingestion of cocoa bean or coffee bean waste in the form of hulls used as bedding, or as landscaping mulch.

Mechanism of Action

- Generally, methylxanthines are competitive inhibitors of intracellular phosphodiesterase, antagonize adenosine receptors, and activate histone deacetylase.
- Phosphodiesterase inhibition leads to increases in intracellular cAMP and cGMP, resulting in CNS stimulation, cardiac stimulation, diuresis, and bronchial smooth muscle relaxation.
- Adenosine receptor antagonism results in CNS stimulation and calcium uptake in muscles, which results in increased force of contraction.
- Histone deacetylase activation results in an anti-inflammatory effect.

Blackwell's Five-Minute Veterinary Consult Clinical Companion: Equine Toxicology,
First Edition. Edited by Lynn R. Hovda, Dionne Benson, and Robert H. Poppenga.
© 2022 John Wiley & Sons, Inc. Published 2022 by John Wiley & Sons, Inc.
Companion website: www.wiley.com/go/hovda/equine

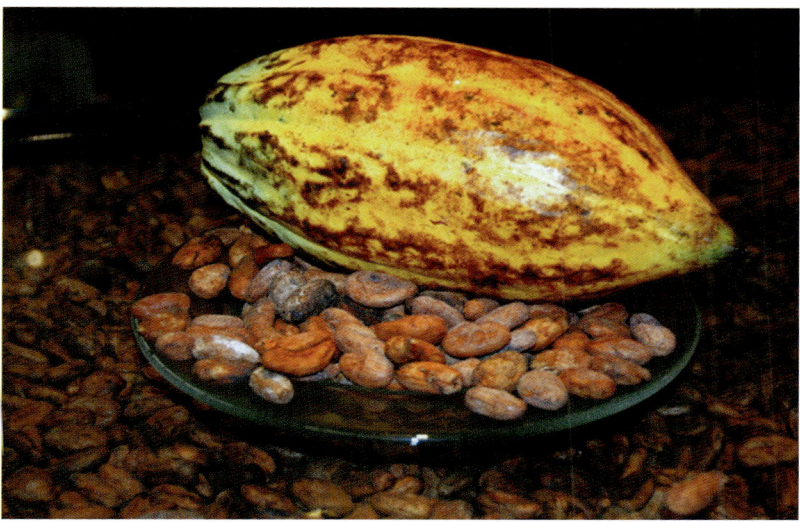

■ **Fig. 22.1.** Cocoa fruit (pod) cut open with roasted cocoa beans placed inside. *Source*: Muninus, https://commons.wikimedia.org/wiki/File:Kakaofrucht_mit_Kakaobohnen.jpg.

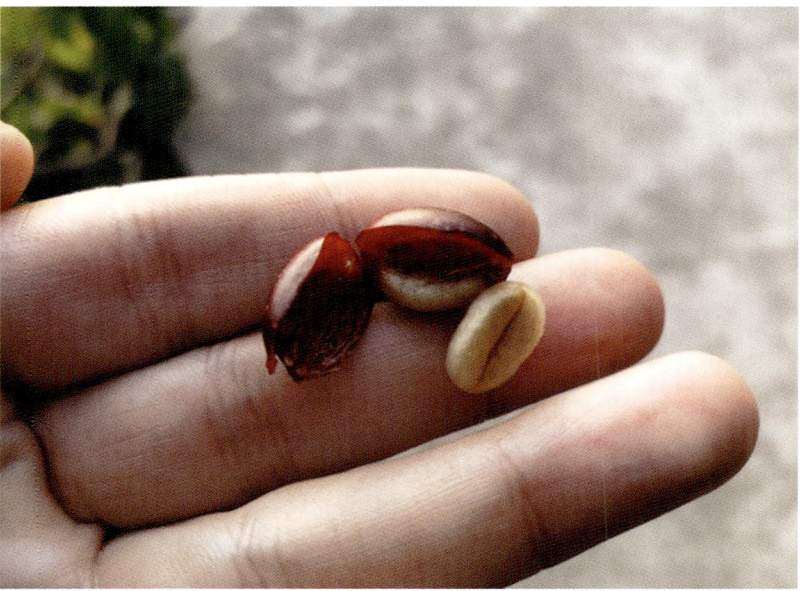

■ **Fig. 22.2.** Coffee cherry open with hull and two raw beans. *Source*: Roger Burger https://commons.wikimedia.org/wiki/File:Open_coffee_cherry.jpg.

Toxicokinetics

- Onset of clinical symptoms of toxicosis usually occur within 1 hour of ingestion.
- Duration of action is variable, but symptoms can resolve within hours to days of removal of the methylxanthine source.
- Methylxanthines are readily absorbed from the GI tract following ingestion and are rapidly distributed throughout the body.

- Metabolism occurs primarily in liver hepatocytes via cytochrome 1A2, N-acetyltransferase and xanthine oxidase.
- Urinary excretion predominates.
- The half-life of caffeine by IV administration is relatively long at 18.2 hours. Following oral administration, caffeine and theobromine can be detected in urine for up to 9 and 10 days, respectively, dependent upon the initial dose.

Toxicity

- Toxicity is lower than in other species (e.g., dogs) but varies by methylxanthine.
- Methylxanthines stimulate the CNS, cardiac and skeletal muscles, promote diuresis and induce smooth muscle relaxation.
- Adverse clinical signs which have been reported in horses can include anorexia, aggressive behavior, excessive sweating, muscle tremors, tremors of the lips and tongue, chewing movements, incoordination, falling, death.
- In severe cases, cardiac arrhythmias can lead to cardiac arrest and death.

Systems Affected

- Cardiovascular – cardiac arrhythmias leading to cardiac arrest.
- Musculoskeletal – stimulation leading to muscle tremors.
- Nervous – stimulation and aggressive behavior.
- Renal/urologic – diuresis.
- Skin/exocrine – sweating.
- Adverse clinical signs can vary depending upon which methylxanthine is involved, dose, duration of exposure, and individual response. Cases in horses are relatively rare, and experimental studies in horses are limited, therefore specifics are not known.

SIGNALMENT/HISTORY

- All Equidae are susceptible to theobromine or caffeine intoxication, but the few reported cases do not allow for determination of breed, age, or sex predilections.
- Adverse clinical signs that have been reported in horses can include anorexia, excitement, aggressive behavior, excessive sweating, muscle tremors, tremors of the lips and tongue, chewing movements, incoordination, falling, death.
- Adverse clinical signs of toxicosis reported in other species (primarily dogs) include hyperactivity, diarrhea, diuresis, muscle tremors, ataxia, cardiac arrhythmias, and death.

Risk Factors

Cases in horses are relatively rare, therefore specific risk factors are not known.

Historical Findings

- History of exposure to methylxanthines through food, treats, bedding.
- See adverse clinical signs above.

Location and Circumstances of Poisoning

- Theobromine and, in lower amounts, caffeine and theophylline are found in cocoa bean hulls, chocolate, and chocolate-containing bakery waste.

- Caffeine is found in coffee husks, coffee beans and coffee, and some pharmaceuticals. It is also found in tea, chocolate, energy drinks, and other products.
- Toxicoses and deaths have been reported through ingestion of cocoa bean hulls or coffee husks used as bedding or in feed.

CLINICAL FEATURES

- Cases in horses are relatively rare, therefore other than the adverse clinical signs listed above, additional specific abnormalities have not been reported.

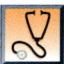

DIFFERENTIAL DIAGNOSIS

- Other causes of toxicity in horses with similar adverse clinical signs include:
  - Accidental ingestion of ionophore feed supplements (test for ionophores in the feed).
  - Ingestion of white snakeroot [*Ageratina altissima* (formerly *Eupatorium rugosum*), based on history; evidence of ingestion and myocardial necrosis].
  - Ingestion of bark and leaves of *Robinia pseudoacacia* or black locust (based on history; evidence of ingestion).
  - Fumonisin ingestion in feed can result in tremors, chewing movements and incoordination, and death can be seen associated with leukoencephalomalacia.
- Rabies can cause aggression.

DIAGNOSTICS

- Diagnosis of theobromine or caffeine intoxication is established based on a history of ingestion and determination of theobromine or caffeine in feedstuffs, serum, plasma, urine, or stomach contents.
- ECG – for possible cardiac arrhythmias.
- LC-MS testing on urine and blood can be helpful for diagnosis, but the time delay would hinder therapeutics.

Pathological Findings

- No gross or histopathologic abnormalities have been reported.
- No blood, serum chemistry, or urinalysis abnormalities have been reported.
- Diagnosis of theobromine or caffeine toxicosis is established based on clinical history, evidence of ingestion, and presence of theobromine or caffeine in serum, plasma, urine, or stomach contents.

THERAPEUTICS

- The goal of therapy is to eliminate exposure, decrease absorption, and provide supportive care.

Detoxification

- Activated charcoal 1–4 g/kg BW PO in watery slurry if appropriate and not contraindicated.

Drugs of Choice

- Intravenous fluids as needed for dehydration and volume expansion; may be helpful to increase elimination.
- Beta-blocker administration has been used in humans to decrease adverse cardiac events.
- Information regarding specific pharmacologic intervention in equine theobromine toxicosis has not been evaluated due to the limited number of cases.

Precautions/Interactions

- Restrict activity because of the possibility of cardiac arrhythmias.
- Because of the limited number of reported cases, specific drug interactions have not been evaluated.

Client Education

- Do not use cocoa bean hulls or coffee bean husks/hulls as bedding for horses. Do not use cocoa bean hull mulch around barns.

Patient Monitoring

- May require long-term ECG monitoring for cardiac effects.

Prevention/Avoidance

- Do not allow horses to eat cocoa bean hulls, chocolate products, coffee husks, or products containing caffeine.

Expected Course and Prognosis

- The relative rarity of methylxanthine toxicosis precludes generalization to all prospective equine cases, however, when less than toxic amounts are ingested and ECG abnormalities are not present, the prognosis is very good.

Abbreviations

See Appendix 1 for a complete list.

Suggested Reading

Blakemore F, Shearer GD. The poisoning of livestock by cacao products. Vet Rec 1943; 55:165.
Benezoli AZ, Goncalves SP, Rondon DA, et al. Equine poisoning by coffee husk (*Coffea canephora*) in Northern Espirito Santo, Brazil. Acta Scientiae Vet 2019; 47(Suppl 1):465.
Gottwalt B, Tadi P. Methylxanthines. [Updated 8 July 2020]. In: StatPearls [Internet]. Treasure Island (FL): StatPearls Publishing; 202. Available at: https://www.ncbi.nlm.nih.gov/books/NBK559165/.
Harkins JD, Rees WA, Mundy GD, et al. An overview of the methylxanthines and their regulation in the horse. Equine Pract 1998; 20:10–16.
Hooser, SB. Methylxanthine (theobromine, caffeine, theophylline) toxicosis in animals – a review of 1984 cases at the NAPCC [Abstract]. Vet Human Toxicol 1985; 28(4):313.
Hooser SB, Beasley VR. Methylxanthine poisoning (chocolate and caffeine toxicosis). In: Kirk, RW, ed. Current Veterinary Therapy for Small Animal Practice IX, 9th edn. Philadelphia, PA: WB Saunders, 1986; pp. 191–192.

Author: Stephen Hooser, DVM, PhD, DABVT
Consulting Editor: Dionne M. Benson, DVM, JD

Endnote

1 I acknowledge that chocolate is tasty for humans and that cocoa bean hulls smell nice when used as mulch. **But be warned:** chocolate and cocoa waste, including cocoa bean hulls, should never be fed to horses, used as bedding in stalls, as mulch around horse barns, or in areas where horses could eat any of the aforementioned theobromine-containing products.

Chapter 23

Nonsteroidal Anti-inflammatory Drugs (NSAIDs)

DEFINITION/OVERVIEW

- Class of medications used for suppression of inflammation and preventing platelet aggregation.
- Some drugs in this class are naturally derived (e.g., salicylates) while others are manufactured.
- NSAIDs have antipyretic, analgesic, and antiplatelet effects.
- FDA-approved versions for the horse include phenylbutazone, ketoprofen, flunixin meglumine, firocoxib, and diclofenac.
- Combining systemic NSAIDs increases likelihood of toxicosis.
- Two general mechanisms of action – COX-selective and non-COX-selective inhibitors.
- COX-1 inhibition is important for platelet aggregation but is also responsible for many of the clinical signs of toxicosis.
- COX-2 inhibition is important to control the signs of inflammation.
- Available in tablet, paste, topical, and injectable formulations. IM administration of injectable formulations should be avoided regardless of routes of administration recommended on the packaging. If IM administration occurs, skin sloughing may result.
- It is important to instruct clients clearly with paste administration. Improper dosing of an entire tube of medication has occurred.
- Controlled medication under ARCI, USEF, FEI, and AQHA regulations.

ETIOLOGY/PATHOPHYSIOLOGY

Mechanism of Action

- COX-selective inhibitors (e.g., firocoxib) preferentially inhibit COX-2 enzyme.
- Non-selective COX inhibitors (e.g., phenylbutazone, flunixin meglumine, etc.) inhibit both COX-1 and COX-2 enzymes.
- Inhibition of prostaglandin production through COX inhibition (especially COX-1) causes GI and renal effects.

Blackwell's Five-Minute Veterinary Consult Clinical Companion: Equine Toxicology, First Edition. Edited by Lynn R. Hovda, Dionne Benson, and Robert H. Poppenga.
© 2022 John Wiley & Sons, Inc. Published 2022 by John Wiley & Sons, Inc.
Companion website: www.wiley.com/go/hovda/equine

Pharmacokinetics

- Onset of action varies with each compound but most often with administration of several days to weeks – however, fatalities have been reported after as few as 4 days of treatment at 4× therapeutic doses of phenylbutazone. Acute toxicity can occur with intra-arterial administration or accidental overdose.
- Duration of action is 12–24 hours.
- Generally good oral bioavailability with PO administration for phenylbutazone, flunixin meglumine, and firocoxib. Poor oral bioavailability for ketoprofen.
- Highly bound to plasma proteins.
- Hepatic metabolism.
- Excretion is primarily in the urine.

Toxicity

- Toxicity varies by NSAID. Phenylbutazone > flunixin meglumine > ketoprofen. Non-selective COX inhibitors are more likely to be associated with toxicity than COX-2-selective inhibitors.

Systems Affected

- Neurological – if accidentally administered intra-arterially: ataxia, muscle weakness; chronic administration: lethargy.
- Cardiovascular – if administered intra-arterially: hyperventilation; if chronic/overdose: dehydration and increased CRT.
- Gastrointestinal – GI ulcers, oral ulcers, RDC, diarrhea, anorexia, colic.
- Renal – acute kidney injury.
- Hepatic – hepatitis.
- Musculoskeletal – edema, localized tissue swelling/sloughing if administered IM.
- Lymphatic – ventral edema.

SIGNALMENT/HISTORY

Risk Factors

- Iatrogenic.
- Accidental over administration by client.
- Horses with musculoskeletal injuries requiring long-term NSAID treatment.

Historical Findings

- History of administration of one or more NSAIDs – particularly long-term administration.

Location and Circumstances of Poisoning

- Accidental intra-arterial administration.
- Accidental overdose – especially with paste products.
- Long-term treatment with NSAIDs associated with musculoskeletal injuries.

CLINICAL FEATURES

- Dependent upon cause of toxicosis (acute intra-arterial versus chronic/overdose).

DIFFERENTIAL DIAGNOSIS

- Bacterial: *Salmonella, Clostridium perfringens, Clostridium difficile. Clostridium botulinum* (botulism).
- Protozoal: *Neorickettsia risticii* (Potomac horse fever).
- Viral: coronavirus.
- Antibiotic toxicity.
- Inflammatory bowel disease.
- Plant toxicities:
  - Oak – *Quercus* spp.
  - Oleander – *Nerium oleander*.
  - Buttercup – *Ranunculus* spp.
  - Nightshade – *Solanum* spp.
  - Rhododendron – *Rhododendron* spp.
  - Pokeweed – *Phytolacca americana*.
- Neoplasia.

DIAGNOSTICS

CBC/Serum Chemistry/Urinalysis

- Routine laboratory work including serum chemistry and urinalysis:
  - Hypoalbuminemia.
  - Hypoproteinemia.
  - Slight anemia.
- BUN, creatinine and creatine kinase for evidence of acute kidney injury.

Other Diagnostic Tests

- Fecal red blood cell.
- Ultrasound of the right dorsal colon to detect thickening.
- Gastroscopy for GI ulcers.
- Presence in serum and urine:
  - LC-MS useful for diagnosis, but the time delay would hinder therapeutics.

Pathological Findings

- Renal tubular necrosis.
- Gastric ulcers

THERAPEUTICS

- The goal of therapy is to limit toxin absorption and provide supportive care for chronic/overdose NSAID toxicity.
- The goal of therapy for accidental intra-arterial administration is supportive care and prevent injury.

Detoxification

- Reflux with NG tube if recent overdose.
- Administer AC (1–3 g/kg) by NG tube as a slurry in water.
- Follow with magnesium sulfate (Epsom salts) 250–500 mg/kg dissolved in 2–4 L of warm water.

Appropriate Health Care

- IV fluids.
- Hospitalization for severe cases.

Antidotes

- No specific antidote.

Drugs of Choice

- Intravenous fluids as needed for dehydration and volume expansion; may be helpful to increase elimination.
- GI protectants:
  - Omeprazole 2–4 mg/kg PO q24h.
  - Sucralfate 22 mg/kg PO q6–8h.
  - Misoprostol 5 µg/kg PO q8–12h (may worsen diarrhea).
  - Metronidazole 15 mg/kg PO q12h for 5 days.
  - Psyllium hydrophilic mucilloid – 1 g/kg PO (NG tube) q12h.

Precautions/Interactions

- If accidentally administered intra-arterially, horse may flip or become ataxic – ensure owner/trainer/groom/veterinarian safety.
- If horse develops RDC, meals should be small amounts and low bulk. Any subsequent diet change should be gradual.

COMMENTS

Client Education

- Educate clients regarding long-term NSAID use.
- Provide clear instruction with prescribing paste forms of NSAIDs to ensure proper dosing.

Prevention/Avoidance

- Consider COX-selective NSAIDs for long-term pain management.

Possible Complications

- Acute kidney injury.
- Acute tubular necrosis.
- RDC adhesions.
- Gastric adhesions.

Expected Course and Prognosis

- For acute intra-arterial administration – prognosis is usually good provided the horse does not injure itself. Recovery should occur within 1–2 hours.
- For chronic/overdose cases – prognosis depends upon clinical signs. Long-term monitoring is necessary to ensure healing.

Abbreviations

See Appendix 1 for a complete list.

Suggested Reading

Black H. Renal toxicity of non-steroidal anti-inflammatory drugs. Toxicol Pathol 1986; 14(1):83–90.

D'Arcy-Moskwa E, Noble GK, Weston LA, et al. Effects of meloxicam and phenylbutazone on equine gastric mucosal permeability. J Vet Intern Med 2012; 26:1494–1499.

Lees P, Toutain PL. Pharmacokinetics, Pharmacodynamics, metabolism, toxicology, and residues of phenylbutazone in humans and horses. The Vet J 2013; 196:294–303.

McConnico RS, Morgan TW, Williams CC, et al. Pathophysiologic effects of phenylbutazone on the right dorsal colon in horses. AJVR 2008; 69(11):1496–1505.

Moses VS, Bertone AL. Non-steroidal anti-inflammatory drugs. Vet Clin Equine 2002; 18 21–37.

Author: Dionne M. Benson, DVM, JD
Consulting Editor: Dionne M. Benson, DVM, JD

Chapter 24

Levothyroxine

DEFINITION/OVERVIEW

- T_4 is a naturally occurring substance in the horse.
- Toxicity is related to the synthetic version of T_4.
- Purchased as prescription levothyroxine for supplementation in horses that suffer from hypothyroidism, equine metabolic syndrome, or insulin resistance.
- Horse owners and trainers often treat this as a supplement instead of a prescription drug. This may increase the likelihood of overuse in horses and overdosing in an individual horse.
- Long-term use will interfere with normal thyroid function in healthy horses (euthyroid).
- Restricted use in several racing jurisdictions; controlled under FEI and USEF regulations.
- Limited information on clinical toxicology in horses; unpublished studies only.

ETIOLOGY/PATHOPHYSIOLOGY

Mechanism of Action

- Replaces naturally occurring source of T_4 in the body. T_4 is necessary to create T_3.
- T_3 is responsible for multiple physiological processes in horses, including metabolism, cardiac functions, and CNS functions.
- Bioavailability reportedly varies among preparations.

Pharmacokinetics

- Acute toxicity is unreported.
- Chronic toxicity is generally responsible for clinical signs.
- Duration of action for cardiac abnormalities may be extended.
- Excretion – primarily via kidneys with secondary excretion in feces.

Toxicity

- Variable toxicity – may be a genetic sensitivity component.

Blackwell's Five-Minute Veterinary Consult Clinical Companion: Equine Toxicology, First Edition. Edited by Lynn R. Hovda, Dionne Benson, and Robert H. Poppenga.
© 2022 John Wiley & Sons, Inc. Published 2022 by John Wiley & Sons, Inc.
Companion website: www.wiley.com/go/hovda/equine

Systems Affected

- Cardiovascular – tachycardia, tachypnea, and arrhythmias including atrial fibrillation reported.
- Metabolism – cachexia/weight loss.
- Neurological – hyperactive behavior.

SIGNALMENT/HISTORY

Risk Factors

- Thyroid supplementation in horse with functioning thyroid.

Historical Findings

- History of supplementation with levothyroxine.
- Difficult to find in blood or urine testing – may observe transient increase in T_3/T_4.
- Findings often consist of sudden death, especially during exercise.

Location and Circumstances of Poisoning

- Worldwide concern.
- Intentional exposure by adding to feed.

CLINICAL FEATURES

- Tachycardia.
- Tachypnea.
- Cardiac arrhythmia, atrial fibrillation.
- Sudden death, particularly during exercise.

DIFFERENTIAL DIAGNOSIS

- Embolism.
- Aortic rupture.
- Potassium imbalance.
- Colic (rupture).
- Underlying heart disease.
- Exercise induced pulmonary hemorrhage.
- Anaphylaxis.

DIAGNOSTICS

CBC/Serum Chemistry/Urinalysis

- T_3/T_4 blood test.

Other Diagnostic Tests

- Auscultation for cardiac abnormalities.
- ECG as needed.

Pathological Findings

- None reported in horses – often a diagnosis of exclusion.

THERAPEUTICS

- Therapy is centered around discontinuation of use and restriction of exercise during cardiac abnormalities.

Detoxification

- Discontinue use of levothyroxine; normal thyroid concentrations should return in approximately 21 days.

Appropriate Health Care

- If discontinuation of levothyroxine does not resolve cardiac issues, consider conversion for atrial fibrillation using quinidine, amiodarone, or transvenous electrical cardioversion.

Antidotes

- None.

Drugs of Choice

- No known treatment.

Precautions/Interactions

- Multiple drug interactions can artificially depress T_3/T_4 concentrations and interfere with testing:
  - Phenylbutazone.
  - Anabolic steroids.
  - Corticosteroids.
  - Diazepam.
  - Salicylates.
  - Sulfa drugs.
  - Phenytoin.
- Horses that are exceptionally fit (e.g., racehorses) will have a naturally depressed T_3/T_4.

COMMENTS

Client Education

- Education of clients regarding the rarity of hypothyroidism in horses is crucial.
- It is important to address significant risks associated with inappropriate use of levothyroxine.

Prevention/Avoidance
- Educate owners and trainers about the adverse effects in horses.
- Perform appropriate testing to identify hypothyroid horses prior to prescribing levothyroxine.

Possible Complications
- Atrial fibrillation resistant to conversion.

Expected Course and Prognosis
- If identified as arrhythmia, prognosis is favorable with discontinuation of levothyroxine.
- Most identified as potential causative agent of death postmortem.

Abbreviations
See Appendix 1 for a complete list.

Internet Resources
Zions J. Study Reveals Thyroxine Detrimental to Racing Performance and Horse Health, University of Guelph E-news; 2019. Available at: https://www.equineguelph.ca/news/index.php?content=610

Suggested Reading
Bertin F, Forsythe L, Kritchevsky J. Effects of high doses of levothyroxine sodium on serum concentrations of triiodothyronine and thyroxine in horses. Am J Vet Res 2019; 80(6):565–571

McGurrin M. The diagnosis and management of atrial fibrillation in the horse. Vet Med (Auckl). 2015; 6:83–90.

Author: Dionne Benson, DVM, JD
Consulting Editor: Dionne Benson, DVM, JD

Chapter 25

Vitamin D (Calciferol)

DEFINITION/OVERVIEW

- Vitamin D toxicosis in horses is often a condition of oversupplementation.
- Two natural sources are cholecalciferol (D3) – synthesized in skin from sun exposure – and ergocalciferol (D2), occurring in plants
- Horses can obtain vitamin D endogenously, via sunlight exposure, and through diet via supplements or certain types of roughag.
- Toxicity is cumulative and can develop over the course of weeks to months.
- An excessive amount of vitamin D supplementation can lead to excessive calcium uptake over time.
- Clinical signs include, weight loss, lethargy, cardiac arrhythmias, exercise intolerance and limb stiffness.
- Treatment is removing source of vitamin D.

ETIOLOGY/PATHOPHYSIOLOGY

Mechanism of Action

- Vitamin D, whether ingested or produced in the skin, is transformed to calcidiol by the liver, or calcitriol by the kidneys. These hormones facilitate the absorption of calcium and phosphorus via the intestines and the kidneys, and the release of calcium and phosphorus from bone.
- Vitamin D metabolites are excreted in the kidney.

Pharmacokinetics

- Vitamin D3 – synthesized in skin and is metabolized by liver.
- Ingested vitamin D (D2 and D3) is absorbed in the distal small intestine and then metabolized by the liver.
- Half-life of metabolites is 10–20 days.
- Metabolites are excreted in the urine.

Toxicity

- 10× recommended dose over a prolonged period causes toxicity.
- Recommended daily dose is 44 IU/kg for long-term feeding (> 60 days).

Blackwell's Five-Minute Veterinary Consult Clinical Companion: Equine Toxicology,
First Edition. Edited by Lynn R. Hovda, Dionne Benson, and Robert H. Poppenga.
© 2022 John Wiley & Sons, Inc. Published 2022 by John Wiley & Sons, Inc.
Companion website: www.wiley.com/go/hovda/equine

Systems Affected

- Cardiovascular – calcification of soft tissues, tachycardia, heart murmur.
- Musculoskeletal – decreased exercise tolerance, weight loss, limb stiffness.
- Gastrointestinal – decreased appetite.
- Renal/urologic – calcification of soft tissues, PU/PD.

SIGNALMENT/HISTORY

Risk Factors

- Horse supplemented with vitamin D.

Historical Findings

- Signs develop slowly over time and may persist for years after the initial episode.
- Horse has a history of supplementation.

CLINICAL FEATURES

- Horse may be stiff and reluctant to move, with a short, choppy gait.
- Elevated pulse and elevated respiratory rate.
- Flexor tendons and suspensory ligaments are sensitive to palpation.
- Slight to moderate kyphosis.
- Weight loss (over the course of several months).

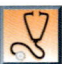
DIFFERENTIAL DIAGNOSIS

- IV calcium administration.
- Hyperparathyroidism (primary or secondary).
- Lymphosarcoma.
- Chronic renal failure.

DIAGNOSTICS

- Patient history and clinical signs:
    - Oversupplementation of Vitamin D.
    - Dystrophic calcification of soft tissues.

CBC/Serum Chemistry/Urinalysis

- Hypercalcemia
- ± hyperphosphatemia depending on the stage and severity of the disease.
- Elevated plasma vitamin D, more than 20–50 ng/mL.
- Hypercalciuria.

Pathological Findings

- Mineralization of the soft tissues, most notably the heart, flexor tendons, and ligaments.

THERAPEUTICS

- The goal of treatment is to decrease intestinal absorption. All feed sources of vitamin D should be removed immediately.
- Because vitamin D increases intestinal calcium absorption, limiting dietary calcium will reduce tissue calcium deposition.
- Supportive care for secondary effects:
  - fluid therapy.

Precautions/Interactions

- Avoid calcium supplementation.
- Avoid strenuous exercise for several weeks due to effects on soft tissue (especially heart).

COMMENTS

Client Education

- Ensure no feed supplements contain vitamin D.

Patient Monitoring

- Serum chemistry for Ca, P and renal values.
- ECG as needed.

Prevention/Avoidance

- Remove all sources of vitamin D from the diet.
- Check ingredient list in all feed supplements.

Possible Complications

- Poor performance.
- Emaciation.
- Cardiac failure.
- Renal failure.

Expected Course and Prognosis

- Toxicity is cumulative and not necessarily due to a single event.
- It may take several weeks for clinical signs to appear.
- Prognosis for recovery, once severe clinical signs are seen, is poor.

Abbreviations

See Appendix 1 for a complete list.

Suggested Reading

Harrington DD, Page EH. Acute vitamin D3 toxicosis in horses: case reports and experimental studies of the comparative toxicity of vitamins D2 and D3. J Am Vet Med Assoc 1983; 182(12):1358–1359.

Hymøller, L, Søren KJ. We know next to nothing about vitamin D in horses! J Equine Vet Sci 2015; 35:785–792.

Talcott P. Disorders of Specific Body Systems: Toxicologic problems. In: Reed SM et al. Equine Internal Medicine-E-book. Elsevier Health Sciences, 2017; 21:1507.

Author: Casille Batten, DVM
Consulting Editor: Dionne M. Benson, DVM, JD

Insecticides, Herbicides and Farm Chemicals

Amitraz

Chapter 26

DEFINITION/OVERVIEW

- Amitraz is a broad-spectrum formamidine insecticide/acaricide used in agriculture (fruit trees and cotton) and in veterinary medicine to control ticks, mites and lice.
- It is registered for use in livestock and dogs, but is toxic to cats and equids (horses, ponies and donkeys).
- Trade names include: Certifect, Francodex, Mitaban, Mitac, Ovasyn, Preventic, Taktic, Triatix and Triatox.
- Application is topical, consisting of sprays or dips (up to 0.2 lb active ingredient/50 gallons of water). Dips for cattle and sheep contain 0.025% amitraz.
- Available formulations for livestock include an emulsifiable concentrate (12.5% and 19.8%) and a wettable pour-on powder (50%).
- Despite no recommendations for use in horses, intoxications occur following intentional dermal application to control ectoparasites.
- Accidental oral exposure may occur.
- Clinical signs mostly involve the central nervous and GI systems, consisting of drowsiness, depression, ataxia and large intestine impaction colic. Milder changes are noted in the respiratory and cardiac systems.
- As noted in multiple species, clinical presentation depends on dose. At low doses, amitraz tends to cause CNS stimulation, while depression is noted at higher doses.

ETIOLOGY/PATHOPHYSIOLOGY

Mechanism of Action

- Although the mechanism of action is not completely understood, amitraz is an $alpha_2$-adrenergic receptor agonist structurally similar to the neurotransmitter norepinephrine, with effects on the central and peripheral nervous systems.
- Other known effects of formamidines include:
  - Monoamine oxidase (MAO) inhibition – the enzyme is necessary for metabolism of the CNS mediators norepinephrine and serotonin. This effect may cause neurotoxicity.

Blackwell's Five-Minute Veterinary Consult Clinical Companion: Equine Toxicology, First Edition. Edited by Lynn R. Hovda, Dionne Benson, and Robert H. Poppenga.
© 2022 John Wiley & Sons, Inc. Published 2022 by John Wiley & Sons, Inc.
Companion website: www.wiley.com/go/hovda/equine

- Decreased prostaglandin E$_2$ synthesis.
- Weak inhibition of platelet aggregation.
- Local anesthetic effect.

Toxicokinetics

- Amitraz is highly lipophilic (fat-soluble) and is absorbed following dermal application and oral ingestion.
- It is distributed throughout multiple tissues, with relatively high concentrations found in liver, bile, intestine and the eye.
- Amitraz is rapidly metabolized in the stomach and liver to multiple active and inactive metabolites, including the highly toxic N-3,5-dimethylphenyl N-methyl formamidine derivative.
- Metabolism is slower in horses than in other mammals, which might account for the increased susceptibility in this species.
- Excretion of metabolites is mainly through the kidneys (60–80% over first 48 hours) with no parent/unchanged molecule present in urine. Smaller excretion occurs in feces (10–40%).

Toxicity

- Acute toxicosis in horses commonly occurs after dermal application of amitraz-containing products, either at the safe concentration for livestock (0.025%) or at higher than recommended concentrations due to improper dilution.
- Clinical signs have been consistently reproduced by spraying horses with 0.1–0.2% solutions.
- Presentation may be complex with formulations containing other substances/solvents (e.g., xylene).
- Information on acute toxicity for horses is lacking. Values from laboratory animals and other species are unlikely to be predictable of toxicity in horses due to higher sensitivity of this species.
- Pharmacokinetic studies in dogs showed that the elimination half-life (time required to produce a 50% reduction in blood or plasma concentration) is about 24 hours. As amitraz metabolism in horses appears to be slower than in other species, drug levels in blood may remain longer.

Systems Affected

- Cardiovascular – tachycardia or bradycardia (at high doses); hypotension due to peripheral vascular dilation.
- Endocrine/metabolic – hypothermia.
- Gastrointestinal – reduced intestinal sounds and motility. Large intestine impaction colic. Rectal muscle relaxation was observed within 30 minutes after IV injection of amitraz at 0.10 mg/kg.
- Hemic/lymphatic/immune – hemoconcentration, acidosis, hyperglycemia and hypoinsulinemia.
- Nervous – somnolence/sedation, depression, ataxia and convulsions (high doses).
- Neuromuscular – muscular weakness.

- Ophthalmic – mydriasis.
- Respiratory – tachypnea is commonly reported but decreased respiratory rate occurs with high doses.
- Skin/exocrine – subcutaneous edema, facial swelling, increased sweating.

SIGNALMENT/HISTORY

Risk Factors

- Concentration of the product, application frequency, environmental temperature and condition of the skin may influence absorption and therefore toxicity.
- Spontaneous hydrolysis of amitraz to the highly toxic 3,5-dimethylphenyl N-methyl formamidine occurs when the product is dissolved or diluted in water at a pH lower than neutrality and stored. Application of the "aged" product appears to have higher toxicity.

Historical Findings

- History of amitraz application to horses by the owner within 2–3 days of developing compatible clinical signs.
- Improper storage of amitraz-containing products creates opportunities for oral exposure.

Location and Circumstances of Poisoning

- Most intoxications occur after topical applications. Despite contraindications for use on horses, amitraz is still frequently used in some parts of the world due to low cost, availability and efficacy to control ectoparasites.
- Inadvertent oral exposure is possible.
- Amitraz has been injected IV due to tranquilizing/sedation effect.

CLINICAL FEATURES

- Onset of clinical signs depends on route of exposure and concentration of the product:
  - After dermal application at the recommended concentration for livestock (0.025%), signs of intoxication in horses may develop within 2–3 days and may remain for up to 10 days.
  - Clinical signs are observed within 2 hours following oral ingestion or after accidental application of preparations with higher concentrations.
- Commonly reported clinical signs include drowsiness, depression, incoordination and decreased intestinal noises:
  - Decreased peristalsis is due to impaired smooth muscle contractility.
  - Reduction of intestinal blood flow has been noted in horses and ponies.
  - Colic and progressive large intestine impaction may develop.
- Tachycardia – due to alpha$_2$-adrenergic agonist effect and pain.
- Tachypnea or bradypnea depending on dose.

- Hypothermia.
- Increased sweating.
- Dehydration.
- Increased capillary filling time and congested mucous membranes.
- Death has been reported after oral administration due to ileus.

DIFFERENTIAL DIAGNOSIS

- Gastrointestinal signs must be differentiated from other causes of colic with large intestine impaction (e.g., coarse feed, teeth problems, decreased water intake)
- With neurological signs, other causes of ataxia must be considered:
  - Infectious agents (rabies, herpesvirus myeloencephalopathy, equine viral encephalomyelitis, protozoan myeloencephalitis).
  - Idiopathic inflammatory diseases.
  - Degenerative conditions and/or compression of tissue.
  - Neoplasia.
  - Toxic agents – ionophores, ivermectin, propylene glycol, heavy metals, acute selenium toxicosis and fumonisin mycotoxins.

DIAGNOSTICS

- Detailed clinical history indicating exposure to amitraz within the last 2–3 days of an animal with compatible clinical signs is crucial to establish a presumptive diagnosis.

CBC/Serum Chemistry/Urinalysis

- Baseline CBC and biochemistry:
  - Dehydration – increased red blood cell parameters and elevated serum albumin.
  - Acidosis – decreased tissue perfusion and respiratory changes.
  - Hyperglycemia – decreased insulin secretion (alpha$_2$-adrenergic effect).

Other Diagnostic Tests

- Rectal palpation may reveal firm consistency of large intestine and small amounts (or absence) of dry feces.
- GC-MS of gastric contents, serum/plasma, and hair can confirm exposure. Due to presumptive long half-life, determination of residues in serum/plasma seems practical; however, laboratories with validated methods may not be readily available and turnaround times can be long.

Pathological Findings

- No specific macroscopic or microscopic lesion are expected.
- Impacted feces may be present in large intestine.

THERAPEUTICS

Detoxification

- For topical application, skin should be washed thoroughly with running water and mild grease-cutting detergent to remove any residual unabsorbed chemical.
- If ingested, activated charcoal (2–4 g/kg) via NG tube may be used; however, this is not recommended for animals that have developed ileus, as retained charcoal may release amitraz for further absorption.

Appropriate Health Care

- Analgesics to control pain if colic is present; walking the animal may help.
- IV and/or oral fluids to maintain adequate hydration and correct any imbalances.
- Soften impacted feces by administration of laxatives (mineral oil, Epsom salts, psyllium) via NG tube every 12–24 hours.
- Saline cathartics may also be helpful.

Antidotes

- Effects of amitraz can be reversed by administration of alpha$_2$-receptor antagonists, such as yohimbine and atipamezole:
    - Yohimbine: 0.15 mg/kg IV slowly.
    - Atipamezole: 0.1 mg/kg IV.

Drugs of Choice

- Sedation and pain relief:
    - Detomidine 0.02–0.04 mg/kg IV or IM prn.
    - Xylazine (1 mg/kg) IV every 3 hours.
- Pain relief:
    - Flunixin meglumine 1.1 mg/kg IV or PO q12–24h.
- IV and/or oral fluids to maintain hydration and re-establish tissue perfusion to control acidosis.

Precautions/Interactions

- Atropine is contraindicated due to sensitivity of horses to anticholinergic effects on GI mobility. It may also increase the heart rate and cause hypertension.
- Adverse reactions to xylazine and benzodiazepines may occur.

Surgical Considerations

- Severe cases with colic impaction may not respond to symptomatic treatment to restore fecal flow and may require surgical intervention.

COMMENTS

Client Education

- Do not use amitraz for control of ectoparasites in horses.

Patient Monitoring

- Check body temperature, intestinal sounds, evidence/frequency of defecation and maintain hydration status.

Possible Complications

- Severe unresponsive colic with compromised circulation, leading to shock, sepsis and death.

Expected Course and Prognosis

- With prompt symptomatic treatment and decontamination most animals recover and prognosis is good. Horses with severe colic/ileus have a guarded prognosis.

Abbreviations

See Appendix 1 for a complete list.

Suggested Reading

Duarte MD, Peixoto PV, Junior PSB et al. Natural and experimental poisoning by amitraz in horses and donkey: clinical aspects. Pesq Vet Bras 2003; 23(3):105–118.

Filazi A, Yurdakok-Dikmen B. Amitraz. In: Gupta RC, ed. Veterinary Toxicology: Basic and Clinical Principles, 3rd edn. Academic Press, 2018; pp. 525–531

Queiroz-Neto A, Carregaro AB, Zamur G, et al. Effect of amitraz and xylazine on some physiological variables of horses. Arq Bras Med Vet Zootec 2000; 52(1):27–32.

Author: Felipe Reggeti, DVM, PhD, DACVP
Consulting Editor: Robert H. Poppenga, DVM, PhD, DABVT

Chapter 27

Cholinesterase-Inhibiting Carbamate Pesticides

DEFINITION/OVERVIEW

- Acetylcholinesterase (AChE)-inhibiting carbamate pesticides can cause muscarinic and nicotinic cholinergic overstimulation in exposed horses.
- Carbamate pesticides are commonly used insecticides.
- Horses can be exposed via accidental access to improperly stored or used products or through contaminated feed material from accidental application errors or drift.
- Not all pesticides labeled "carbamate" pesticides inhibit the AChE enzyme, so it is important to know the exact chemical name of the compound.
- Examples of AChE-inhibiting carbamate pesticides include aldicarb, bendiocarb, carbaryl, carbofuran, carbosulfan, ethinenocarb, fenobucarb, methiocarb, methomyl, oxamyl, pirimicarb, and propoxur.

ETIOLOGY/PATHOPHYSIOLOGY

Mechanism of Action

- The carbamate pesticides inhibit the enzyme AChE by occupying both the anionic and esteratic sites, thus leading to excessive stimulation of the sympathetic and parasympathetic ganglia, parasympathetic muscarinic junctions, sympathetic fibers in sweat glands, and nicotinic receptors at the skeletal neuromuscular junctions.
- The AChE–carbamate complex is not stable and the carbamyl moiety can be split from the enzyme by spontaneous hydrolysis and therefore carbamates are considered reversible AChE inhibitors.

Toxicokinetics

- Most carbamate compounds are thought to be absorbed from the skin, lungs, conjunctiva, mucous membranes, and GI tract.
- This group of compounds are not known to accumulate extensively in tissues, and half-lives for most carbamates are relatively short, leading to clinical signs that typically do not last longer than 36–48 hours.
- Some lipophilic compounds may redistribute into fat leading to a prolonged clinical syndrome.

Blackwell's Five-Minute Veterinary Consult Clinical Companion: Equine Toxicology,
First Edition. Edited by Lynn R. Hovda, Dionne Benson, and Robert H. Poppenga.
© 2022 John Wiley & Sons, Inc. Published 2022 by John Wiley & Sons, Inc.
Companion website: www.wiley.com/go/hovda/equine

- Carbamates are removed from circulation mostly through spontaneous hydrolysis of the AChE–carbamate complex and renal elimination.

Toxicity

- The carbamate pesticides are a group of structurally similar compounds; the toxicity of compounds can range from low to high.

Systems Affected

- Central and peripheral nervous system: persistently elevated acetylcholine levels due to AChE inhibition lead to increased neurotransmitter signaling and reflect both muscarinic and nicotinic cholinergic overstimulation:
  - Muscarinic cholinergic overstimulation may include colic (sweating, abdominal discomfort, diarrhea), excessive salivation and lacrimation and urination, miosis, altered respiratory and heart rate:
    - The DUMBBELS mnemonic ascribed to carbamate poisonings in all animals refers to "defecation, urination, miosis, bradycardia, bronchoconstriction, emesis, lacrimation and salivation".
    - Coughing can be seen due to excessive respiratory secretions.
    - Rarely does one see all of these signs in affected animals; one should look for a preponderance of signs consistent with a cholinergic toxidrome. Sometimes tachycardia and mydriasis are reported.
  - Nicotinic cholinergic overstimulation can range from generalized muscle twitching in mild cases to flaccid paralysis in severe poisonings.
  - Central nervous system signs can include depression although seizures have been reported in high-dose exposures.

SIGNALMENT/HISTORY

- No reported breed, age or sex predilections.
- The onset of clinical signs will vary depending on the individual compound, exposure dose, route of exposure, and length of exposure; this means that clinical signs can occur within minutes or be delayed for a few hours.
- Clinical signs appear to start abruptly, and signs associated with overstimulation of the parasympathetic system appear to predominate.

Historical Findings

- Owners might describe recent feed change or agricultural spraying in the area.

Location and Circumstances of Poisoning

- Poisonings can occur through accidental access to the product (inappropriate use or storage) or consumption through contaminated feed material as a result of direct treatment or drift.

CLINICAL FEATURES

- Colic.
- Diarrhea.
- Excessive salivation, lacrimation, urination.
- Cough.
- Serous nasal discharge.
- Dyspnea and tachypnea.
- Bradycardia (or tachycardia).
- Generalized muscle twitching.
- Stiff and rigid gait.
- Anxiety, restlessness, or hyperactivity.
- Miosis (or mydriasis).
- Central nervous system depression.
- Seizures (rare).

DIFFERENTIAL DIAGNOSIS

- Organophosphate poisoning.
- Muscarine-containing mushrooms.
- Nicotine poisoning.
- Poison hemlock (*Conium* sp.).
- Lupine (*Lupinus* sp.).
- Infectious gastroenteritis.

DIAGNOSTICS

- History of exposure.
- Compatible clinical toxidrome (cholinergic overstimulation).

CBC/Serum Chemistry/Urinalysis

- No significant or specific complete blood count, serum chemistry panel and urinalysis changes.

Other Diagnostic Tests

- Inhibition of blood (possibly brain) AChE activity (lack of inhibition does not rule out exposure due to the reversibility of the AChE–carbamate complex binding).
- Finding of chemical residue (stomach contents, liver, urine, blood, suspect feed, environmental samples).
- Muscarinic signs resolve after atropine use.

Pathological Findings

- No consistent or specific gross and histopathologic findings.
- Look for evidence of diarrhea, pulmonary edema.

THERAPEUTICS

- Decontamination to prevent further absorption, reactivate the enzyme, control cholinergic overstimulation that is present, correct respiratory failure and hypoxemia (ultimate cause of death due to bronchoconstriction, build-up of respiratory fluid, muscular weakness and depression of the respiratory drive), control seizures and agitation if necessary.

Detoxification

- Bathe in cases of dermal exposure (warm water with mild detergent).
- Oral activated charcoal if exposure was oral, within 1–4 hours after exposure, and patient is not significantly symptomatic and can protect their airway.
- AC 1–4 g/kg in a water slurry PO.

Appropriate Health Care

- Maintain adequate respiratory support and ventilation.
- Safe environment to avoid self-induced injuries if flaccid paralysis is present.
- Maintain adequate cardiovascular and hydration support.

Drugs of Choice

- Atropine sulfate, 0.2 mg/kg BW (initial dose: ¼ IV, ¾ SC or IM; repeated doses may be required, but use with caution to avoid GI stasis) – use mydriasis and absence of salivation as therapy endpoints.
- Benzodiazepines for seizures or agitation, if necessary.

Precautions/Interactions

- Avoid drugs that are respiratory depressants or exhibit AChE inhibition (e.g., physostigmine, neostigmine).
- Succinylcholine, phenothiazine, and procaine should be avoided.

Alternative Drugs

- Pralidoxime chloride (2-PAM) is of questionable value given the reversibility of the enzyme–carbamate bound complex, lack of efficacy data in horses, and cost of use. 20 mg/kg, as a 20% solution, slow IV over several minutes, repeat every 4–6 hours if necessary.

COMMENTS

Client Education

- Patient should recover in a quiet, safe environment.
- Change feed and water source, clean the environment – prevent further exposure.

Patient Monitoring

- Signs should improve over a 24-hour period.

Prevention/Avoidance

- Store and dispose of pesticides appropriately to prevent accidental exposure.

Possible Complications

- Avoid self-exposure through wearing of personal protective equipment.

Expected Course and Prognosis

- Prognosis is good, and signs resolve in less than 48 hours.
- Patients exhibiting flaccid paralysis or seizure have a guarded prognosis.

See Also

Cholinesterase-Inhibiting Organophosphate Pesticides

Abbreviations

See Appendix 1 for a complete list.

Suggested Reading

Plumb DC. Plumb's Veterinary Drug Handbook, 9th edn. Wiley Blackwell, 2018.
Silberman J, Taylor A. StatPearls Publishing. Available at: https://www.ncbi.nlm.nih.gov/books/NBK482183/ (accessed November 27, 2020).
Talcott, P. Toxicologic problems. In: Reed SM, Bayly WM, Sellon DC, eds. Equine Internal Medicine, 4th edn. St Louis: Elsevier, 2018; pp. 1471–1472.

Author: Patricia A. Talcott, MS, DVM, PhD, DABVT
Consulting Editor: Robert H. Poppenga, DVM, PhD, DABVT

Chapter 28

Cholinesterase-Inhibiting Organophosphate Pesticides

DEFINITION/OVERVIEW

- Acetylcholinesterase (AChE)-inhibiting organophosphate (OP) pesticides can cause muscarinic and nicotinic cholinergic overstimulation in exposed horses.
- OP pesticides are commonly used insecticides.
- Horses can be exposed via accidental access to improperly stored or used products or through contaminated feed material from accidental application or drift.
- Examples of AChE-inhibiting OP pesticides include azamethiphos, azinphos-methyl, chlorpyrifos, diazinon, dichlorvos, fenitrothion, malathion, methyl parathion, parathion, phosmet, terbufos, and tetrachlorvinphos.

ETIOLOGY/PATHOPHYSIOLOGY

Mechanism of Action

- The OP pesticides inactivate the enzyme acetylcholinesterase by phosphorylating the serine hydroxyl group of the esteratic site, thus leading to excessive stimulation of the sympathetic and parasympathetic nervous systems.
- The AChE–OP complex is mostly stable, and OPs are considered irreversible AChE inhibitors.

Toxicokinetics

- Horses can be affected through dermal, inhalation and oral exposure.
- This group of compounds are not known to accumulate extensively in tissues although some heavily chlorinated compounds can redistribute to fat leading to longer half-lives.
- Many OPs require hepatic microsomal activation to become toxic.
- OPs are removed from circulation mostly through serum and liver esterases, and the parent compound along with metabolites are primarily excreted in the urine.

Blackwell's Five-Minute Veterinary Consult Clinical Companion: Equine Toxicology, First Edition. Edited by Lynn R. Hovda, Dionne Benson, and Robert H. Poppenga. © 2022 John Wiley & Sons, Inc. Published 2022 by John Wiley & Sons, Inc. Companion website: www.wiley.com/go/hovda/equine

Toxicity

- As the OP insecticides are a group of structurally similar compounds, their toxicity can range from low to high.
- Toxicity of some compounds (e.g., parathion, malathion, fenthion) can be enhanced through bioactivation.

Systems Affected

- Central and peripheral nervous systems – persistently elevated acetylcholine levels due to AChE inhibition leads to increased neurotransmitter signaling and reflects both muscarinic and nicotinic cholinergic overstimulation:
    - Muscarinic cholinergic overstimulation may include colic (sweating, abdominal discomfort, diarrhea), excessive salivation and lacrimation and urination, miosis, altered respiratory and heart rate:
        - The DUMBBELS mnemonic ascribed to OP poisonings in all animals refers to 'defecation, urination, miosis, bradycardia, bronchoconstriction, emesis, lacrimation and salivation'.
        - Coughing can be seen, due to excessive respiratory secretions.
        - Rarely does one see all these signs in affected animals; one should look for a preponderance of signs consistent with a cholinergic toxidrome. Sometimes tachycardia and mydriasis occur.
    - Nicotinic cholinergic overstimulation can range from generalized muscle twitching in mild cases to flaccid paralysis in severe poisonings.
    - Central nervous system signs can include depression although seizures are reported following high dose exposures.
    - An intermediate syndrome has been reported in humans and other animal species 24 to 96 hours post-exposure. Clinical features include profound weakness, respiratory insufficiency, and neck flexion.

SIGNALMENT/HISTORY

- No reported breed, age or sex predilections.
- The onset of clinical signs will vary depending on the individual compound, exposure dose, route of exposure, and length of exposure; this means that clinical signs can occur within minutes or be delayed for a few hours.
- Clinical signs appear to start abruptly, and signs associated with overstimulation of the parasympathetic system appear to predominate.

Historical Findings

- Owners might describe recent feed change or agricultural spraying in the area.

Location and Circumstances of Poisoning

- Poisonings can occur through accidental access to the product (inappropriate use or storage), malicious events, or consumption through contaminated feed material as a result of treatment or drift.

CLINICAL FEATURES

- Colic.
- Diarrhea.
- Excessive salivation, lacrimation, urination.
- Cough.
- Serous nasal discharge.
- Dyspnea and tachypnea.
- Bradycardia (or tachycardia).
- Generalized muscle twitching.
- Stiff and rigid gait.
- Anxiety, restlessness, or hyperactivity.
- Miosis (or mydriasis).
- Central nervous system depression.
- Seizures (rare).

 ## DIFFERENTIAL DIAGNOSIS

- Carbamate poisoning.
- Muscarine-containing mushrooms.
- Nicotine poisoning.
- Poison hemlock (*Conium* sp.).
- Lupine (*Lupinus* sp.).
- Infectious gastroenteritis.

 ## DIAGNOSTICS

- History of exposure.
- Compatible clinical toxidrome (cholinergic overstimulation).

CBC/Serum Chemistry/Urinalysis

- No significant or specific complete blood count, serum chemistry panel or urinalysis changes.

Other Diagnostic Tests

- Inhibition of blood (possibly brain) cholinesterase activity.
- Finding of chemical residue (stomach contents, liver, urine, blood, suspected, environmental samples).
- Muscarinic signs resolve after atropine use.

Pathological Findings

- No consistent or specific gross and histopathologic findings.
- Look for evidence of diarrhea, pulmonary edema.

THERAPEUTICS

- Decontamination to prevent further absorption, reactivate the enzyme, control cholinergic overstimulation that is present, correct respiratory failure and hypoxemia (ultimate cause of death due to bronchoconstriction, build-up of respiratory fluids, muscular weakness and depression of the respiratory drive), control seizures and agitation.

Detoxification

- Bathe in cases of dermal exposure (warm water with mild detergent).
- Oral activated charcoal if exposure was oral, within 1–4 hours post-exposure, and patient is not significantly symptomatic and can protect their airway:
  - Activated charcoal: 1–4 g/kg in a water slurry PO.

Appropriate Health Care

- Maintain adequate respiratory support and ventilation.
- Safe environment to avoid self-induced injuries if flaccid paralysis is present.
- Maintain adequate cardiovascular and hydration support.

Antidotes

- Pralidoxime chloride (2-PAM) may be of value but may not be economically feasible: 20 mg/kg, as a 20% solution, slow IV over several minutes, repeat every 4–6 hours if necessary.

Drugs of Choice

- Atropine sulfate, 0.2 mg/kg (initial dose ¼ IV, ¾ SC or IM; repeated doses may be required but use with caution to avoid GI stasis) – mydriasis and absence of salivation can be used as therapy endpoints.
- Benzodiazepines for seizures or agitation, if necessary.

Precautions/Interactions

- Avoid drugs that are respiratory depressants or exhibit AChE inhibition (e.g., physostigmine, neostigmine).
- Avoid succinylcholine, phenothiazine, and procaine.

COMMENTS

Client Education

- Patient should recover in a quiet, safe environment.
- Change feed and water sources and clean the environment to prevent further exposure.

Patient Monitoring

- Signs should improve over 24–48 hours.

Prevention/Avoidance
- Store and dispose of pesticides appropriately to prevent accidental exposure.

Possible Complications
- Avoid self-exposure through wearing of personal protective equipment.

Expected Course and Prognosis
- Prognosis is good, and most signs resolve in less than 48–72 hours.
- Patients exhibiting flaccid paralysis or seizures have a guarded prognosis.

See Also
Cholinesterase-Inhibiting Carbamate Insecticides

Abbreviations
See Appendix 1 for a complete list.

Suggested Reading
Plumb DC. Plumb's Veterinary Drug Handbook, 9th edn. Wiley Blackwell, 2018.
Robb EL, Baker MB. StatPearls Publishing. Available at: https://www.ncbi.nlm.nih.gov/books/NBK-532233/ (accessed November 28, 2020).
Talcott, P. Toxicologic problems. In: Reed SM, Bayly WM, Sellon DC, eds. Equine Internal Medicine, 4th edn. St Louis, MO: Elsevier, 2018; pp. 1472–1473.

Author: Patricia A. Talcott, MS, DVM, PhD, DABVT
Consulting Editor: Robert H. Poppenga, DVM, PhD, DABVT

Fertilizers – Nitrates, Urea, Phosphates, and Others

Chapter 29

DEFINITION/OVERVIEW

- Fertilizers are compounds applied to soil that provide nutrients to plants to encourage and enrich growth.
- Nitrate (ammonium, calcium, potassium)-, urea-, and phosphate (diammonium, mono-ammonium)-based fertilizers are the most commonly used.
- Poisonings associated with fertilizers are commonly associated with ruminant species due to increased susceptibility and sensitivity but are relatively rare in horses – a potassium nitrate fertilizer was believed to be associated in the deaths of several horses following ingestion of forage material after recent application of the product.
- Poisoning is most likely to occur following ingestion of large amounts of product directly. Ingestion of recently fertilized forage or water from runoff may also serve as potential sources although this does not carry as large a risk.

ETIOLOGY/PATHOPHYSIOLOGY

Mechanism of Action

- Fertilizer salts can act as direct irritants to GI mucosa.
- Nitrate oxidizes ferrous iron (Fe^{2+}) to ferric iron (Fe^{3+}) to form methemoglobin. Methemoglobin is unable to carry oxygen, resulting in cell death and asphyxiation.
- Urea is converted to ammonia by the enzyme urease. Excessive amounts of ammonia enter the blood stream and cross the BBB, resulting in neurological signs.

Toxicokinetics

- Nitrate and urea can be metabolized in the cecum of horses.
- Ammonia that is produced from the metabolism of urea in the cecum is converted to urea in the liver and excreted through the urine.
- Due to the limited capacity to metabolize urea and nitrate in comparison to ruminants, the toxic metabolites (nitrite and ammonia) of these compounds are produced at relatively low concentrations.

Blackwell's Five-Minute Veterinary Consult Clinical Companion: Equine Toxicology,
First Edition. Edited by Lynn R. Hovda, Dionne Benson, and Robert H. Poppenga.
© 2022 John Wiley & Sons, Inc. Published 2022 by John Wiley & Sons, Inc.
Companion website: www.wiley.com/go/hovda/equine

Toxicity

- There are very few data regarding the toxicity of fertilizers in horses.
- Horses are less sensitive to nitrate poisoning in comparison to ruminant species.
- Horses may tolerate up to approximately 2% nitrate (20,000 ppm) in forage in comparison to ruminants which may safely tolerate up to 0.5% (5,000 ppm) on a dry matter basis.
- Oral administration of 450 g (approximately 3,308 mg/kg) of urea to ponies was observed to be lethal.

Systems Affected

- Cardiovascular – tachycardia.
- Gastrointestinal – direct irritation of the GI mucosa by fertilizer salts may result in abdominal pain and discomfort.
- Hemic/lymphatic/immune – excessive methemoglobin formation may lead to buish to brown-colored mucous membranes.
- Nervous – both nitrate and urea may result in CNS signs.
- Neuromuscular – tremors may be observed.
- Reproductive – abortion may occur in pregnant mares due to decrease oxygen to fetus.
- Respiratory – respiratory distress and labored breathing can be observed with excessive nitrate/nitrite.

SIGNALMENT/HISTORY

Risk Factors

- There are no breed, sex, or age predilections.
- Direct consumption of fertilizer products.
- Consumption of forages following recent or excessive application of fertilizer to forages.
- Accidental spills or application of fertilizer compounds.
- Consumption of water from sources exposed to potential runoff following application and rainfall should also be considered as a potential source of exposure.

Historical Findings

- History of consuming either recently treated forage or concentrated product.

Location and Circumstances of Poisoning

- Poisonings are more likely to occur during early spring when fertilizers are applied to encourage the growth of new vegetation./

CLINICAL FEATURES

- Ataxia and incoordination.
- Respiratory difficulty/acute dyspnea.
- Colic.
- Tremoring.

- Convulsions.
- Head pressing.
- Death.
- Nitrate – brown to chocolate-colored blood and cyanotic membranes may be observed.
- Urea – pupillary light, palpebral, and corneal reflexes were noted to be depressed in a reported urea case.

DIFFERENTIAL DIAGNOSIS

- Poisonous plants – identification of plant material or, in the case of yews, detection of taxine alkaloids in the stomach content.
- Cyanobacteria – exposure to algal blooms, identification of toxin-producing algal species, or detection of cyanotoxins in tissue or GI tract.
- Ionophores – myocardial or skeletal muscle necrosis, detection of ionophores in feed, GI contents or tissues.
- Fumonisins – detection of fumonisins in feedstuffs and evaluation for leukoencephalomalacia (necrosis of the white matter) in brain tissue.
- Hepatic encephalopathy – microscopic evaluation of the liver as well as enzyme values.

DIAGNOSTICS

CBC/Serum Chemistry/Urinalysis
- None in particular.

Other Diagnostic Tests
- Nitrate analysis of serum, ocular fluid, forage, and suspect material.
- Urea analysis of forage or suspect material.
- Ammonia analysis of serum, ocular fluid, or cecal content.
- Samples should be collected in an air-tight container and frozen immediately.

Pathological Findings
- Gross and histological lesions, aside from potential discoloration of blood, are not commonly observed.

THERAPEUTICS

Appropriate Health Care
- Further exposure to the fertilizer product should be eliminated.

Antidotes
- 1% Methylene blue 4–22 mg/kg IV for nitrate.

COMMENTS

Client Education

- Poisonings associated with fertilizers rarely occur in horses due to their limited capability of metabolizing the compounds of concern.
- Intoxication is likely to occur only following direct ingestion of large quantities of fertilizer products.

Patient Monitoring

- Patients should be monitored for GI distress, respiratory difficulty, and progression of neurologic signs.

Prevention/Avoidance

- Avoid turning out horses onto pastures where fertilizers have been recently applied.
- Fully disclose information about compounds used and application rates.
- Proper storage of fertilizer products.

Expected Course and Prognosis

- Recovery and prognosis are considered good following ingestion of low concentrations.
- Direct ingestion of large amounts carries a poor prognosis due to the acute onset of clinical signs.

Abbreviations

See Appendix 1 for a complete list.

Suggested Reading

Hintz HF, Lowe JE, Clifford AJ, et al. Ammonia intoxication resulting from urea ingestion in ponies. J Am Vet Med Assoc 1970; 157:963–966.

Oruc HH, Akkoc A, Uzunoglu I, et al. Nitrate poisoning horses associated with ingestion of forage and alfalfa. J Equine Vet Sci 2010;30:159–162.

Thompson LJ. Overview of nitrate and nitrite poisoning. In: Aiello SE, Moses MA, eds. Merck Veterinary Manual, 11th edn. Kenilworth, NJ: Merck Sharp & Dohme Corp., 2016.

Author: Scott L. Radke, DVM, MS
Consulting Editor: Robert H. Poppenga, DVM, PhD, DABVT

Chapter 30

Herbicides

DEFINITION/OVERVIEW

- Herbicide poisoning is not a common occurrence in horses. Exposure to herbicide residues is of little concern as poisonings are likely to occur only following ingestion of large amounts of these products.
- Older and less selective herbicide compounds, including but not limited to sodium arsenite, sodium chlorate, and arsenic trioxide, are not as commonly used as they were in the past.
- The majority of current herbicide products are selective for plants and are of low toxic concern for mammalian species, with GI irritation being the most frequent complication.
- Of the newer organic products, dipyridyls (diquat, paraquat) pose the greatest threat.
- Although not as commonly used, arsenical (MSMA) herbicides still pose potential threats to horses.
- Organophosphate compounds such as products containing the active ingredient glyphosate are far less toxic than their insecticide counterparts as they do not inhibit acetylcholinesterase.
  - There is no good evidence that glyphosate, at normal use levels, causes adverse effects.
- Intoxication following ingestion of noxious vegetation is more likely to occur following application of herbicides as these products can increase palatability of plants.
- See Appendix 2: Herbicides.

ETIOLOGY/PATHOPHYSIOLOGY

Mechanism of Action

- The mechanism of action varies depending on the compound.
- Paraquat – free radicals that damage tissue are formed through cyclic redox reactions (reduction and oxygenation) of the compound.
- Arsenicals – depending on the valence, arsenic decreases ATP through either blocking cellular respiration (3^+) or uncoupling oxidative phosphorylation (5^+). Arsenical products have corrosive effects on the GI mucosa.
- Dinitrophenols – increase oxygen consumption, leading to decreasing glycogen stores.

Blackwell's Five-Minute Veterinary Consult Clinical Companion: Equine Toxicology,
First Edition. Edited by Lynn R. Hovda, Dionne Benson, and Robert H. Poppenga.
© 2022 John Wiley & Sons, Inc. Published 2022 by John Wiley & Sons, Inc.
Companion website: www.wiley.com/go/hovda/equine

Toxicokinetics

- Paraquat is poorly absorbed and remains in the GI tract for an extended period. Paraquat concentrates in the lungs and is excreted in the urine.
- Arsenic is readily absorbed from the GI tract. Portions of the pentavalent form (5+) are metabolized in the kidney to the more toxic trivalent (3+) form. Arsenic is rapidly excreted through feces.

Toxicity

- Little information is available in relation to horses regarding toxic and lethal doses of herbicide compounds.

Systems Affected

- Gastrointestinal – GI irritation is common for the majority of herbicides following consumption. Arsenicals result in sloughing of the GI tract.
- Hemic/lymphatic/immune – the herbicide propanil may cause hemolysis.
- Nervous – parasympathetic signs of increased salivation, lacrimation, urination, and defecation may be observed with carbamate and thiocarbamate herbicides.
- Ophthalmic – irritation, corneal edema, and blindness may occur following direct contact.
- Renal/urologic – renal insufficiency and tubular necrosis may be observed with arsenical and dipyridyl products.
- Respiratory – dyspnea and labored breathing are commonly associated with paraquat intoxication due to extensive damage to the lungs.
- Skin/exocrine – irritation following direct contact.

SIGNALMENT/HISTORY

Risk Factors

- There are no breed, sex, or age predilections.
- Recently applied or excessive application of herbicides to forages.
- Consumption of forages prior to the end of the recommended graze-out period.
- Access to accidental spills.
- Consumption of water from sources exposed to potential runoff following application and rainfall should also be considered as a potential source of exposure.

Historical Findings

- History of consuming either recently treated forage or a concentrated product or the animal being sprayed.

Location and Circumstances of Poisoning

- Intoxications are more likely to occur during the spring and summer when herbicides are applied to growing vegetation.
- Exposure may occur during the fall if defoliation products are used.

CLINICAL FEATURES

- The majority of herbicides, aside from the mentioned exceptions, are unlikely to cause significant clinical complications, and horses are most likely to present with only GI signs. Clinical presentation may include feed refusal, colic, and diarrhea.
- Arsenicals – colic and abdominal discomfort, GI hemorrhage and diarrhea, CNS depression, and hypovolemia.
- Paraquat – difficulty breathing and oral ulcerations. Polyuria/polydipsia may also be observed.

DIFFERENTIAL DIAGNOSIS

- Ionophores – detection of ionophores in feed and observation of cardiac and skeletal muscle necrosis.
- Noxious plants – history of consumption, identification of plant material in the GI tract, detection of plant toxins.

DIAGNOSTICS

CBC/Serum Chemistry/Urinalysis

- Renal indices and hepatic enzymes as needed.

Other Diagnostic Tests

- Collection of urine for further testing should be considered due to its ease of collection and the ability to test for a number of herbicides.

Pathological Findings

- Arsenicals – hemorrhagic gastroenteritis, renal tubular necrosis. Liver and kidney should be submitted for analysis. Hair may be used to evaluate for chronic exposures.
- Paraquat – pulmonary edema, necrosis and fibrosis, renal tubular necrosis. Paraquat may be detected in the urine within the first 30 hours following exposure.

THERAPEUTICS

Detoxification

- Eliminate further exposure.
- Paraquat – bentonite or Fuller's earth at 5 g/kg BW PO. These possess greater adsorption capabilities than AC.
- If bentonite or Fuller's earth is unavailable, AC can be used at 1–4 g/kg PO in a water slurry (1 g of AC in 5 mL of water).

Appropriate Health Care

- Continual monitoring for GI distress following dilution with water.
- Administration of IV or PO fluids and forced diuresis.
- Symptomatic and supportive care if renal or hepatic impairment occurs.

Antidote

- Arsenic – chelation using dimercaprol at 2.5–5 mg/kg IM every TID for 2 days followed by BID for 10 days.

Drugs of Choice

- Sucralfate 12–20 mg/kg PO TID.

Precautions/Interactions

- Arsenic within the GI tract must be removed prior to chelation treatment. Administration of a chelator prior to removal will increase arsenic absorption.
- Oxygen is contraindicated following paraquat exposures because administration of oxygen perpetuates redox reactions, leading to more tissue damage.

COMMENTS

Client Education

- Herbicides are suspected as causes of health complications due to past use of highly toxic products that are no longer available.
- Most herbicides are selective for plants and possess low toxicity for mammalian species including horses. The likelihood that an herbicide will severely affect horses is relatively low.
- Sprayed pastures to be grazed should be evaluated for toxic plants due to potentially increased palatability. Toxic plants should be removed if feasible.
- Fully disclose information about compounds used and application rates.
- It is difficult to diagnose chronic herbicide poisoning as the effects may be subtle and develop over months to years.

Patient Monitoring

- Patients should be monitored closely for GI distress.
- Monitor electrolytes and renal function.

Prevention/Avoidance

- Follow labeled application rates and graze-out guidelines.
- Properly store herbicide compounds and limit access.

Expected Course and Prognosis

- A good prognosis and recovery are associated with exposure to the majority of herbicides.
- Arsenicals – guarded to poor prognosis depending on the amount ingested and clinical signs.
- Paraquat – poor prognosis following onset of clinical signs.

See Also

Arsenic
Cholinesterase-Inhibiting Carbamate Pesticides
Cholinesterase-Inhibiting Organophosphate Pesticides
Paraquat and Diquat

Abbreviations

See Appendix 1 for a complete list.

Suggested Reading

Gupta PK. Overview of herbicide poisoning. In: Aiello SE, Moses MA, eds. Merck Veterinary Manual, 11th edn. Kenilworth, NJ: Merck Sharp & Dohme Corp., 2016.
Gupta PK. Toxicity of herbicides. In: Gupta RC ed. Veterinary Toxicology: Basic and Clinical Principles, 3rd edn. Boston, MA: Academic Press, 2018.
Gwaltney-Brant S. Herbicide toxicosis. In: Wilson DA, Gaskill CL ed. Clinical Veterinary Advisor: The Horse. St Louis, MO: Elsevier Inc., 2012.
Osweiler GD, Carson TL, Buck WB, Van Gelder GA. Clinical and Diagnostic Veterinary Toxicology, 3rd edn. Dubuque, IA: Kendall/Hunt Publishing Company, 1985.
Plumlee KH. Clinical Veterinary Toxicology. St Louis, MO: Mosby Inc., 2004.

Author: Scott L. Radke, DVM, MS
Consulting Editor: Robert H. Poppenga, DVM, PhD, DABVT

Chapter 31

Paraquat and Diquat

DEFINITION/OVERVIEW

- Reported equine paraquat and diquat poisoning cases in the literature are rare; the information provided here is what might be expected to be seen based on exposures in other animals and humans.
- Paraquat and diquat are both non-selective dipyridyl contact herbicides and preharvest (desiccant) defoliants.
- Both herbicides have widespread uses throughout the United States.
- A coloring agent, odor agent, and emetic are present in US liquid paraquat formulations to limit ingestion and absorption.
- Horses can be exposed via accidental access to improperly stored or used products, recently treated feed material, or malicious events.
- The more toxic paraquat primarily affects the gastrointestinal, respiratory, and renal systems, while the less toxic diquat's major effects are on the renal and central nervous systems (pulmonary injury is less prominent).
- Oral exposures are likely to lead to acute poisoning.

ETIOLOGY/PATHOPHYSIOLOGY

Mechanism of Action

- The toxic effects of paraquat and diquat are similar – they both cause multiple organ system damage through the generation of oxygen free radicals, leading to cell death and tissue destruction via lipid peroxidation.

Toxicokinetics

- Both herbicides are rapidly, but incompletely, absorbed from the gastrointestinal tract; approximately 70% of the parent compounds are excreted unchanged in the feces.
- Inhalation exposures are uncommon and dermal absorption is poor through intact skin.
- Peak concentrations occur within 2 hours of ingestion.
- Both herbicides have a wide range of tissue distribution, and paraquat is selectively taken up and concentrated by pulmonary alveolar cells (hence it is considered a selective pneumotoxin).

Blackwell's Five-Minute Veterinary Consult Clinical Companion: Equine Toxicology, First Edition. Edited by Lynn R. Hovda, Dionne Benson, and Robert H. Poppenga.
© 2022 John Wiley & Sons, Inc. Published 2022 by John Wiley & Sons, Inc.
Companion website: www.wiley.com/go/hovda/equine

- Most absorbed paraquat and diquat is eliminated unchanged in the urine within the first 24 hours. However, as renal failure develops, renal clearance is reduced, increasing plasma half-lives and prolonging the clinical syndrome.

Toxicity

- Both herbicides are extremely toxic; the oral median lethal dose (LD_{50}) for paraquat for various animal species ranges between 22 and 290 mg/kg BW.

Systems Affected

- Gastrointestinal tract – following oral exposures, severe edema, swelling, necrosis and ulceration of the mucosa occur.
- Pulmonary – paraquat accumulates in type I and type II pneumocytes, causing severe necrosis, edema, and hemorrhage acutely; progressive pulmonary fibrosis will lead to impairment of gas exchange, hypoxemia and death. Diquat causes mild reversible damage to the type I pneumocytes but no progressive pulmonary fibrosis occurs.
- Renal – damage to the proximal renal tubules occurs with both paraquat and diquat (diquat typically causes greater kidney damage). As this is the major route of excretion, impairment of renal function will exacerbate the clinical syndrome.
- Focal necrosis of the striated muscle (myocardium and skeletal muscle) is reported following paraquat intoxication.
- Cerebral edema and brain lesions have been reported in both paraquat and diquat intoxications.
- Irritation (contact dermatitis) can be observed following dermal exposure to either herbicide.

 # SIGNALMENT/HISTORY

- There are no reported breed, age or sex predilections.
- The onset of clinical signs following oral exposure is acute, within minutes.

Risk Factors

- No known risk factors.

Historical Findings

- Owners might describe recent feed change or agricultural spraying in the area.

Location and Circumstances of Poisoning

- Intoxications can occur through accidental access to the product (inappropriate use or storage) or consumption of contaminated feed material via direct application or environmental drift; often a cause of malicious poisoning in animals.

 # CLINICAL FEATURES

- Severe colic and abdominal pain.
- Diarrhea (± hemorrhage).

- Pain, swelling, and oral ulcerations may be visible.
- Aphagia.
- Cough, dyspnea, and tachypnea, which progressively worsens.
- Hyperexcitability, depression, irritability, disorientation.
- Cardiogenic shock in high-dose exposures.
- Localized discoloration or transverse band of white discoloration of the nail plate in dermal exposures.

DIFFERENTIAL DIAGNOSIS

- Infectious or antibiotic-related gastrointestinal disease.
- General pulmonary and cardiac disease.

DIAGNOSTICS

- History of exposure.
- Compatible clinical toxidrome – oral lesions, gastroenteritis, pulmonary abnormalities, renal necrosis.

CBC/Serum Chemistry/Urinalysis

- Evidence of hemoconcentration; renal disease leads to proteinuria, hematuria, azotemia, oliguria/anuria.
- Hepatic disease indicated by hyperbilirubinemia, elevations in AST, ALT, LDH, and alkaline phosphatase.

Other Diagnostic Tests

- Thoracic radiography – pneumomediastinum, fibrosis, edema, interstitial pattern.
- Plasma and urine (postmortem – urine, kidney, lung) paraquat and diquat concentrations.
- Colorimetric test of urine utilizing 1% sodium dithionite – not readily available and questionable sensitivity (blue or green color indicates presence of paraquat or diquat > 0.5 ppm).

Pathological Findings

- Gross – oral and GI ulceration and necrosis, diarrhea, pulmonary edema and hemorrhage and necrosis, contact dermatitis, cerebral edema.
- Histopathologic – pulmonary edema, hemorrhage, necrosis and fibrosis; corrosive dermatitis; edema, necrosis and ulceration of the mucosal lining of the GI tract; centrilobular hepatocellular degeneration and necrosis; proximal renal tubule necrosis, focal necrosis of the myocardium and skeletal muscle and adrenal glands; cerebral edema; brain stem infarction.

THERAPEUTICS

Decontamination to prevent further absorption, along with basic symptomatic and supportive care.

Detoxification

- Bathe in cases of dermal exposure (warm water with mild detergent); flush eyes if conjunctivitis is present.
- Oral activated charcoal if exposure was oral, within 1–4 hours after exposure, and patient is not significantly symptomatic and can protect their airway (bentonite and Fuller's earth are highly effective but often not available).
- Activated charcoal: 1-4- g/kg in a water slurry PO.

Appropriate Health Care

- Maintain adequate respiratory support and ventilation – oxygen therapy should be used cautiously, especially in the early stages, because of the potential to worsen the respiratory changes.
- IV fluid therapy – maintain adequate cardiovascular and hydration support along with maintaining adequate renal output.
- Monitor organ system function.
- Hemoperfusion (and less effective hemodialysis) is unlikely to be available for equine patients.

Antidotes

- No proven antidotes have been identified although many have been tried – early and aggressive decontamination procedures and symptomatic and supportive care are essential.

Drugs of Choice

- Analgesia for pain control.
- Cyclophosphamide and methylprednisolone have been shown to be effective in humans in reducing mortality rates.

Precautions/Interactions

- Early oxygen therapy is often considered contraindicated due to the possibility of causing more pulmonary damage, particularly with paraquat exposures.

COMMENTS

Client Education

- Prepare the client for a poor prognosis.

Prevention/Avoidance

- Store and dispose of pesticides appropriately to prevent accidental exposure.

Possible Complications

- Avoid self-exposure through wearing of personal protective equipment.
- Clean up environmental spills and discard contaminated feed.

Expected Course and Prognosis

Prognosis is extremely poor to grave.

Abbreviations

See Appendix 1 for a complete list.

Suggested Reading

Chapter 12: Paraquat and Diquat, pp. 110–117, 2018. www.epa.gov (accessed November 29, 2020).

Geller RJ. Chapter 122. Paraquat and diquat. In: Olson KR, ed. Poisoning and Drug Overdose. McGraw Hill Education, 6th edn, 2012.

Oehme FW, Mannala S. Chapter 68. Paraquat. Veterian Key. https://veteriankey.com/paraquat (Accessed November 28, 2020).

Author: Patricia A. Talcott, MS, DVM, PhD, DABVT
Consulting Editor: Robert H. Poppenga, DVM, PhD, DABVT

Pentachlorophenol (PCP)

Chapter 32

DEFINITION/OVERVIEW

- PCP is highly lipid-soluble and volatile with a pungent phenol type odor.
- Primarily used as a wood preservative, fungicide, and herbicide. Exposure occurs through inhalation of vapors, GI absorption, or dermal absorption.
- Acute and chronic intoxication syndromes have been described in animals. The chronic syndrome may be due to PCDD and PCDF isomers found in PCP.
- Current restrictions on the use of PCP owing to environmental and toxicity concerns make exposure and toxicosis unlikely.
- PCP is still used in industrial settings by certified applicators as a wood preservative/pesticide for railroad ties, underwater dock/wharf pilings, utility poles and fence posts.

ETIOLOGY/PATHOPHYSIOLOGY

Mechanism of Action

- PCP causes uncoupling of oxidative phosphorylation and direct irritation to the skin and the respiratory tract.
- In humans, some chronic effects believed to be due to impurities (PCDD and PCDF) in PCP formulations.

Toxicokinetics

- Well absorbed by oral, dermal and inhalation routes and distributed to the liver, lungs, kidneys, blood, fat tissues, and brain.
- Rapid hepatic metabolism and renal elimination.

Toxicity

- Acute and chronic effects are possible.
- Not well defined for horses but acute oral LD_{50} dosages in laboratory animals are in the 30–300 mg/kg range.

Systems Affected

- Gastrointestinal.
- Integument (dermal).

Blackwell's Five-Minute Veterinary Consult Clinical Companion: Equine Toxicology,
First Edition. Edited by Lynn R. Hovda, Dionne Benson, and Robert H. Poppenga.
© 2022 John Wiley & Sons, Inc. Published 2022 by John Wiley & Sons, Inc.
Companion website: www.wiley.com/go/hovda/equine

- Respiratory.
- Nervous.

SIGNALMENT/HISTORY

- There is no sex, age, or breed predilection.

Risk Factors

- Most likely sources of exposure are treated wood used for fences or stalls, bedding from treated wood, or old railroad ties used around buildings.
- Contaminated soil.
- High ambient temperatures might increase volatilization.
- Poor body condition.

CLINICAL FEATURES

- Acute – hyperthermia, restlessness, tachypnea, increased GI motility, weakness, seizures, and collapse.
- Chronic – anorexia, weight loss, dependent edema, alopecia, skin cracks and fissures, colic, joint stiffness, recurrent hoof problems, conjunctivitis, hematuria, and secondary opportunistic infections.

DIFFERENTIAL DIAGNOSIS

- Acute – infectious causes of pyrexia (CBC, bacterial culture, serology).
- Chronic – *Vicia villosa* toxicosis (skin biopsy).

DIAGNOSTICS

CBC/Serum Chemistry/Urinalysis

- Acute – no specific abnormalities.
- Chronic – changes consistent with hepatic dysfunction, anemia, and thrombocytopenia.

Other Diagnostic Tests

- Acute – antemortem detection of PCP in blood, serum/plasma, or urine; PCP is rapidly cleared so measurement is useful only in acute intoxications; postmortem detection of PCP in skin, liver, or kidney.
- Chronic – measurement of PCDD or PCDF isomers in plasma/serum or tissues.

Pathological Findings

- Acute – not reported for horses.

- Chronic:
  - Gross – emaciation; alopecia; crusty, scaly dermatitis; cracks or fissures of the skin that exude clear serum-like fluid; splenomegaly.
  - Histopathologic – chronic nonsuppurative dermatitis; hepatic bile duct proliferation, inflammation, and focal necrosis; splenic hemosiderosis; multifocal renal tubular necrosis; nonregenerative bone marrow.

THERAPEUTICS

Detoxification

- Acute – activated charcoal at 1–4g/kg in water slurry (1 g AC in 5 mL water) PO and either magnesium sulfate at 250 mg/kg PO or sorbitol (70%) at 3 mL/kg PO, given once with AC.
- Chronic – none.

Appropriate Health Care

- Acute:
  - Remove from source.
  - If recent oral exposure, consider GI decontamination.
  - Wash exposed skin.
  - Control hyperthermia.
  - Symptomatic and supportive care.
- Chronic:
  - Remove from source of exposure.
  - Provide symptomatic and supportive care.

Antidotes

- There is no antidote.

Drugs of Choice

- NSAIDS for inflammation, hyperthermia, and pain control:
  - Flunixin 1.1 mg/kg IV or PO q12–24h.
  - Phenylbutazone 2.2–4.4 mg/kg IV or PO q12–24h.
  - Ketoprofen 2.2 mg/kg IV q24h.

COMMENTS

Client Education

- This is a restricted-use product no longer allowed in residential and most commercial settings, so toxicosis would be rare.
- Use care, however, if you purchase old dock/wharf pilings, railroad ties, or utility poles as they are all potential sources of intoxication.

Prevention/Avoidance

- Avoid use of treated wood where animal contact is possible.
- Don't use old railroad ties around out buildings or store them where horses have access.

Possible Complications

- Chronic intoxication of pregnant horses with PCDD and PCDF can result in birth of weak foals susceptible to opportunistic infections.

Expected Course and Prognosis

- Poor prognosis and prolonged recovery in chronic intoxication due to dioxin.

Abbreviations

See Appendix 1 for a complete list.

Internet Resources

Agency for Toxic Substances and Disease Registry. Division of Toxicology. Tox FAQs: Pentachlorophenol. Available at: https://www.atsdr.cdc.gov/toxfaqs/tfacts51.pdf

Agency for Toxic Substances and Disease Registry, Division of Toxicology. Toxicological Profile for Pentachlorophenol. Available at: https://www.atsdr.cdc.gov/toxprofiles/tp51.pdf

Suggested Reading

Kerkvliet NI, Wagner SL, Schmotzer WB, et al. Dioxin intoxication from chronic exposure of horses to penta-chlorophenol-contaminated wood shavings. J Am Vet Med Assoc 1992; 201:296–302.

Authors: Arya Sobhakumari, DVM, PhD, ERT, DABT, DABVT; Robert H. Poppenga, DVM, PhD, DABVT
Consulting Editor: Lynn R. Hovda, RPh, DVM, MS, DACVIM

Pyrethrins and Pyrethroid Insecticides

Chapter 33

DEFINITION/OVERVIEW

- *Pyrethrins* are natural insecticides extracted from the flowers of some species of Chrysanthemum.
- *Pyrethroids* are manufactured insecticides with similar chemical structures to pyrethrins but are often more toxic to insects and mammals.
- Pyrethrins and pyrethroids are the most common products to control ectoparasites on horses.
- Effective against horn flies, face flies, stable flies, house flies, horse flies, black flies, eye gnats, mange mites, scabies mites, ticks, lice and fleas.
- Available as sprays, wipes, granules and spot-ons (roll-ons and dust), as well as residual products specially formulated to spray premises.
- Dermal exposure is most common but accidental ingestion or inhalation may occur.
- Pyrethrins and pyrethroids act primarily on the nervous system and can cause allergic skin reactions.

ETIOLOGY/PATHOPHYSIOLOGY

- Natural pyrethrins include six compounds: pyrethrins I and II, cinerins I and II, and jasmolins I and II. These are rapidly degraded (photosensitive) and effects last for only a few hours.
- Pyrethroids are synthetic compounds chemically derived from pyrethrins to increase stability and prolong insecticidal effects and are classified as type I or type II.
- Type I and type II pyrethroids have different molecular structures (type II contain an alpha-cyano group) and biological effects (type II are generally considered more toxic that type I):
  - Type I: allethrin, permethrin, phenothrin, resmethrin, bifenthrin, tefluthrin, and tetramethrin.
  - Type II: cyfluthrin, cyhalothrin, cypermethrin, cyphenothrin, deltamethrin, esfenvalerate, fenvalerate, flumethrin, lambda-cyhalothrin, and tralomethrin.
- Some products contain multiple active ingredients, such as combinations of pyrethrins and synthetic pyrethroids, different insecticides (e.g., organophosphate) and/or synergists to increase insecticidal activity (piperonyl butoxide).

Blackwell's Five-Minute Veterinary Consult Clinical Companion: Equine Toxicology, First Edition. Edited by Lynn R. Hovda, Dionne Benson, and Robert H. Poppenga.
© 2022 John Wiley & Sons, Inc. Published 2022 by John Wiley & Sons, Inc.
Companion website: www.wiley.com/go/hovda/equine

- Trade names of common pyrethroid-containing insecticides registered for horse are:
  - Cypermethrin – Bite Free Biting Fly Repellent, Endure Sweat-Resistant Fly Spray for Horses, Repel-X Lotion, Tri-tec 14 Spray, Endure Roll-On for Horses, Python Dust, Prozap Insectrin Dust for Livestock & Poultry.
  - Permethrin – Bronco, Equine Fly Spray Plus, Prozap Final Fly-T Horse, Flysect Super-C Repellent Concentrate, Ambush Insecticide & Repellent, Mosquito Halt Repellent Spray for Horses, Durvet Fly Rid Plus, Horse Lice Duster II, Bug Block Easy Wipe, Ultra Shield Towelettes.
  - Pyrethrins + piperonyl butoxide (synergist) – Equisect Fly Repellent, Flysect Citronella Spray.

Mechanism of Action

- Pyrethrins and pyrethroids act by disrupting the voltage-gated sodium channels, causing repeated nerve firing and cellular hyperexcitability. In mammals, sodium channels are present in muscle fibers, salivary glands and the CNS.
- At high concentrations, pyrethroids act on gamma-aminobutyric acid (GABA)-gated chloride channels, causing decreased synaptic inhibition and a strychnine-like effect.
- Direct action on terminal sensory nerves may cause paresthesia (burning, itching sensation). This is more likely to occur with type II pyrethroids.
- Mechanism of toxicity may be more complex when formulations contain more than one insecticide, such as organophosphates, causing anticholinesterase effects.

Toxicokinetics

- Dermal absorption is poor. Intradermal metabolism occurs further limiting absorption.
- Rapidly absorbed via ingestion (> 50%) or inhalation.
- Widely distributed throughout tissues (including CNS) due to high lipophilicity
- Rapidly metabolized in the liver, kidney, intestine and other tissues via hydrolysis reactions and conjugation to inactive metabolites.
- Excretion is via urine and feces.

Toxicity

- Pyrethrins and pyrethroids are relatively safe when used according to label instructions.
- Acute toxicity varies significantly but it is in general considered to be low to moderate
  - Pyrethrins:
    - Oral LD50 (rats): 260 to more than 600 mg/kg.
    - Dermal LD50 (rats): 1350 mg/kg.
  - Pyrethroids:
    - Permethrin oral LD50 (rats): 540–2,690 mg/kg
    - Tefluthrin oral LD50 (rats): 22 mg/kg.
- Information on acute toxicity in horses is lacking, but effects are probably similar to other mammals (cats are more sensitive).

Systems Affected

- Endocrine/metabolic – lactic acidosis due to dehydration and decreased tissue perfusion (seizures); hyperthermia.
- Gastrointestinal – salivation.
- Hemic/lymphatic/immune – hemoconcentration due to dehydration.

- Musculoskeletal – myopathy due to tremors and seizure activity.
- Nervous – paresthesia, seizures.
- Neuromuscular – tremors, repetitive movements.
- Ophthalmic – irritant to the eyes.
- Renal/urologic – potential for myoglobinuric nephrosis if significant muscle damage and dehydration.
- Respiratory – nasal and respiratory irritation after inhalation of dust or spray particles.
- Skin/exocrine – hypersensitivity reactions

SIGNALMENT/HISTORY

Risk Factors

- As with other species, young or advanced age and overall health condition may predispose horses to toxicosis.
- Skin sensitivity reactions and physical activity increasing blood flow and environmental temperature may increase dermal absorption.

Location and Circumstances of Poisoning

- Excessive exposure may result from repeated applications or inappropriate use of products.
- Accidental oral ingestion, inhalation, and/or ocular contact may occur.

CLINICAL FEATURES

- Clinical signs are noted within minutes to hours and commonly last for 2–3 days depending on dose and type of exposure (dermal, oral or inhalation).
- Changes are mostly related to the CNS, including hyperexcitability, hyperesthesia, salivation, tremors, seizures and death.
- Hyperthermia and shock (tremors and seizures).
- Type I and II pyrethroids differ in molecular structure and biological effects, with type II generally more toxic than type I:
  - Type I: tremors.
  - Type II: repetitive but coordinated (choreiform) movements of the forelimbs, seizures and salivation.
- Pyrethroids cause a dose-dependent reduction in motor function.
- May cause eye, nose and/or lung irritation.
- Application to the skin may cause sensitivity, itchiness, redness, rash and hair discoloration/loss at site of application. Anaphylactic allergic reactions are possible.

DIFFERENTIAL DIAGNOSIS

- Organophosphate, carbamate and organochlorine insecticides.
- Strychnine.
- Cyanide.

- Metaldehyde.
- Locoweed.
- Bromide.

DIAGNOSTICS

- History of exposure and compatible clinical signs.

CBC/Serum Chemistry/Urinalysis

- CBC – dehydration, underlying conditions.
- Biochemistry – acidosis, increased serum muscle enzymes, elevated renal parameters.
- Urinalysis – specific gravity, proteinuria.

Other Diagnostic Tests

- Identification of pyrethrins and pyrethroids by GC-MS in GI contents, hair, tissue (skin, liver, fat, brain, milk) and/or suspect material to confirm exposure.
- Postmortem determination of acetylcholinesterase activity in brain may be helpful to rule out organophosphate and carbamate toxicoses, as pyrethrins and pyrethroids show similar clinical presentation but lack anticholinesterase activity.

Pathological Findings

- Effects are primarily on the nervous system.
- Toxicosis does not cause specific anatomical lesions; however, secondary injury to tissues from hypoxia (shock), muscle damage due to seizure activity and myoglobinuric tubular nephrosis may occur.

THERAPEUTICS

Detoxification

- For dermal exposure, wash the skin thoroughly with abundant running water and a mild detergent to prevent further absorption. Using a detergent is important because pyrethrins and pyrethroids do not dissolve well in water (lipophilic). Avoid warm water, as it may increase circulation and absorption. Control tremors and seizures prior to skin decontamination, as bathing may cause overstimulation aggravating clinical signs.
- If there is accidental ocular exposure, wash the affected eye(s) with abundant water or normal saline and/or apply an ointment.
- If large amounts ingested within 12 hours, decontaminate with gastric lavage and activated charcoal (1–4 g/kg).

Appropriate Health Care

- Control tremors and seizures with muscle relaxants and anticonvulsants. Seizures may cause irreversible brain damage and care should be taken to avoid additional injuries to the horses and/or caretakers.

- IV fluids to maintain proper hydration.
- Paresthesia commonly resolves spontaneously within 24 hours and usually does not require symptomatic treatment.
- If skin sensitivity develops:
  - Discontinue application of the product and decontaminate, as above. For future treatments, try a different product or assess skin reactions in a small area.
  - Topical vitamin E may help – open a soft capsule and apply onto the affected skin area.
  - Antihistamines if necessary.

Antidote

- There is no specific antidote.

Drugs of Choice

- To control seizures:
  - Diazepam (GABA agonist): 0.05–0.2 mg/kg in 25–100 mg doses IV or IM, as needed.
  - Phenobarbital: 12–20 mg/kg initial dose (diluted in saline over 30 min), then 1–9 mg/kg IV, every 12 hours after initial dose.
  - Dexamethasone (to prevent cerebrocortical edema): 0.1–0.25mg/kg IV, q6–24h
- Tremors: muscle relaxants – methocarbamol 4–22 mg/kg slow IV for moderate conditions.
- Skin sensitivity reactions: cetirizine or diphenhydramine.

Precautions/Interactions

- Phenothiazine tranquilizers are contraindicated, as pyrethroids cause extrapyramidal stimulation.
- Some formulations contain a synergist (piperonyl butoxide) and/or additional insecticides (e.g., organophosphates) increasing toxicity (organophosphates inhibit pyrethroid metabolism and have anticholinesterase activity).
- Ivermectin and pentobarbital have been observed to antagonize pyrethroid-induced salivation, choreoathetosis (repetitive coordinated movements) and myotonia.

COMMENTS

Client Education

- Always follow label instructions for safe application, avoid human exposure and protect the environment (pyrethroids are toxic to fish and invertebrates).

Prevention/Avoidance

- Avoid application of concentrated/residual products formulated for premises on horses.
- Protect water and feed when applying insecticides to walls, ceilings and rafters in barns and sheds.

Possible Complications

- Seizures and death in severe cases.

Expected Course and Prognosis

- Prognosis depends on type of compound, dose and route of exposure.
- Prognosis is good, with mild intoxications treated soon after exposure.
- For severe cases presenting with uncontrolled seizures, prognosis worsens.

Abbreviations

See Appendix 1 for a complete list.

Suggested Reading

Anadon A, Martinez-Larranaga MR, Martinez MA. Use and abuse of pyrethrins and synthetic pyrethroids in veterinary medicine. Vet J 2009; 182(1):7–20.

Author: Felipe Reggeti, DVM, PhD, DACVP
Consulting Editor: Robert H. Poppenga, DVM, PhD, DABVT

Ionophores and Growth Promotants

Chapter 34

Ionophores

DEFINITION/OVERVIEW

- Ionophores are carboxylic antibiotics that are commonly added to livestock feeds to control coccidiosis, improve growth rate in beef cattle, and prevent ketosis in dairy cattle.
- Ionophores commonly used in livestock feeds include monensin, lasalocid, and salinomycin.
- Although relatively safe for use at FDA-approved levels in intended species, toxicity can occur when non-intended species gain access to ionophore supplemented feeds. Horses are the species most sensitive to the toxic effects of ionophores.
- Poisoning is usually caused by accidental feeding of ionophore-containing cattle, swine, and poultry feed, or contamination of horse feed at the feed mill or during feed delivery.
- On a mg/kg ingested basis, salinomycin and monensin are the most toxic of the ionophores while lasalocid is five- to 10-fold less toxic.
- Monensin poisoning is the most common ionophore toxicity reported in horses.

ETIOLOGY/PATHOPHYSIOLOGY

Mechanism of Action

- Ionophores' mode of action is from enhanced membrane permeability and by forming complexes with cations. The lipid-soluble complexes are transported across membranes into excitable cells where their adverse effects occur. Excitable cells, skeletal, muscle, and nerve cells are predominantly affected.
- Sufficient ingestions and intestinal absorption of an ionophore can disrupt transmembrane ion gradients for Na^+, K^+, Mg^{2+} and Ca^{2+}, causing cellular Ph changes and, importantly, increased intracellular Ca^{2+}. Mitochondrial damage, decreased ATP, and necrosis/apoptosis can be the cellular end result.

Toxicokinetics

- Intestinal bioavailability studies of the different ionophores have not been performed in horses.

Blackwell's Five-Minute Veterinary Consult Clinical Companion: Equine Toxicology,
First Edition. Edited by Lynn R. Hovda, Dionne Benson, and Robert H. Poppenga.
© 2022 John Wiley & Sons, Inc. Published 2022 by John Wiley & Sons, Inc.
Companion website: www.wiley.com/go/hovda/equine

- Intestinal absorption of these highly lipophilic ionophores may be affected by the amount of and type of food in the stomach.
  - Oils in the feed may enhance absorption.
- Ionophores are metabolized by the liver, excreted in bile and then eliminated in the feces.

Toxicity

- The LD_{50} of monensin is reported to be 2–3 mg/kg (non-fasted horses).
  - All fasted horses administered 1.2–1.5 mg/kg monensin mixed in complete diet.
- The LD_{50} of lasalocid is estimated to be 21.5 mg/kg. The LD_{50} of salinomycin in horses may be as low as 0.6 mg/kg.
- A threshold level of ingestion is believed to be necessary to produce disease. Therefore, it is common that some horses exposed to ionophores do not develop a disease.
- Feeds containing monensin at ≥ 125 ppm would likely be toxic to horses.

Systems Affected

- Cardiovascular – acute death, congestive heart failure, collapse, exercise intolerance.
- Neurological – ataxia, weakness, tremors, lethargy.
- Gastrointestinal – colic, diarrhea, anorexia.
- Musculoskeletal – sweating, muscle atrophy, weakness

SIGNALMENT AND HISTORY

Risk Factors

- Horses ingesting concentrate feeds that have been manufactured in a feed mill where other species' feed is also prepared.
- Horses ingesting concentrate feeds that have been transported in a truck where feed intended for other livestock is also transported.
- Horses gaining access to feeds manufactured for other livestock that have ionophores as an ingredient.

Historical Findings

- Recent change in feed or a new delivery of feed.
- Feed manufactured at a local feed mill where ionophores are kept to be added to other livestock feeds.

Location and Circumstances of Poisoning

- Horses that are fed manufactured feed which is unintentionally contaminated with ionophores.
- Horse that ingests ionophore-containing feed intended for other species.

CLINICAL FEATURES

- Anorexia and lethargy are the most common initial signs with ionophore toxicity.
- Colic, diarrhea and profuse sweating can occur in some horses within an hour after ingestion of an ionophore:

- Intestinal signs may be a result of the antibiotic's effect on intestinal flora.
- In one report, a horse developed fatal *Clostridium difficile* colitis following monensin administration.
■ Neurologic and neuromuscular signs (ataxia, weakness, tremors) may occur within 12–36 hours after ingestion of an ionophore at a toxic dose. Muscle atrophy and weakness may be seen later (days to weeks) in some cases.
- Neurologic signs, although not as commonly reported as GI and cardiac signs, have been reported with monensin, lasalocid, and salinomycin.
■ Cardiac signs are the best-known signs of monensin poisoning in horses:
- Cardiac signs could include acute death, signs of congestive heart failure, collapse, and exercise intolerance.
- Necrosis of cardiac myocytes and signs of cardiac disease commonly occur 12 hours or more after ingestion of a toxic dose of ionophore.
- Myocardial fibrosis may result in chronic signs of cardiac disease.

DIFFERENTIAL DIAGNOSIS

■ Cantharidin toxicosis (multiple horses demonstrating colic and signs of cardiac disease).
■ Selenium toxicity or deficiency.
■ Myocarditis.
■ Serum electrolyte abnormalities, especially abnormalities in K^+ and Ca^{2+}.
■ Anaphylaxis, lightning stroke, hemorrhage, botulism or other causes of acute death.
■ Exertional and non-exertional myopathies or myositis.
■ EHV-1 or botulism when multiple horses are affected.
■ Electrolyte abnormalities

DIAGNOSTICS

■ Patient history and possible exposure to ionophores.
■ Clinical signs comparable with ionophore toxicity.

CBC/Serum Chemistry

■ Measure serum plasma or whole blood concentrations of cTnI. Increases may occur 24 hours after ingestion of a cardiotoxic dose of an ionophore.

Other Diagnostic Tests

■ Echocardiography revealing dilated chambers, thinning of the cardiac wall and decreased fractional shortening of the left ventricle.
■ Collect suspect feed for analysis.

Pathological Findings

■ Necropsy findings:
- Gross findings may include pale areas in the myocardium, chamber dilatation.
- Collection of stomach contents, heart, muscle, liver, blood, and urine to test for ionophore exposure.
- Microscopic examination of heart or nervous tissue may be required to detect lesions.

THERAPEUTICS

Detoxification

- Gastric lavage if ingestion of ionophore has occurred within the last 10 hours
- Gastric administration of activated charcoal and/or magnesium sulfate:
  - Magnesium sulfate should not be administered if serum magnesium is abnormally high.
- Fluid therapy with potassium and phosphorus supplementation.

Appropriate Health Care

- Clinically affected horses often require hospitalization.

Antidotes

- No specific antidote.

Drugs of Choice

- Acute exposure:
  - Vitamin E/Selenium 1 ml of E-SE®/45.5 kg (100 lb; Merck Animal Health) IM.
- Mitochondrial support:
  - Co-enzyme Q10 (ubiquinol) -15 G/454.5 kg (1,000 lb) daily mixed in feed or PO.
- Cardiovascular (ventricular arrythmias):
  - Lidocaine 0.5 mg/kg IV over 2 minutes, repeat every 5–10 minutes as needed for a maximum of three treatments.
  - Magnesium sulfate 50–100 mg/kg mixed in 1 L of 0.9% saline and administered IV over 10 minutes.

Precautions/Interactions

- Digoxin, chloramphenicol, and sulfonamides are contraindicated.
- Mineral oil could be contraindicated as this might increase absorption of the ionophore.

COMMENTS

Prevention/Avoidance

- Most cases occur on farms where cattle are housed. Extreme caution should be used to avoid horses having access to the cattle feed!
- Always purchase feed from a separate source. Horse feed should be manufactured in a facility that does not produce feeds that contain ionophores. Transportation of large quantities of horse feed should not occur in vehicles that are also used for deliveries for cattle or poultry feed.
- If horses refuse eating a new batch of feed, always consider the possibility of an impurity such as monensin in the feed. In general, horses do not like to taste monensin-contaminated feed.

Possible Complications

- Previously clinically affected but now normal-appearing horses along with subclinical horses that were possibly exposed to a toxic dose should be monitored for ongoing cardiac and neuronal damage:
    - cTnI should be evaluated at rest and 1–2 hours following exercise.
    - Heart rate recovery following exercise should also be performed. Resting heart rate may be normal in some diseased horses.
    - If either of these are abnormal or if there are any signs of cardiorespiratory dysfunction or a concerning arrhythmia is detected upon auscultation, a 24-hour Holter monitor should be performed along with an echocardiography.

Expected Course and Prognosis

- Toxicity with clinical signs is often fatal
- Horses with signs of fulminant heart failure and/or having very high levels of cTnI in serum collected 0.5–5.0 days following exposure have a poor prognosis.
- cTnI levels will usually decrease after several days even in severely affected and eventually fatal cases. Serum/plasma/blood levels of cTnI and heart rate may increase dramatically following mild exercise in sub-acutely diseased horses.

Abbreviations

See Appendix 1 for a complete list.

Suggested Reading

Aleman M, Magdesian KG, Peterson TS, et al. Salinomycin toxicosis in horses. J Am Vet Med Assoc 2007; 230(12):822–1826.
Bautista AC, Tahara J, Mete A, Gaskill CL, Bryant UK, Puschner B. diagnostic value of tissue monensin concentrations in horses following toxicosis. J Vet Diagn Invest. 2014; 26(3):423–427.
Decloedt A, Verheyen T, De Clercq D, et al. Acute and long-term cardiomyopathy and delayed neurotoxicity after accidental lasalocid poisoning in horses. J Vet Intern Med 2012; 26(4):1005–1011.
Divers TJ, Kraus MS, Jesty SA, et al. Clinical findings and serum cardiac troponin i concentrations in horses after intragastric administration of sodium monensin. J Vet Diagn Invest 2009; 21(3):338–343.
Gy C, Leclere M, Bélanger MC, et al. Acute, Subacute and chronic sequelae of horses accidentally exposed to monensin-contaminated feed. [published online ahead of print, 2020 Mar 7]. Equine Vet J 2020; 10.1111/evj.13258.
Hughes KJ, Hoffmann KL, Hodgson DR. Long-term assessment of horses and ponies post exposure to monensin sodium in commercial feed. Equine Vet J 2009; 41(1):47–52.
Peek SF, Marques FD, Morgan J, et al. Atypical acute monensin toxicosis and delayed cardiomyopathy in belgian draft horses. J Vet Intern Med 2004;18(5):761–764.

Author: Thomas J. Divers, DVM, DACVIM, DACVECC
Consulting Editor: Dionne Benson, DVM, JD

Chapter 35

Ractopamine

DEFINITION/OVERVIEW

- Beta$_2$-adrenergic approved by the FDA as a feed additive to improve leanness for use in US swine (Paylean®), cattle (Optaflexx®), and turkeys (Topmax®).
- Over 160 countries have banned the use of ractopamine in food-producing animals. When permitted, a maximum residue level of 10–50 ppb is applied to muscle cuts of beef and pork.
- Causes stimulation of lipolysis and protein synthesis, while downregulating lipogenesis.
- Commercial preparation is a racemic mixture of the four stereoisomers (RR, RS, SR and SS). The RR isomer (butopamine) is a potent cardio-stimulant in humans and is likely the functional and most active stereoisomer mediating the growth response in pigs.
- Toxic exposures in horses likely occur through accidental ingestion of feed containing or contaminated with ractopamine and through illegal use to enhance performance in competition.
- Not FDA-approved for use in the horse.
- Prohibited under ARCI, USEF, FEI, and AQHA.

ETIOLOGY/PATHOPHYSIOLOGY

Mechanism of Action

- Beta$_2$-adrenergic receptor agonist. Also has beta$_1$ activity.
- Causes smooth muscle relaxation in bronchi and reflex tachycardia.
- May see an increase in skeletal muscle contractility and resultant muscle tremors.
- Increases intracellular cAMP which results in decreased adiposity and increased muscle growth in animals.
- Ractopamine also increases protein synthesis and activates the downregulation of lipogenesis.

Pharmacokinetics

- Equine pharmacokinetics have not been extensively described.
- Horses fed ractopamine at 10× toxic dose of zilpaterol did not show clinical signs.
- Studies in other species indicate that ractopamine HCl is rapidly and well absorbed from the GI tract, with peak plasma concentrations occurring from 0.5 to 2 hours after administration. The half-life was about 6–7 hours.

Blackwell's Five-Minute Veterinary Consult Clinical Companion: Equine Toxicology, First Edition. Edited by Lynn R. Hovda, Dionne Benson, and Robert H. Poppenga.
© 2022 John Wiley & Sons, Inc. Published 2022 by John Wiley & Sons, Inc.
Companion website: www.wiley.com/go/hovda/equine

- Studies in several species indicate that the significant first pass metabolism occurs after oral administration, leading to lower systemic drug concentrations. Consequently, urine and blood concentrations of ractopamine will be comparatively higher after IV administration than after oral administration.
- Major metabolites of ractopamine are sulfates and glucuronides. The relatively large amount of glucuronide metabolites has effects on the detectability of ractopamine. Compared with other β-agonists, ractopamine is found at lower levels in ocular tissue and clears the blood more rapidly.

Toxicity

- Toxicity is lower in horses than other beta$_2$ agonists.
- Ractopamine is associated with health problems in food-producing animals, such as "Downer syndrome" in pigs.

Systems Affected

- Cardiovascular – tachycardia, high intra-arterial blood pressure.
- Neurological – sweating, stiff gait, excitation, hyperactivity, tremors.
- Gastrointestinal – colic, NG reflux. Other risks include significant cardiovascular, musculoskeletal, reproductive, and endocrine issues.

SIGNALMENT/HISTORY

- History of exposure to ractopamine along with clinical signs.

Risk Factors

- Equine exposure to feed containing ractopamine or contaminated with ractopamine residue.
- Intentional administration to performance horse.

Historical Findings

- History of exposure or access to ractopamine.
- Recent new feed/new lot of feed from manufacturer that also makes other species' feeds.

CLINICAL FEATURES

- Sweating, agitation, skeletal muscle tremors, and tachycardia are common with beta$_2$-agonist exposure.

DIFFERENTIAL DIAGNOSIS

- Colic of other etiology.
- Ionophore toxicity (monensin).
- Other beta agonists (e.g., clenbuterol, albuterol, zilpaterol).
- CNS stimulants – cocaine, amphetamines.

- Drugs affecting cardiovascular system – alpha$_1$-adrenergic agonists (tricyclic antidepressants), alpha$_2$-adrenergic agonists (xylazine, detomidine).

DIAGNOSTICS

- History of exposure to ractopamine, clinical signs.

CBC/Serum Chemistry/Urinalysis

- Serum chemistry:
  - Hyponatremia.
  - Hypochloremia.
  - Elevated LDH, AST, CK.

Other Diagnostic Tests

- ECG as needed for tachycardia.
- Colic work-up.
- LC-MS for detection of ractopamine/metabolites in blood, urine, hair, muscle, liver or eye fluid.
  - Cattle fed ractopamine HCl for 8 consecutive days had detectable levels in urine for up to 5 days after the last feeding.
- ELISA detection: in at least one study in horses, a 300 mg oral dose resulted in urine detection 24 hours after administration.
- If suspect contamination to horse feed, consider sampling and testing of feed.

Pathological Findings

- None reported in horses.

THERAPEUTICS

- Limited information exists for ractopamine – recommendations are based upon zilpaterol toxicosis.

Detoxification

- Prevent further exposure to ractopamine and provide supportive care.

Appropriate Health Care

- Intravenous fluid therapy.

Antidotes

- None.

Drugs of Choice

- Sinus tachycardia:
  - Propranolol 0.3 mg/kg PO; repeated administration as needed.
  - Potassium chloride (0.08 mEq/kg/h) IV.
  - IV crystalloid fluids.

- Anxiety and muscle tremors (treatment has had mixed success):
  - Methocarbamol 4.4–22.2 mg/kg IV to effect. Administer ½ estimated dose and pause until animal has relaxed. Administer remainder of dose to effect. Repeat as needed, not to exceed 330 mg/kg/day.
  - Butorphanol tartrate 0.1 mg/kg IV q3–4h for up to 48 hours.
  - Xylazine 1.1 mg/kg IV prn.
  - Phenylbutazone 1–2 g IV per 454 kg q12h.

Precautions/Interactions

- Nursing care for clinical signs.

COMMENTS

Client Education

- Limited data on ractopamine toxicosis exists – history of exposure to ractopamine is important for diagnosis.
- LC-MS testing useful in legal cases.

Prevention/Avoidance

- Prevent exposure to feed of other species.
- Purchase feed made in an equine-specific manufacturing facility.

Possible Complications

Possible cardiac damage.

Expected Course and Prognosis

- Clinical signs in mild cases likely to resolve within weeks and prognosis is good.
- As clinical signs worsen, prognosis worsens, and long-term monitoring becomes important.

Synonyms

Ractopamine, Ractopamine HCl, Paylean, Optaflexx, Topmax

Abbreviations

See Appendix 1 for a complete list.

Internet Resources

Kriewald RD. Effects of Ractopamine HCl on Physical and Reproductive Parameters in the Horse(Doctoral dissertation, Texas A&M University) 2008. Available at: https://oaktrust.library.tamu.edu/bitstream/handle/1969.1/ETD-TAMU-2008-05-3/KRIEWALD-THESIS.pdf?sequence=2&isAllowed=y (accessed February 13, 2021).

Suggested Reading

Lehner AF, Hughes GC, Harkins JD, et al. Detection and confirmation of ractopamine and its metabolites in horse urine after paylean administration. J Anal Toxicol 2004; 28(4):226–238.
Yaeger MJ, Mullin K, Ensley SM, et al. Myocardial toxicity in a group of greyhounds administered ractopamine. Vet Pathol 2012; 49(3): 569–573.

Author: Petra Hartmann-Fischbach, MS, FAORC
Consulting Editor: Dionne Benson, DVM, JD

Zilpaterol

DEFINITION/OVERVIEW

- Beta$_2$-adrenergic agonist approved by the FDA as a feed additive for cattle to improve weight gain and improve carcass leanness and sold under the trade name Zilmax (zilpaterol hydrochloride).
- Zilmax is composed of 4.8% w/w zilpaterol hydrochloride as the active ingredient.
- Toxic exposures in horses have occurred through accidental ingestion of cattle feed containing zilpaterol and through illegal use of zilpaterol to enhance performance in competition.
- Not FDA-approved for use in horses.
- Prohibited under ARCI, USEF, FEI, and AQHA.

ETIOLOGY/PATHOPHYSIOLOGY

Mechanism of Action

- Beta$_2$-adrenergic receptor agonist.
- Causes smooth muscle relaxation, including smooth muscles in the lung and dilation of bronchial airways. Can result in peripheral vasodilation with subsequent hypotension and reflex tachycardia.
- May result in increased skeletal muscle contractility and subsequent muscle tremors, excessive sweating, and agitation. Potentially causes insulin release.
- Side effects such as tremor, tachycardia, and ventricular arrhythmias may be partially mediated by the beta$_1$ receptor.
- Beta-adrenergic receptor effects elevate cAMP which results in decreased adiposity and increased muscle growth in animals.

Pharmacokinetics

- Equine pharmacokinetics have not been extensively described.
- Onset of clinical signs in limited research occurred minutes after exposure and peaked 20–30 minutes post ingestion.
- Duration of action in limited research indicated clinical signs resolve within 2–3 weeks; may be longer with more severe clinical signs.

Blackwell's Five-Minute Veterinary Consult Clinical Companion: Equine Toxicology,
First Edition. Edited by Lynn R. Hovda, Dionne Benson, and Robert H. Poppenga.
© 2022 John Wiley & Sons, Inc. Published 2022 by John Wiley & Sons, Inc.
Companion website: www.wiley.com/go/hovda/equine

- Like rat and cattle data, the equine data suggests that most zilpaterol is excreted primarily in the urine unchanged.
- After 5 days post-dosage, urinary zilpaterol elimination markedly slowed, but zilpaterol was detected in the urine after 21 days post-dosage.

Toxicity

- Toxic effects observed after a single therapeutic dose for cattle (0.17 mg/kg fed in grain).
- Adverse effects of sweating, agitation, and signs of possible abdominal pain (flatulence and pawing) occurred, with a marked tachycardia observed about 20–30 minutes post-exposure.

Systems Affected

- Limited data available based upon existing research.
- Cardiovascular – severe tachycardia (HR > 150 beats/min), HR can remain elevated for weeks post-exposure.
- Neurological – sweating across the neck, shoulder, and foreleg, ± depressed behavior, tremors (for up to 1 week).
- Gastrointestinal – flatulence, colic, ± inappetence.
- Renal – brownish urine with high levels or protein, bilirubin, and heme compounds

SIGNALMENT/HISTORY

Risk Factors

- Equine exposure to cattle feed containing zilpaterol.
- Intentional administration to performance horse.

Historical Findings

- Onset of sweating, agitation, colic-like behavior, muscular tremors, tachycardia based upon single research study.
- History of exposure/access to zilpaterol.

CLINICAL FEATURES

- Profuse sweating, restlessness and agitation, skeletal muscle tremors, and marked, prolonged tachycardia that may take days to weeks to resolve are suggestive of zilpaterol exposure.
- Clinical signs of laminitis have been observed in one case.
- Discolored, brownish urine in more severe cases.

DIFFERENTIAL DIAGNOSIS

- Colic of other etiology.
- Ionophore toxicity (monensin/rumensin).

- Cantharidin or blister beetles.
- Oleander (*Nerium oleander*).
- Summer pheasant's eye (*Adonis aestivalis*).
- Other beta agonists (i.e., ractopamine, clenbuterol, albuterol, cimaterol)

DIAGNOSTICS

- History of use of zilpaterol (Zilmax or a beta$_2$-adrenergic agonist) on the premises where equine is located, or possible doping of equine is extremely important for diagnosis.

CBC/Serum Chemistry/Urinalysis

- Serum chemistry:
  - Elevated LDH, AST, CK.
  - Elevated BUN and creatinine.
  - Hyperglycemia.
  - Hyponatremia.
  - Hypochloremia.
- Urinalysis:
  - Discolored, brownish urine in severe cases.
  - Proteinuria.
  - ± Azotemia.
  - ± Bilirubinuria.
  - ± RBCs/heme.

Other Diagnostic Tests

- ECG as needed for tachycardia.
- cTnI to determine cardiac muscle damage.
- Colic work-up.
- LC-MS helpful for diagnosis but time delay would hinder therapeutics.
  - Note: urine concentrations decline rapidly below 3,000 ng/mL within 24 hours post-dosage.

Pathological Findings

- None reported in horses.

THERAPEUTICS

- The goal of therapy is to limit toxin absorption and provide supportive care.

Detoxification

- Prevent further exposure to possible contaminated feed or determine if doping incident

Appropriate Health Care

- Intravenous fluid therapy with correction of electrolyte imbalances (e.g., hypertonic sodium chloride and potassium chloride were utilized in one case).

Antidotes

- None

Drugs of Choice

- Sinus tachycardia:
  - Propranolol 0.3 mg/kg PO; repeated administration may be necessary.
- Potassium chloride 0.08 mEq/kg/h IV.
- IV crystalloid fluids as needed.
- Anxiety and muscle tremors (treatment has had mixed success):
  - Methocarbamol 4.4–22.2 mg/kg IV to effect. Administer ½ estimated dose and pause until animal has relaxed. Administer remainder of dose to effect. Repeat as needed not to exceed 330 mg/kg/day.
  - Butorphanol tartrate 0.1 mg/kg IV q3–4h for up to 48 hours.
  - Xylazine 1.1 mg/kg IV prn.
  - Phenylbutazone 1–2 g IV per 454 kg q12h.

Precautions/Interactions

- Adequate nursing care for clinical signs.
- Monitor for signs of laminitis.

COMMENTS

Client Education

- There are limited data available regarding long-term effects following exposure to toxic concentrations of zilpaterol.
- May recommend long-term ECG monitoring.
- Education regarding possibility of laminitis post-exposure.

Prevention/Avoidance

- Prevent horse exposure to cattle feed with Zilmax® and caution against use as doping agent in horses.

Possible Complications

- Possible cardiac damage.
- Laminitis.

Expected Course and Prognosis

- Clinical signs in mild cases resolve within weeks without treatment and prognosis is good.
- In more severe cases, prognosis is guarded based upon heart function and laminitis. These horses should be monitored for months post-exposure.

Abbreviations

See Appendix 1 for a complete list.

Suggested Reading

Hepworth-Warren KL. Alcott CJ. Case report. Treatment and Resolution of zilpaterol hydrochloride toxicity in a quarter horse gelding. Equine Vet Educ 2014; 26:81–85.

Shelver, WL, Thorson JF, Hammer CJ, Smith DJ. Depletion of urinary zilpaterol residues in horses as measured by ELISA and UPLC-MS/MS. J Agric Food Chem 2010; 58:4077–4083.

Wagner SA, Mostrom MS, Hammer CJ, Thorson JF, Smith DJ. Adverse effects of zilpaterol administration in horses: three cases. J Equine Vet Sci 2008; 28:238–243.

Author: Michelle Mostrom, DVM, MS, PhD, DABVT, DABT
Consulting Editor: Dionne Benson, DVM, JD

Metals

Arsenic

Chapter 37

DEFINITION/OVERVIEW

- Intoxication results from excessive exposure to arsenic-containing pesticides (most removed from use, but legacy pesticides such as lead arsenate can still be present and accessible by animals), Fowler's solution, arsenic-contaminated soils, burn piles, and water or feed.
- Similar to arsenic-containing pesticides, organic arsenicals (e.g., arsanilic acid and 3-nitro-4-hydroxyphenylarsonic acid [roxarsone], nitarsone and carbasone) for use in swine and poultry feeds have been banned, so exposure to arsenic-containing feeds is unlikely.
- Ashes from chromated copper arsenate (CCA)-treated lumber are high in arsenic.

ETIOLOGY/PATHOPHYSIOLOGY

Mechanism of Action

- Trivalent inorganic arsenicals inhibit cellular respiration and damage capillaries.
- Pentavalent inorganic arsenicals uncouple oxidative phosphorylation, leading to deficits in cell energy.

Toxicokinetics

- Many factors influence the absorption of arsenicals, such as form of arsenic, particle size, and solubility.
- Distribution occurs to all organs although it accumulates in the liver before wider distribution to other organs such as the spleen, kidneys and lungs.
- Arsenic can cross the placenta.
- Metabolism is complex and relatively poorly understood.
- Excretion is form-dependent: pentavalent arsenicals are eliminated predominately via the kidneys while trivalent arsenicals are eliminated primarily via the bile.

Blackwell's Five-Minute Veterinary Consult Clinical Companion: Equine Toxicology,
First Edition. Edited by Lynn R. Hovda, Dionne Benson, and Robert H. Poppenga.
© 2022 John Wiley & Sons, Inc. Published 2022 by John Wiley & Sons, Inc.
Companion website: www.wiley.com/go/hovda/equine

Toxicity

- Toxicity depends on the form of arsenic ingested.
- Trivalent inorganic forms (e.g., arsenic trioxide; sodium, potassium and calcium salts of arsenite) are 10-fold more toxic than inorganic pentavalent forms (e.g., sodium, potassium, and calcium salts of arsenate).
- Toxicity of organic pentavalent forms used as growth promoters in livestock feeds has not been determined for horses.

Systems Affected

- Cardiovascular – capillary damage leading to blood loss and circulatory collapse.
- Gastrointestinal – congestion, edema, hyperemia, necrosis, hemorrhagic fluid contents.
- Nervous – primarily reported for organic arsenicals, necrosis of myelin-supporting cells, degeneration of myelin sheaths and axons, gliosis of affected cells reported for other species.
- Renal/urologic – renal tubular degeneration.

SIGNALMENT/HISTORY

- No breed or sex predilections.
- Peracute or acute syndromes are most likely.
- Peracute – patient often found dead; death caused by cardiovascular collapse.

Risk Factors

- Ingestion of arsenic-containing products or arsenic-contaminated soils, water, or feed.
- Access to burn piles containing CCA-treated lumber ash.

CLINICAL FEATURES

- Acute – intense abdominal pain, hypersalivation, severe watery diarrhea, decreased abdominal sounds, muscle tremors, weak and rapid pulse with signs of circulatory shock, ataxia, depression, and recumbency; if the animal survives for several days, oliguria and proteinuria secondary to renal damage.
- Chronic – not described in horses.

DIFFERENTIAL DIAGNOSIS

- Lead toxicosis – evidence of neurologic dysfunction is likely.
- Mercury toxicosis.
- NSAID toxicosis – history of previous use.
- Cantharidin toxicosis – evidence of cystitis.
- Salmonellosis.
- Colitis X.
- Acute cyathastomiasis.
- Clostridial colitis.

DIAGNOSTICS

CBC/Serum Chemistry/Urinalysis

- Reflect circulatory shock and possible liver and kidney damage.
- Hemoconcentration – elevated PCV and plasma total protein.
- Leukopenia with degenerative changes in polymorphonuclear leukocytes (neutrophils).
- Azotemia.
- Hematuria.
- Electrolytes – hypokalemia, hyponatremia, hypochloremia.
- Hyperglycemia.
- Hyperbilirubinemia.
- Elevated LDH and CK.

Other Diagnostic Tests

- Antemortem – measurement of arsenic in urine, whole blood or GI contents.
- Postmortem – measurement of arsenic in liver or kidney.
- Chronic exposures – arsenic can be measured in hair to reflect arsenic exposure over time.
- Arsenic is rapidly excreted after exposure ceases, so length of time between exposure and sample collection can impact detection of arsenic in biological samples.

Pathological Findings

Gross findings

- GI hemorrhage, mucosal congestion, edema, and erosion, either localized or throughout the GI tract, which may be filled with watery, dark-green, black, or hemorrhagic ingesta, with necrotic material from mucosal sloughing.
- Pulmonary edema and epicardial and serosal hemorrhage.

Histopathologic findings

- Necrotizing, hemorrhagic typhlocolitis, with necrotizing vasculitis, renal tubular necrosis, and hepatic fatty degeneration.

THERAPEUTICS

- Emergency treatment is necessary.
- Remove animal from known or potential source of exposure.
- Treat circulatory shock and acidosis.
- Appropriate fluid therapy.

Detoxification

- GI decontamination generally not rewarding but if animal is asymptomatic gastric lavage might be of benefit.

Antidotes

- Chelators can bind arsenic and hasten its elimination:

- Dimercaprol (British anti-Lewisite) is the classic arsenic chelator (loading dose of 4–5 mg/kg given by deep muscular injection, followed by 2–3 mg/kg q4h for 2+ hours and then 1 mg/kg q4h for 2 days); adverse reactions include tremors, convulsions, and coma.
- 2,3-Dimercaptosuccinic acid is a less toxic chelator (equine dose not established, but 10 mg/kg PO q8h is suggested).

Drugs of Choice

- Control abdominal pain:
  - Flunixin meglumine (1.1 mg/kg IV or IM q12h or as needed) or butorphanol tartrate (0.1–0.2 mg/kg IV q3–4h up to 48 hours).
  - Xylazine hydrochloride (0.3–0.4 mg/kg IV) may be used in conjunction with butorphanol (0.01–0.02 mg/kg IV).
- Demulcents – mineral oil or kaolin-pectin

Precautions/Interactions

- Use NSAIDs cautiously because of possible adverse GI and renal effects.
- IM injections of dimercaprol can be painful, particularly if not administered deeply.

COMMENTS

Client Education

- Identify potential sources of exposure, and properly dispose of sources.

Patient Monitoring

- Monitor renal and hepatic function.
- Provide a bland diet, containing reduced amounts of high-quality protein.
- Dehydration and fluid loss are major factors in mortality.

Prevention/Avoidance

- Ensure that any arsenic-containing products are properly identified and removed or properly stored.

Expected Course and Prognosis

- Expected course and prognosis depend on the severity of clinical signs.
- If the animal survives, recovery should be complete.

Abbreviations

See Appendix 1 for a complete list.

Suggested Reading

Casteel SW. Metal toxicosis in horses. Vet Clin N Am: Equine Practice 2001; 17(3):517–527.
Pace LW, Turnquist SE, Casteel SW, Johnson PJ, Frankeny RL. Acute arsenic toxicosis in five horses. Vet Pathol 1997; 34:160–164.

Author: Robert H. Poppenga, DVM, PhD, DABVT
Consulting Editor: Robert H. Poppenga, DVM, PhD, DABVT

Fluoride

Chapter 38

DEFINITION/OVERVIEW

- Fluoride is readily consumed and an important dietary component in horses.
- Dietary allowance in horses is 40–60 ppm.
- Fluorine rarely exists in its elemental form but commonly exists as fluoride combined with other elements.
  - Calcium fluoride is the most common form found in soil
- Fluoride is present in the environment as well as in dietary ingredients:
  - Natural sources include rock phosphate deposits, volcanic ash, iron ores, and deep wells.
  - Other significant sources occur during refining of iron or aluminum ores.
  - Fluorine discharged during refining of metal ores combines with atmospheric water and particulates, eventually settling on the surface of forages.
  - Plant uptake is usually not a significant concern.
  - Rock phosphates used as feed supplements should be de-fluorinated, but due to cost some are used in their natural form and can be a significant source for livestock.
  - Rock phosphate supplements should have a phosphorous:fluorine ratio of more than 100:1.
- Chronic intoxication is more common than acute intoxication.
- Fluoride toxicosis (fluorosis) primarily affects teeth and bones.

ETIOLOGY/PATHOPHYSIOLOGY

Mechanism of Action

- Fluoride substitutes for the hydroxyl groups in hydroxyapatite, altering the mineralization process and altering the crystalline structure of bone.
- Fluoride damages ameloblasts and odontoblasts in developing teeth, resulting in abnormal mineralization of both dentine and enamel.

Toxicokinetics

- The form of fluoride ingested greatly impacts its bioavailability.
- Approximately 50% of ingested fluoride is excreted by the kidneys with the remainder deposited in bone and teeth.

- 95% of the total bodily fluoride is contained in bones and teeth.
- If dietary fluoride decreases, fluoride will slowly be released from bone.

Toxicity

- There are rare reports of acute fluoride intoxication related to ingestion of pesticides that are no longer used in the United States.
  - There remains a chance for illegal importation and use of these pesticides.
- Toxicity of fluoride depends on a number of variables including duration of exposure, bioavailability, species, age and diet of the animal involved.
- Depending on the duration of exposure and species susceptibility, concentrations in the diet in the range from 100–300 mg/kg can produce chronic poisoning.
- Water concentrations > 30 mg/L are considered to be toxic.
- Chronic fluorosis in horses is usually associated with grazing contaminated pastures.

Systems Affected

- Skeletal.
- Gastrointestinal.
- Musculoskeletal.
- Hematopoietic.

SIGNALMENT/HISTORY

Risk Factors

- Daily dosage – fluoride is cumulative during constant intake.
- Source/form of fluoride – some forms are much more bioavailable than others and can contribute to the total body burden to a greater degree.
- Age of the animal – younger animals are at higher risk due to active bone and tooth formation.
- Nutrition – nutritional interrelationships are complicated, but a calcium deficient diet can exacerbate fluoride accumulation.

Location and Circumstances of Poisoning

- Animals pastured near refining plants or volcanoes are at higher risk of excessive exposure.
- Poorly defluorinated rock phosphate supplements are more commonly associated with chronic intoxication in horses.

CLINICAL FEATURES

Acute fluorosis
- Acute fluorosis is seen when large amounts of soluble fluoride are ingested.
- These sources are not readily available so acute fluoride poisoning is uncommon.
- Clinical signs include excitation, seizures, diarrhea, vomiting, weakness, excessive salivation, depression, and death.

Chronic fluorosis
- Chronic fluorosis occurs from excessive dietary intake.
- The most common sources are forage contamination and poorly defluorinated rock phosphate supplements.
- Dental fluorosis only occurs in actively forming teeth; once teeth have erupted, they are not susceptible to damage by fluoride:
  - Clinical signs associated with dental lesions include difficult mastication, decreased feed intake, poor growth, and excessive dental wear.
- Skeletal damage results in clinical signs related to lameness:
  - Periodic lameness, abnormal hoof wear, generalized stiffness, and abnormal locomotion.
- Secondary effects include poor reproduction, reduced milk production, and general wasting.

DIFFERENTIAL DIAGNOSIS

Acute
- Organophosphate/carbamate insecticides, heavy metals, anatoxin-a(s).

Chronic
- Common causes of dental pain – abnormal wear, overgrowth, fractured teeth, tooth root abscess, retained deciduous teeth, blind wolf teeth.
- Common causes of lameness – pain, bone disease, metabolic, circulatory, infectious.

DIAGNOSTICS

Other Diagnostic Testing
- Diagnosis is typically based on confirmed exposure to fluorides, dental and skeletal lesions, and excessive fluoride levels in bone and urine.
- Plasma concentrations ranging from 0.7 to 1.9 mg/L are consistent with poisoning.
- Toxic urinary concentrations based on recent exposure lie in the range 14–120 mg/L.
- Bone and teeth fluoride concentrations in the ranges 6,000–13,000 and 7,500–11,000 mg/kg, respectively, are consistent with a diagnosis of chronic fluorosis in livestock.
- Plasma concentrations may rise substantially once the skeletal concentrations of fluoride approach saturation.
- Radiographs can aid in visualization of palpable growths of bone.
- Bone assays can be performed on biopsies or postmortem bone samples.
- Feed, forage, water, and supplements can be analyzed to approximate total daily intake.

Pathological Findings
- Affected teeth will have hypoplastic enamel and the surface will be mottled with debris in pits causing a brown or black discoloration.
- Teeth will show excessive wear, and exposure of pulp will cause dental pain.
- Grossly, bones are thickened and rough beginning at the proximal one-third of metatarsals and progressing to metacarpals, mandible, and ribs.

- The articular surfaces are unaffected.
- Microscopically, hyperostosis, irregular mineralization, endosteal reabsorption, and excessive osteoid tissue are common lesions.

THERAPEUTICS

Appropriate Health Care

- Symptomatic therapy aimed at pain abatement may help prolong life.
- Limited grazing and easily masticated feeds should be offered.
- All excess fluoride should be removed from the diet.

Antidotes

- There are no specific antidotes for acute or chronic fluoride toxicosis.

COMMENTS

Prevention/Avoidance

- Producers/owners should be aware of the quality and sources of their minerals.
- Phosphate products not designed for animal rations should not be used.
- Forage and water analysis can provide information to help estimate the risk.

Expected Course and Prognosis

- Acute:
  - Prognosis is guarded at best for acute toxicity, luckily acute fluorosis is uncommon
- Chronic:
  - Prognosis for chronic fluorosis is heavily based on the degree of clinical signs.
  - Animals can recover from mild disease provided all fluoride is removed from the diet.
  - Mildly affected animals maintained on NSAIDs can have a productive life.
  - Severely affected animals may mandate euthanasia due to welfare

Abbreviations

See Appendix 1 for a complete list.

Suggested Reading

Thompson LJ. Fluoride. In: Gupta RC, ed. Veterinary Toxicology: Basic and Clinical Principles 3rd edn. San Diego, CA: Elsevier, 2018; pp. 429–431.

Livesey C, Payne J. Diagnosis and investigation of fluorosis in livestock and horses. In Practice. 2011; 33: 454–461.

Osweiler, G. Fluoride. In: Plumlee KH, ed. Clinical Veterinary Toxicology. St Louis, MO: Mosby, 2004; pp. 197–200.

Author: Scott Fritz, DVM
Contributing Editor: Robert H. Poppenga, DVM, PhD, DABVT

Chapter 39

Iron

DEFINITION/OVERVIEW

- Iron is an essential mineral required for a variety of physiologic functions involving oxidation–reduction reactions.
- Horses often are supplemented with iron, either in their feed or via parenteral administration.
- Oral forms include ferrous fumarate, ferrous sulfate, ferrous gluconate, ferrous carbonate, and ferric phosphate.
- Injectable forms include ferric ammonium citrate and iron–dextran complexes.
- Acute intoxications have been reported in neonates given ferrous fumarate.
- Chronic hepatopathies associated with increased hepatic iron concentrations have also been reported in adult horses.

ETIOLOGY/PATHOPHYSIOLOGY

Mechanism of Action

- After absorption, ferrous iron (Fe^{2+}) is converted to ferric iron (Fe^{3+}), releasing an unbuffered hydrogen ion and causing metabolic acidosis.
- Intracellularly, iron disrupts oxidative phosphorylation and causes free-radical formation and lipid peroxidation, resulting in cell death.
- Iron toxicosis is associated with both local and systemic effects.
- Ingestion of iron salts causes corrosive damage to the GI mucosa, resulting in edema, ulceration, and hemorrhage.
- Iron can result in a coagulopathy from inhibition of thrombin.
- The cause of chronic hepatopathy associated with apparent liver iron accumulation is unknown.

Toxicokinetics

- Iron absorption from the GI tract is poor.
- Excretion of iron is limited, and absorption is balanced against the need of the animal.

Blackwell's Five-Minute Veterinary Consult Clinical Companion: Equine Toxicology,
First Edition. Edited by Lynn R. Hovda, Dionne Benson, and Robert H. Poppenga.
© 2022 John Wiley & Sons, Inc. Published 2022 by John Wiley & Sons, Inc.
Companion website: www.wiley.com/go/hovda/equine

- Iron is absorbed by enterocytes in the small intestine as ferrous iron (Fe^{2+}) and transferred to the serum where it is converted to ferric iron (Fe^{3+}) and bound primarily to the transport glycoprotein transferrin, with lesser amounts bound to ferritin.
- Serum iron forms a pool that fluctuates due to the synthesis and breakdown of hemoglobin, ferritin, cytochromes and other iron-containing proteins.
- Daily iron loss is minimal unless RBCs are lost due to bleeding.

Toxicity

- Toxicity of iron salts depends on the amount of elemental iron present – ferrous sulfate is 20% elemental iron; ferrous gluconate is 12% elemental iron.
- The toxicity of elemental iron to horses has not been firmly established but toxic doses for neonates are estimated to be 25-fold less than those for adults.
- The sensitivity of neonates is believed to result from their lower capacity to bind iron to transferrin and their increased absorption of orally administered iron.

Systems Affected

- Cardiovascular – cardiotoxicity results in decreased cardiac output and hypovolemia from GI fluid loss; decreased cardiac output contributes to circulatory shock.
- Gastrointestinal – ingestion of iron salts causes corrosive damage to the GI mucosa, resulting in edema, ulceration, and hemorrhage.
- Hemic/lymphatic/immune – coagulopathy from inhibition of thrombin.
- Hepatobiliary – periportal hepatocytes are especially vulnerable to damage and necrosis with acute exposures; iron-associated hepatopathy results in cirrhosis and hemochromatosis.

SIGNALMENT/HISTORY

- Iron toxicosis in horses is most often associated with oral exposure to iron-containing supplements, with most documented cases occurring in neonates < 3 days of age from oral administration of a digestive inoculant containing ferrous fumarate.
- Recent reports have implicated high iron concentrations in water as a potential cause of hepatic iron overload and associated hepatopathy.

Risk Factors

- Increased iron bioavailability in young animals might predispose to overexposure following oral administration of an iron supplement.
- Iron is more toxic in selenium- or vitamin E-deficient individuals

CLINICAL FEATURES

- Early signs associated with oral ingestion of iron salts include colic, diarrhea, and melena.
- Intoxicated horses often present with anorexia, lethargy, and icterus
- Signs of hepatoencephalopathy (e.g., ataxia, head pressing, and coma) can be seen.

DIFFERENTIAL DIAGNOSIS

Adult horses
- Other hepatotoxicants – aflatoxins (detection in feed, histopathologic lesions), blue-green algae toxins (presence of algal bloom, detection of toxins, histopathologic lesions), PAs (evidence of PA-containing plant consumption, histopathologic lesions).
- Theiler's disease – history of equine immune serum administration.
- Causes of hemolytic anemia – red-maple ingestion (evidence of plant consumption, Heinz bodies, methemoglobinemia); equine infectious anemia (positive Coggins test).
- Immune-mediated thrombocytopenia–positive Coombs' test.
- DIC – detection of underlying disease, thrombocytopenia, moderately prolonged PT and APTT, and increased serum FDPs.
- Bacterial cholangiohepatitis – liver biopsy.
- Lymphosarcoma – evaluation of blood smears, cytologic evaluation of bone marrow, and enlarged lymph nodes or tumor masses.

Foals
- Septicemia – fever, neutrophilia.
- Neonatal isoerythrolysis – low PCV, positive Coombs' test.
- Tyzzer's disease – histopathologic examination.
- Equine herpes virus – histopathologic lesions, serology, virus identification or isolation.

DIAGNOSTICS

CBC/Serum Chemistry/Urinalysis
- Thrombocytopenia, lymphopenia, and prolonged PT and APTT.
- Increased serum GGT, ALP, total and conjugated bilirubin, bile acids, fibrinogen, FDP, and ammonia.
- Anion gap metabolic acidosis.

Other Diagnostic Tests
- High serum iron concentration, high saturation of iron binding (as assessed by TIBC), and high free iron in tissues.
- Liver biopsy for histopathologic evaluation and possible determination of iron concentration.
- Postmortem interpretation of high liver iron concentrations is difficult in the absence of compatible histopathological lesions as liver iron concentrations above an expected "normal" range are common in horses.

Pathological Findings

Gross findings
- Lesions include icterus, small livers with dark red areas or tan discoloration and uneven surfaces, GI hemorrhages, and thymic atrophy in foals.

Histopathological findings
- Lesions include hepatocellular necrosis, which may be primarily periportal or panlobular, varying degrees of bile duct proliferation, fibrous connective tissue proliferation, mixed inflammatory cell infiltration, and cholestasis.
- There may be multifocal to locally extensive areas of necrosis and hemorrhage in the gastric glandular mucosa and areas of necrosis in the lamina propria of the small intestine.
- Mild to severe lymphoid lesions, including thymic lymphoid necrosis and necrosis in splenic lymphoid follicles.
- In chronic iron overload cases, fibrosis and hemosiderin accumulation in hepatocytes can be pronounced.

THERAPEUTICS

- Stabilize the patient, paying particular attention to cardiovascular support and acid–base status.
- Use of the specific iron-chelator deferoxamine mesylate is possible. Appropriate dosage regimens have not been definitively determined, however, and efficacy and safety studies in horses are lacking.
- Therapeutic phlebotomy has also been used in chronic iron overload.

Detoxification
- GI decontamination is unlikely to be beneficial after oral ingestion of iron because of the delay in presentation and inability of AC to bind iron.

Antidote
- Chelation considered to be antidotal.
- Chelator of choice – deferoxamine mesylate, which forms a stable, water-soluble compound readily excreted by the kidneys; veterinary experience is limited.
- A recommended dose of deferoxamine is 40 mg/kg every 4–8 hours; can also be given as a continuous infusion at the rate of 15 mg/kg/hour. Chelation should continue until serum iron concentrations fall below 300 µg/dL (3 ppm) or below the TIBC.
- For mild acute intoxications, chelation therapy probably offers little advantage compared with supportive care.

Precautions/Interactions
- Do not give deferoxamine to patients with renal impairment.
- Rapid administration of deferoxamine can cause cardiac dysrhythmias and exacerbate existing hypotension.
- Do not give deferoxamine to pregnant animals because of possible fetal skeletal abnormalities.
- Do not give corticosteroids to iron-intoxicated patients because of possible increased serum free-iron concentrations.

COMMENTS

Patient Monitoring

- Monitor serum iron concentrations, liver function, and cardiovascular status.
- Following oral exposure, monitor for damage to esophagus or other portions of the GI tract.

Prevention/Avoidance

- Do not over-supplement iron in individuals without confirmed iron deficiency.
- A normal dietary requirement of iron in adult horses is 40 ppm.
- Assess iron concentrations in water sources to avoid over exposure.

Possible Complications

- Following oral exposure to iron salts scarring in the GI tract with subsequent stenosis and obstruction is possible.

Expected Course and Prognosis

- Individuals with mild liver pathology have a good prognosis with good supportive care.
- Individuals with severe liver pathology or hepatoencephalopathy have a guarded prognosis.

Abbreviations

See Appendix 1 for a complete list.

Suggested Reading

Edens LM, Robertson JL, Feldman BF. Cholestatic hepatopathy, thrombocytopenia and lymphopenia associated with iron toxicity in a thoroughbred gelding. Equine Vet J 1993; 25:81–84.
Gummery L, Johnston PEJ, Sutton DGM, Raferty AG. Two cases of hepatopathy and hyperferraemia managed with deferoxamine and phlebotomy. Equine Vet Educ 2019; 31:575–581.
Mullaney TP, Brown CM. Iron toxicity in neonatal foals. Equine Vet J 1988; 20:119–124.
Pearson EG, Hedstrom OR, Poppenga RH. Hepatic cirrhosis and hemochromatosis in three horses. J Am Vet Med Assoc 1994; 204:1053–1056.

Author: Robert H. Poppenga, DVM, PhD, DABVT
Consulting Editor: Robert H. Poppenga, DVM, PhD, DABVT

Chapter 40

Lead

DEFINITION/OVERVIEW

- Lead toxicosis (plumbism) affects the nervous, musculoskeletal, GI, hematopoietic, and renal systems.
- Horses are less susceptible to plumbism than cattle or dogs. Lead intoxication in horses is relatively uncommon in the USA.
- Acute (rare) and chronic forms result from exposures to lead-contaminated forages in habitats adjacent to mines and smelters or environments with buildings or fences built prior to 1977 (with lead pipes) and coated with lead-based paints.
- Ingestion of lead from lead acid batteries, soil contaminated with lead-containing products, or the ashes of combusted older buildings also poses a risk of lead intoxication in horses.

ETIOLOGY/PATHOPHYSIOLOGY

Mechanism of Action

Lead binds to sulfhydryl groups and mimics calcium, thereby disrupting heme synthesis, neurotransmission, and vitamin D metabolism.

Toxicokinetics

- Toxicosis is rare in the horse.
- Onset of action depends upon whether exposure is chronic or acute.
- Absorption of lead is greater in foals than adult horses.
- Lead is sequestered in organs and tissues, and excretion is via urine.

Toxicity

- Acute exposures to greater than 500 to 750 mg.
- Chronic exposures to greater than 1.7–7.0 mg/kg/day.

SIGNALMENT/HISTORY

- No breed predilections.
- Horses have history of exposure to lead.

Blackwell's Five-Minute Veterinary Consult Clinical Companion: Equine Toxicology,
First Edition. Edited by Lynn R. Hovda, Dionne Benson, and Robert H. Poppenga.
© 2022 John Wiley & Sons, Inc. Published 2022 by John Wiley & Sons, Inc.
Companion website: www.wiley.com/go/hovda/equine

- Young, growing foals are most susceptible as they absorb 10–20% of ingested lead.
- Pregnant and lactating mares also have enhanced GI absorption of lead and transfer lead to the fetus or neonate.

Location and Circumstances of Poisoning

- Habitats near smelting or mining operations.
- Housing in or around barns or fences built prior to 1977 that contain lead-lined pipes and/or walls painted with lead-based paints.
- Premises contaminated with lead-containing batteries, shot, solder, gasoline, oil, or ashes of combusted older buildings.
- Diets deficient in calcium, zinc, iron, or vitamin D.
- Trauma from lead-containing objects.

Systems Affected

- Nervous – laryngeal hemiplegia, ataxia, dysphagia, stiffness, agitation, seizures.
- Gastrointestinal – colic, impaction, anorexia.
- Hematological – anemia.
- Musculoskeletal – muscle fasciculations, weakness, decreased muscle tone, lameness, swollen joints.
- Dermatological – roughened hair coat.

CLINICAL FEATURES

- Peripheral neuropathies including abnormal lip and tongue movements, laryngeal hemiplegia ("roaring") or paralysis, dysphagia, esophageal obstruction ("choke"), aspiration pneumonia.
- Weakness, depression, ataxia
- Muscle fasciculations.
- Hyperesthesia.
- Anorexia, weight loss, diarrhea, colic.
- Lameness and swollen joints (young, growing horses or lead-containing foreign bodies near joint surfaces).
- Anemia.
- Seizures.
- Death.

DIFFERENTIAL DIAGNOSIS

- Laryngeal hemiplegia or paralysis ("roaring"), esophageal obstruction ("choke"), and exercise-induced pulmonary hemorrhage not associated with plumbism – physical examination, endoscopy, radiography, no identified sources of lead exposure, history of trauma.
- Rabies and other viral encephalitides.
- Equine motor neuron disease and equine degenerative myeloencephalopathy.
- Fumonisin B_1 intoxication ("moldy corn poisoning" or equine leukoencephalomalacia).
- Botulism.

- Intoxications by *Centaurea* sp.
- Arsenic toxicosis.

DIAGNOSTICS

CBC/Serum Chemistry/Urinalysis
- Anemia.
- Nucleated red blood cells.
- Basophilic stippling and Howell–Jolly bodies.
- Proteinuria (uncommon).

Other Diagnostic Tests
- Antemortem – whole-blood concentrations of lead > 0.35 ppm in the presence of appropriate clinical signs, alterations in erythrocyte D-aminolevulinic acid dehydratase (ALAD) activity (decreased), zinc protoporphyrin concentrations (increased), and increased urinary excretion of coproporphyrin and uroporphyrins (ALAD and porphyrin analyses not performed in many veterinary diagnostic laboratories).
- Postmortem – concentrations of lead in liver or kidney > 10 ppm on a wet-weight basis (> 5 ppm in chronic cases), bone concentrations of lead > 40 ppm on a dry-matter basis in chronic cases.
- Endoscopy to diagnose laryngeal hemiplegia or to visualize lead-containing foreign bodies in the stomach.
- Measurement of 24-hour urinary excretion of lead following chelation therapy (logistically challenging).

Imaging
- Radiography to detect lead-containing objects in the GI tract of small foals or around joints.
- Radiographic visualization of "lead lines" at epiphyseal plates of long bones in young, growing horses.

Pathological Findings
- Gross – inconsistent gross pathologic changes in horses, aspiration pneumonia, and emaciation in chronic cases.
- Histologic – peripheral neuropathy with segmental degeneration of axons and myelin in distal motor fibers, pulmonary changes consistent with aspiration pneumonia, reports of renal tubular disease in chronic cases.

THERAPEUTICS

Detoxification
- *No activated charcoal* – it does not bind to lead.
- Administer sulfate-containing cathartics to bind lead in GI tract (decrease absorption) and to increase elimination of lead:
  - Sodium or magnesium sulfate administered by NG tube (250–500 mg/kg).

Appropriate Health Care

- Prevent further lead exposure.
- Identification and removal of lead source.
- Enhance urinary lead excretion with chelation.
- Control pain and hyperexcitability.
- Periodic neurologic assessments.
- Treat aspiration pneumonia with appropriate antibiotics and NSAIDs.
- Provide supportive care for dehydration, circulatory shock, and dysphagia.
- Monitor serum electrolytes and supplement with IV fluids as needed.
- Monitor hemogram and whole-blood lead concentrations.

Antidotes

- Dimercaprol (British anti-Lewisite) to chelate intracellular and extracellular lead at a dimercaprol loading dose of 4–5 mg/kg given by deep IM injection, followed by 2–3 mg/kg every 4 hours for 24 hours and then 1 mg/kg every 4 hours for 2 days; adverse reactions include tremors, convulsions, and coma.
OR
- Calcium-EDTA to chelate lead at a dosage of 75 mg/kg/day divided into two or three equal treatments and administered for 5 days by slow IV infusion as a 6.6% solution in normal saline or 5% dextrose (1.1 mL of 6.6% EDTA solution/kg); if deemed necessary, retreatment with Ca-EDTA after a 2-day "rest"; adverse effects include depletion of zinc and essential electrolytes.
- Recheck lead concentration in whole blood 2 weeks after final chelation dose; repeat chelation if > 0.35 ppm.
- In cattle, thiamine hydrochloride at dosages of 2–10 mg/kg twice daily IM for 2 weeks is used, but dosage and efficacy not clearly established in horse

Drugs of Choice

- Abdominal discomfort:
  - Flunixin meglumine at 0.55–1.1 mg/kg IV every 12–24 hours; *and/or*
  - Butorphanol tartrate at 0.02–0.1 mg/kg IV every 3–4 h up to 48 hours.
- Sedation/severe pain:
  - Xylazine hydrochloride at 0.3–1.1 mg/kg IV alone (higher dosage) or with butorphanol at 0.01–0.02 mg/kg IV (lower dosage of xylazine).
- Seizures:
  - Diazepam administered to adults (25–50 mg IV) or foals (0.05–0.4 mg/kg IV) for hyperesthesia, muscle tremors, and seizures (can repeat in 30 min).

Precautions/Interactions

- Chelators may deplete essential cations and electrolytes.
- Sedatives in ataxic horses.
- Cautious use of NSAIDs in GI and renal disease or dimercaprol if renal disease is present.

COMMENTS

Client Education

- Identify and remove lead sources if possible or limit access if not possible
- Proper disposal of, or limited access to, lead sources
- Appropriate regulatory agencies should be notified of lead-contaminated matrices that could potentially poison children, e.g. soil or water.

Prevention/Avoidance

- Prevent exposure to habitats near smelters or mines.
- Avoid use of lead-containing paints.
- Clean up lead-contaminated pastures, paddocks, or soil.

Possible Complications

- Aspiration pneumonia.
- Concurrent exposure to other toxic metals.
- Lead can cross the placenta and, potentially, have adverse effects on the fetus.

Expected Course and Prognosis

- Long-term neurologic deficits possible following removal from lead source and partial recovery of neurologic function.

Abbreviations

See Appendix 1 for a complete list.

Suggested Reading

Casteel SW. Metal toxicosis in horses. Vet Clin North Am Equine Pract 2001; 17:517–527.
Gwaltney-Brant S. Lead. In: Plumlee KH, ed. Clinical Veterinary Toxicology. St Louis: Mosby, 2004: pp. 204–210.
Kruger K, Saulez MN, Nesser JA, Soldberg K. Acute lead intoxication in a pregnant mare. J S Afr Vet Assoc 2008; 79(1):50–53.
Puschner B, Aleman M. Lead toxicosis in the horse: a review. Eq Vet Educ 2010; 22(10):526–530.
Sojka JE, Hope W, Pearson D. Lead toxicosis in two horses: similarity to equine degenerative lower motor disease. J Vet Int Med 1996; 10(6):420–423.

Authors: Tim J. Evans, DVM, MS, PhD, DACT, DABVT
Consulting editors: Lynn R. Hovda, RPh, DVM, MS, DACVIM; Robert H. Poppenga, DVM, PhD, DABVT

Chapter 41

Selenium

DEFINITION/OVERVIEW

- Selenium has a narrow therapeutic window.
- Selenium is the only regulated mineral with a maximum feed inclusion of 0.3 ppm.
- Deficiency and intoxications both occur; acute and chronic intoxications have been reported.
- The most common cause of selenium intoxication in livestock is iatrogenic.
- Acute selenosis most often occurs as a result of over-supplementation either via miscalculated feed supplementation or parenteral medications:
  - Clinical signs most notably involve the respiratory, cardiovascular, and gastrointestinal systems.
  - The most well-known case of equine acute selenium intoxication involved a miscalculated injectable selenium supplement that resulted in the acute death of 21 Venezuelan polo horses in Florida.
- Chronic selenosis is associated with forages that naturally accumulate selenium:
  - The most obvious clinical signs include hair and hoof abnormalities

ETIOLOGY/PATHOPHYSIOLOGY

Mechanism of Action
- Toxic effects in the body are not clear despite a wealth of research.
- Likely dependent on chemical form.

Acute
- Selenium can react with thiols to produce free radicals, resulting in oxidative tissue damage.
- Depletion of intermediate substrates (glutathione and S-adenosylmethionine) disrupt enzyme pathways.
- Incorporation of selenium in place of sulfur in proteins disrupts normal cellular functions.

Chronic
- Incorporation of selenium in place of sulfur in disulfide bridges that provide structural integrity to keratinized tissues particularly hair and hooves.
- Possibly inhibit DNA methylation by S-adenosylmethionine.

Blackwell's Five-Minute Veterinary Consult Clinical Companion: Equine Toxicology,
First Edition. Edited by Lynn R. Hovda, Dionne Benson, and Robert H. Poppenga.
© 2022 John Wiley & Sons, Inc. Published 2022 by John Wiley & Sons, Inc.
Companion website: www.wiley.com/go/hovda/equine

Toxicokinetics

- Absorption primarily occurs in the small bowel:
  - The chemical form of selenium greatly impacts absorption.
  - Relative absorption ranges from 45% to 95%.
- Tissue distribution is dependent on the chemical form.
- Selenium generally is incorporated into tissue proteins, utilized for selenoprotein synthesis, or eliminated.
- Metabolism occurs in red blood cells and liver via different pathways depending on the chemical form.
- Selenium is mainly eliminated via urine with some fecal elimination.

Systems Affected

- Cardiovascular.
- Gastrointestinal.
- Musculoskeletal.
- Respiratory.
- Integumentary.

SIGNALMENT/HISTORY

- There are no known age, breed, or sex predilections.
- Horses appear to be more sensitive to selenium than ruminants and can show clinical signs on pastures that are safe for cattle to graze.

Risk Factors

- Certain areas in Montana, the Dakotas, Nebraska, Wyoming, Colorado, Kansas, Oklahoma, Arizona, New Mexico, Utah, Nevada, and Idaho are known to have seleniferous soils with increased plant uptake.
- Certain plants require high concentrations of bioavailable selenium to grow and are known as obligate accumulators:
  - *Astragalus* spp., *Oonopsis* spp., *Xylorrhiza* spp., and *Stanleya* spp.
- The presence of these plants indicates high soil selenium concentration.
- These plants are often unpalatable.
- Other plants (including grasses and crops) grown in these soils can accumulate enough selenium from the soil to cause chronic selenosis.
- Water-soluble selenium can leach from the soil into water and be a significant source.

CLINICAL FEATURES

Acute selenosis

- Often presents as sudden death with few to no clinical signs.
- The clinical course is often rapid.
- Dyspnea, weakness, diarrhea, colic, lethargy, and anorexia.

- Tachycardia and dyspnea along with cyanosis and a weak pulse.
- Animals will usually succumb to lethal doses within 12–24 hours.

Chronis selenosis
- This condition is known as "Alkali disease".
- Usually results from chronic (months) exposure to seleniferous forages.
- The most obvious signs are symmetric bilateral alopecia and dystrophic growth of the hooves.
- Alopecia is usually limited to the mane and tail but will occasionally involve other parts of the body.
- Hoof growth abnormalities often result in lameness as well as reddening and swelling of the coronary bands.
- The lesions can progress to circumferential cracking and hoof separation.
- Affected animals become so lame they can't eat or drink normally resulting in emaciation.
- "Blind staggers" has historically been attributed to selenium but is more likely related to excessive sulfur intake.

DIFFERENTIAL DIAGNOSIS

Acute selenosis
- Heavy metal poisoning (arsenic, lead).
- Blister beetle ingestion.
- Endotoxemia.
- Ionophore intoxication.
- Organophosphate or carbamate insecticide intoxication.
- Anthrax.

Chronic selenosis
- Ergotism.
- Laminitis.
- Thallium intoxication.
- Frostbite.
- Fluorosis.

DIAGNOSTICS

- Diagnosis is based on clinical signs, pathological findings, biochemical changes, and chemical analysis of tissues, feed and environmental samples.

CBC/Serum Chemistry/Urinalysis
- Acute selenosis – nonspecific changes indicating damage to the heart, liver, and GI tract.
- Chronic selenosis is not reliably associated with any clinical pathology abnormalities.

Other Diagnostic Tests
- Tissue concentrations can vary considerably with tissue, the chemical form of selenium, type of analysis used, and the presence of other elements that may bind selenium.
- Tissue concentrations do not reliably correlate with tissue damage.

- Samples traditionally recommended for analysis include whole blood, serum, urine, liver, kidney, hoof, and hair.
- Urine and serum concentrations can change relatively quickly.
- Whole blood and liver are better indicators if sampling is delayed.
- Blood and liver concentrations >1 ppm wet weight are suggestive of selenosis.
- Hair and hoof are theoretically more reliable for analysis of selenium intake over time.

Pathological Findings

Acute selenosis
- Pale, mottled, flaccid heart.
- Hydrothorax and ascites indicative of acute congestive heart failure.
- Petechial or ecchymotic hemorrhaging of the myocardium and thoracic viscera.
- Congested lungs with septal edema and froth in the airways.
- Myofiber degeneration and interfascicular hemorrhage.
- Hyperemia or hemorrhage of the GI tract.
- Hepatic centrilobular necrosis and renal proximal tubular necrosis are often seen histologically.

Chronic selenosis
- Classic lesion is alopecia of the main and tail and separation of the hoof wall.
- Atrophy of the primary hair follicles can be seen histologically.
- Keratinocytes near the tips of the primary laminae will be degenerate and have evidence of necrosis.

THERAPEUTICS

- There are no effective treatments for acute intoxication.
- Supportive care and antioxidants (vitamin E) may be helpful.
- Uncomplicated chronic selenosis can be successfully managed.

Detoxification
- Detoxification is likely of little value once clinical signs are observed

Antidotes
- There are no known antidotes.

Drugs of choice
- Antioxidants like vitamin E may be of some use in acute intoxications.
- NSAIDs and analgesics are imperative in chronic cases for pain abatement.

COMMENTS

Client Education
- Clients should be made aware of the potential catastrophic nature of acute selenium intoxication when giving parenteral medications.
- Diets lacking protein can exacerbate selenium toxicity.
- All dietary constituents and water can be analyzed to determine total dietary intake.

Prevention/Avoidance

- Avoiding excess selenium exposure is imperative to preventing intoxication.
- Clients in high-selenium areas should avoid selenium-containing mineral supplements.

Expected Course and Prognosis

- Acute selenium intoxication is often fatal and warrants a poor prognosis.
- Chronic selenosis can be successfully managed but will often be a lengthy recovery process – mainly due to the time it takes to regrow hoof tissue to alleviate lameness.

Abbreviations

See Appendix 1 for a complete list.

Suggested Reading

Hall JO. Selenium. In: Gupta RC, ed. Veterinary Toxicology: Basic and Clinical Principles, 3rd edn. San Diego, CA: Elsevier, 2018; pp. 469–477.
Maldonado G, et al. Acute selenium toxicosis in polo ponies. J Vet Diagn Invest 2011; 23(3):623–628
Raisbeck MF. Selenosis. Vet Clin North Am Food Anim Pract 2000; 16:465–481.

Author: Scott Fritz, DVM
Consulting Editor: Robert H. Poppenga, DVM, PhD, DABVT

Mycotoxins/Fungus

Chapter 42

Aflatoxins

DEFINITION/OVERVIEW

- Aflatoxins are a large group of mycotoxins produced by certain mold species, including *Aspergillus flavus* and *A. parasiticus* under specific environmental conditions.
- Aflatoxin B1 (AFB1) is most toxic and is usually present in the highest concentrations in feedstuffs.
- A wide variety of feedstuffs can be contaminated, including corn, oats, and many other common ingredients in equine feeds, both in the field and during storage.
- Aflatoxins can cause acute or chronic liver disease, depending on the dosage and duration of ingestion.

ETIOLOGY/PATHOPHYSIOLOGY

Mechanism of Action

- The toxic metabolites of aflatoxins are reactive epoxides, which cause hepatocellular dysfunction and necrosis, bile duct hyperplasia, and, in chronic cases, hepatic fibrosis.

Toxicokinetics

- Rapid and complete absorption from the small intestine, primarily the duodenum. Rate is more rapid in young animals.
- Liver primary site of metabolism. In horses, olfactory and respiratory tissues are secondary sites of metabolism.
- Mixed-function oxidases (cytochrome P450, or CYPs) produce reactive epoxides, which bind cellular DNA, RNA, and proteins, impairing cell function.
- Glutathione conjugation is considered the primary detoxification pathway.
- Excretion occurs in bile, feces, urine, and milk.

Toxicity

- Chronic poisoning more common than acute.
- 2 mg/kg administered as a single oral dose was lethal to ponies.
- 3.8 ppm in the diet lethal to some ponies after 37–39 days.
- 0.5 ppm (500 ppb) in the diet produced clinical signs.

Blackwell's Five-Minute Veterinary Consult Clinical Companion: Equine Toxicology,
First Edition. Edited by Lynn R. Hovda, Dionne Benson, and Robert H. Poppenga.
© 2022 John Wiley & Sons, Inc. Published 2022 by John Wiley & Sons, Inc.
Companion website: www.wiley.com/go/hovda/equine

Systems Affected

- Gastrointestinal – anorexia, diarrhea, weight loss, abdominal straining, bloody feces.
- Hepatobiliary – icterus, hyperbilirubinemia, elevated SDH, AST, and GGT.
- Hemic/lymphatic/immune – anemia, coagulopathy, petechiae, ecchymoses, hemorrhage, immunosuppression.
- Musculoskeletal – weakness.
- Endocrine/metabolic – hyperthermia.
- Nervous – depression, obtundation, convulsions.
- Neuromuscular – ataxia, tremors.
- Respiratory – coughing, tracheal exudate.

SIGNALMENT/HISTORY

- There is no age, breed, or sex predilection; however, absorption of toxins is more rapid in young animals.

Risk Factors

- Corn or other grains or grain by-products in the diet.
- Field contamination most likely in areas with warm ambient temperature and high relative humidity. Insect damage, drought, or other crop stress increases risk.
- Storage contamination can occur anywhere feed is not properly stored. Damage to grains during handling increases risk.
- Young animals may be more susceptible.
- Animals on poor-quality diet are at greater risk.

Historical Findings

- Initial clinical signs of chronic aflatoxin poisoning can be subtle.
- Decreased appetite or feed refusal, weight loss, general unthriftiness, and a rough or unkempt haircoat are often reported.
- Multiple animals are usually affected if consuming the same contaminated feed.
- Diet includes corn or other grains or grain by-products.

CLINICAL FEATURES

- Dependent on dosage and duration of exposure.
- Chronic (most common) – anemia, icterus, anorexia, depression.
- Hepatic encephalopathy can cause behavior changes, head-pressing, and somnolence.
- Acute – anorexia, depression, weakness, diarrhea with blood or mucus, icterus, hyperthermia, epistaxis, tremors, ataxia, convulsions.
- Inhaled aflatoxins may result in coughing, tracheal exudate, and chronic obstructive pulmonary disease.

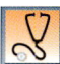

DIFFERENTIAL DIAGNOSIS

- Other causes of liver disease:
    - Toxic – pyrrolizidine alkaloid-containing plants, mushrooms, cocklebur (*Xanthium strumarium*), lantana (*Lantana camera*), alsike clover, blue-green algae, phenolics, coal tar derivatives, and iron.
    - Infectious – viral (Theiler's disease), bacterial (leptospirosis).
    - Inflammatory – hepatitis, cholangitis, cholangiohepatitis.
    - Metabolic – hepatic lipidosis.
    - Cholelithiasis.
    - Neoplasia.

DIAGNOSTICS

CBC/Serum Chemistry/Urinalysis

- CBC – anemia.
- Chemistry – elevated AST with normal CK; elevated GGT, SDH, hyperbilirubinemia.
- Coagulation panel – prolonged aPTT, PTT.

Other Diagnostic Tests

- Liver biopsy – hepatocellular necrosis, megalocytosis, bile duct hyperplasia.
- Aflatoxin testing of feed or biological samples (most helpful in recent exposures):
    - Detection methods include ELISA, GC-MS, and LC-MS.
    - See www.aavld.org for a list of accredited veterinary diagnostic laboratories.
- Urine, liver, and kidney of recently exposed animals may contain detectable aflatoxin residues, but analysis is often unrewarding:
    - Most aflatoxin is excreted within several days of exposure, but onset of clinical signs can be delayed for several weeks.
- Feed testing can also be unrewarding. Contaminated bags of feed may have been entirely consumed by the time clinical signs are apparent.

Pathological Findings

- Icterus.
- Enlarged, pale tan liver.
- Intestinal hemorrhage.
- Multifocal petechiae, ecchymoses, and/or hemorrhage.
- Centrilobular hepatocellular degeneration and necrosis.
- Megalocytosis.
- Bile duct hyperplasia.
- Hepatic fibrosis.
- Cerebral edema.
- Renal tubular necrosis.

THERAPEUTICS

Detoxification

- Activated charcoal may be helpful in recent ingestions, but most exposures are chronic.
  - 1–4 g/kg in a water slurry PO.

Appropriate Health Care

- Remove source. Provide high-quality nutrition, hydration, and liver support.
- Offer a high-quality diet, especially protein, vitamins, and trace minerals
- Maintain perfusion and electrolyte balance with crystalloid IV fluids.
- Supplement with dextrose and/or electrolytes as necessary.
- Monitor liver enzymes; GGT usually remains elevated the longest.

Antidotes

- There is no specific antidote.

Drugs of Choice

- Hepatic support:
  - N-acetylcysteine.
  - SAM-e.
  - Silymarin (milk thistle).

Precautions/Interactions

- Avoid medications metabolized by the liver.

COMMENTS

Prevention/Avoidance

- Never feed moldy feeds or forages.
- Store feed in a clean, dry location protected from rodent and insect damage.
- Screen feeds periodically for mycotoxins.
- Mold retardants such as propionic acid may help to prevent mold growth during storage but do not affect toxin already present.
- Management of insect pests in fields reduces contamination of corn.

Possible Complications

- Animals may never fully regain normal liver function.

Expected Course and Prognosis

- Depends on dosage and duration of exposure. Prognosis worsens with higher dosage and longer exposure.
- Guarded even with treatment once clinical signs of liver disease are apparent.

Abbreviations
See Appendix 1 for a complete list.

Suggested Reading
Bischoff K. Aflatoxin toxicosis. In: Wilson DA, ed. Clinical Veterinary Advisor: The Horse. St Louis: Elsevier, 2012.
Caloni F, Cortinovis C. Toxicological effects of aflatoxins in horses. Vet Journal 2011; 188:270–273.
Meerdink GL. Aflatoxins. In: Plumlee KH, ed. Clinical Veterinary Toxicology. St Louis: Elsevier, 2004.
Riet-Correa F, Rivero R, Odriozola E, et al. Mycotoxicoses of ruminants and horses. J Vet Diagn 2013; 25(6):692–708.

Author: Megan C. Romano, DVM, DABVT
Consulting Editor: Robert H. Poppenga, DVM, PhD, DABVT

Chapter 43

Fescue (Endophyte-Infected Tall Fescue)

DEFINITION/OVERVIEW

- Toxicosis in horses and ruminants associated with ingestion of endophyte-infected tall fescue grass [*Schedonorus arundinaceus* (Schreb.) Dumort or *Lolium arundinaceum* (Shreb.) Darbysh]. This disease syndrome in horses is primarily manifested in late-gestational mares (i.e., post-gestation day 300). Previous names for this grass include *Festuca elatior* L. and *Festuca arundinacea* (Schreb.).
- The endophyte is a fungus (*Epichloë coenophiala* or *Neotyphodium coenophialum*) that lives in a mutualistic relationship within the intercellular spaces of tall fescue grass. Previous names for the fungus include *Acremonium coenophialum* and *Epichloë typhina*.
- The endophyte produces ergot alkaloids, the most prominent being an ergopeptine alkaloid or ergot peptide alkaloid, ergovaline.
- The endophytic ergot alkaloids produced are mycotoxins – secondary fungal metabolites.
- Ergovaline concentrations are highest in seed heads during late spring and early summer months; concentrations are increased by excessive rain and addition of nitrogen containing fertilizers.
- Fescue hay has lower but still potentially toxic concentrations of ergovaline.
- Non-endophyte-infected fescue cannot become infected by the endophyte, however, endophyte-infected (E+) fescue outcompetes non-E+ fescue and will eventually take over a pasture.
- Nontoxic E− (novel E+ or genetically modified E+) varieties of tall fescue have been developed and can greatly reduce the chances of intoxication, until possible repopulation of pastures with E+ tall fescue.

ETIOLOGY/PATHOPHYSIOLOGY

Mechanism of Action

- Ergovaline is a potent D_2-dopamine receptor agonist, suppressing prolactin secretion.
- Prolactin is essential for equine mammary development and milk production as well as for the production of reproductive hormones, especially progestogens, biogenesis, and normal immune function.
- Ergovaline has also been associated with vasoconstriction in horses.

Blackwell's Five-Minute Veterinary Consult Clinical Companion: Equine Toxicology, First Edition. Edited by Lynn R. Hovda, Dionne Benson, and Robert H. Poppenga.
© 2022 John Wiley & Sons, Inc. Published 2022 by John Wiley & Sons, Inc.
Companion website: www.wiley.com/go/hovda/equine

Toxicokinetics

- Ergot alkaloids, including ergovaline, may be absorbed via active transport mechanisms and are almost immediately removed from the peripheral circulation.
- Metabolism occurs in the liver.
- Depending on molecular size, ergot alkaloid excretion occurs via urine and feces.

Toxicity

- Any tall fescue should be considered infected by a toxic endophyte, unless the owner has purposely planted an endophyte-free or a nontoxic endophyte variety, in which case testing for ergopeptine alkaloids or total ergot alkaloids is recommended.
- Lower percentages of E+ tall fescue in mixed pastures decrease the severity of problems; however, minimal toxic concentrations of ergovaline in pastures and hay have not been determined for horses.
- With mammary development and milk production being largely dependent on prolactin, any E+ tall fescue exposure should be considered potentially toxic for mares.

Systems Affected

- Endocrine/metabolic – aglactia/dysgalactia often the first clinical signs observed.
- Reproductive – prolonged gestation, dystocia, retained fetal membranes, and possible abortion in late-gestational mares, as well as prolonged transitional phase in non-pregnant mares and early embryonic death/conception failure. Dysmaturity/over-maturity can also be observed in foals born to mares with fescue toxicosis.
- Musculoskeletal/cardiovascular – laminitis and hyperthermia from vasoconstriction, especially with higher ergovaline concentrations.

SIGNALMENT/HISTORY

- Late gestational mares, especially during the last 30 days of pregnancy (i.e. post-gestation day 300), represent the most susceptible equine population.

Location and Circumstances of Poisoning

- E+ tall fescue is cool season, perennial grass characterized by its resistance to overgrazing, drought, and nematode infections, as well as other plant diseases, and is well suited to the growing conditions in the "fescue belt," as well as the Pacific Northwest where it is grown to produce grass seed.
- States traditionally considered as part of the "fescue belt" include large parts of Missouri, Arkansas, Illinois, Indiana, Kentucky, Tennessee, Ohio, West Virginia, Virginia, North Carolina, and South Carolina, as well as smaller portions of Kansas, Oklahoma, Mississippi, Alabama, Georgia, Maryland, and Pennsylvania.

CLINICAL FEATURES

Historical Findings

- Incomplete breeding history and/or limited records of pregnancy examination.
- Lack of udder development in mare.

- Unexpected parturition without normal mammary development and "waxing."
- Mare past her due date.
- "Red bag" presentation with premature placental separation of chorioallantois preceding foal through birth canal.
- Mare is having foaling problems/dystocia with abnormally large foal.
- Retained fetal membranes and/or metritis in mares.
- Weak, "over-mature" foal with "dummy-like" behavior, and failure of passive transfer.
- Multiple mares exhibiting agalactia, prolonged gestation, dystocia, "red bag," and/or retained fetal membranes, as well as abortion and increased incidence of stillbirths, foal dysmaturity or over-maturity, and/or failure of passive transfer are highly indicative of late-gestational exposure of mares to ergot alkaloids, especially ergopeptine alkaloids from ergot sclerotia and/or toxic E+ tall fescue
- Lower average daily gain is possible in yearlings not supplemented with concentrates.
- Higher incidence of irregular cycling of mares in the early spring, embryonic loss, an increased incidence of laminitis, and increased post-exercise hyperthermia

Physical Examination

- Agalactia or dysgalactia are the earliest and most predominant signs in mares; milk appears brown or straw-colored, rather than white, usually without a premature increase in calcium.
- Larger-than-normal foal or inadequate preparation of the reproductive tract may cause dystocia; foal may be malpositioned in the pelvis with its neck reflected to its side.
- Chorioallantois may be thickened enough that the foal has trouble breaking through and the mare may retain the fetal membranes.
- Foals are stillborn or weak.
- Foals are frequently large and gangly, with long and fine hair coats, poor muscle mass, overgrown hooves, and nonerupted incisor teeth (i.e. dysmature or over mature).
- Foals may be hypothyroid, with signs of incoordination and poor suckling reflex.
- Foals may suffer from failure of passive transfer of antibodies in colostrum, due to mare agalactia or dysgalactia; septicemia in foals is common.
- Potentially, in the early spring, an increased incidence of mares with grape-like clusters of anovulatory follicles on their ovaries, early pregnancy loss, an increased incidence of laminitis in any horses, not just mares, as well as increased hyperthermia after exercise.

 DIFFERENTIAL DIAGNOSIS

- Fescue toxicosis can be mimicked by exposure to ergot alkaloids, including ergopeptine alkaloids, such as ergocornine, ergocriptine, ergocristine, ergosine, and ergotamine associated with dark brown, black, or purplish sclerotia of ergot (*Claviceps purpurea*) in small grains (barley, oats, rye, triticale, wheat, not corn) or pastures or hay containing a wide range of grasses, including brome grass, orchard grass, ryegrass, Timothy grass and, especially, E+ tall fescue.
- Anecdotally, more severe clinical signs, including abortion, with exposure to the total concentrations of ergopeptine alkaloids in ergot sclerotia.

- Limited number of differential diagnoses for agalactia/dysgalactia in mares, other than, perhaps, some maiden mares, malnourished mares, and "idiopathic" causes.
- Other causes of dystocia, placentitis, abortion, stillbirths, and/or dysmature foals.
- Other causes of laminitis, including exposure to shavings produced from *Juglans* species (especially black walnut or butternut).

 ## DIAGNOSTICS

- Note that the following diagnostics and therapeutics focus exclusively on the effects of fescue toxicosis on pregnant mares and foals,.

CBC/Serum Chemistry/Urinalysis

- No major changes are likely, unless a stress leukogram results from prolonged parturition or dystocia, or an abnormal leukogram is caused by septicemia in the mare or foal.

Other Diagnostic Tests

- Mares – decreased serum concentrations of prolactin and progestogen (measured as progesterone by radioimmunoassay because of cross-reactivity with 5α-pregnanes) during the last 30 days of gestation; increased serum estradiol-17β has also been reported.
- Foals – decreased serum triiodothyronine and plasma adrenocorticotropin hormone and cortisol concentrations.
- Pasture or hay concentrations of ergovaline and/or ergopeptine alkaloids from ergot are likely to be > 200 ppb, on a dry-weight basis; however, no minimal toxic concentrations have been established for mares; ergopeptine alkaloid concentrations > 50 ppb are suspect.
- Endophyte contamination can be checked qualitatively by staining plant tillers at plant pathology laboratories or by ELISA testing; however, depending on the type of testing performed, nontoxic endophyte might not be differentiated from toxic endophyte.
- Total ergot alkaloids can be measured by ELISA in urine; however, ergot alkaloids are excreted very rapidly after exposure, and effects can potentially persist after exposure.

Imaging

- Ultrasonography may show a thickened placenta and large foal.

Pathological Findings

- Thickened and edematous fetal membranes without significant bacterial growth.
- Edema is most severe in the chorioallantois at the area of the cervical star.
- The amnion is edematous throughout and the umbilical cord may also be edematous.
- Fetal membranes ("placenta") may be ruptured in the uterine body rather than the typical location at the cervical star.
- Foals may be abnormally large, with overgrown hooves (increased growth of eponychium) and various patterns of incisor eruption, including non-eruption or premature eruption.
- Enlarged thyroid glands foals are not apparent grossly, but large, distended thyroid follicles lined by flat, cuboidal epithelial cells can be observed microscopically.
- If a mare dies post-dystocia, uterine rupture, metritis, and peritonitis may be present.

THERAPEUTICS

Detoxification

- None.

Appropriate Health Care

- Management of dystocia may entail a C-section or a partial fetotomy of a dead foal.
- Other symptomatic and supportive care.
- Monitor serum IgG concentration in foals to assess adequate passive transfer.
- Keep mares away from fescue for around 10–15 days until the mare is lactating well.
- Bucket- or bottle-feeding of milk replacers or a nurse mare may be needed for foal.

Antidotes

- Domperidone (see below) is a physiological antidote for agalactia or dysgalactia.

Drugs of Choice

- Retained fetal membranes:
    - Oxytocin – 10–20 IU IM, IV, or SC q2–3h.
    - Uterine infusion of fluids.
    - ± antibiotics/anti-inflammatories, as indicated by clinical circumstances.
- Domperidone, a D_2-dopamine receptor antagonist, has largely replaced other drugs (ie reserpine and perphenazine) for treating agalactia in mares and is administered as follows:
    - Give 1.1 mg/kg q24 PO for up to 10–15 days before anticipated parturition, if the mare exhibits no signs of milk production.
        - May be continued at 1.1 mg/kg q24h PO for 5–10 days after foaling at the same dosage, if lactational problems persist.
    - A similar treatment protocol for confirmed prolonged gestation, especially if a mare approaching is 360 days of gestation without any mammary development.
    - Agalactia in a mare that has already foaled can be treated q12h at 1.1 mg/kg PO for 2 days and then once a day at 1.1 mg/kg PO for at least 3 more days.
- Stored colostrum or plasma as immunoglobulin sources for foals not receiving enough colostrum; antibiotics for septicemia in foals.

Precautions/Interactions

- Domperidone stimulates GI motility; avoid use in mares with GI blockage or perforation.
- Domperidone may cause leaking of colostrum and elevated calcium in "milk" prior to foaling:
    - If this occurs, administer one-half the regular dose twice daily.
    - If colostrum loss continues, consider giving the half dose only once daily or reduce dose further.
    - Collect and save colostrum; if any colostrum is lost, monitoring serum IgG levels in the foal is essential.
- Domperidone increases calcium in mammary secretions without predicting foaling date.

Alternative Drugs

- Various "binders" are marketed to prevent the absorption of ergovaline from the GI tract

COMMENTS

Prevention/Avoidance

- Prevention is a much better approach than treatment and can be accomplished by removal of mares from E+ tall fescue pastures and/or hay, a minimum of 4 weeks before their foaling date, if there are good breeding records supported by pregnancy examinations.
- Many practitioners recommend removal from E+ tall fescue 6–8 weeks before foaling, especially if the breeding records and history of pregnancy examinations are incomplete. No mares should be exposed to any sources of ergot alkaloids beyond day 300 of gestation.
- It is important to monitor mammary development and to supervise foaling if mares reside anywhere in the "fescue belt, and forages and other feedstuffs fed during late gestation can be analyzed for ergopeptine alkaloids or total ergot alkaloids at several laboratories.
- If removal from fescue pasture is not possible, domperidone can be administered orally at 1.1 mg/kg q24h during the last 10–15 days of gestation.
- Toxic E+ tall fescue pastures can be replaced with other grasses or non-toxic varieties of novel E+ fescue, which do not contain ergovaline but retain the positive attributes of toxic E+ tall fescue; endophyte-free tall fescue is not very hardy or persistent.

Possible Complications

- Mare dystocia, uterine rupture, peritonitis, metritis, laminitis, and rebreeding difficulties.
- Residual health problems in foals following septicemia.

Expected Course and Prognosis

- Generally good if diagnosed and treated prior to foaling; otherwise, prognosis is guarded.

Abbreviations

See Appendix 1 for a complete list.

Internet Resources

Cornell College of Agriculture and Life Sciences. Fescue Toxicosis in Horses. February 28, 2019. Available at: https://poisonousplants.ansci.cornell.edu/toxicagents/fesalk.html (accessed February 20, 2021).
Dechra Equidone® Gel Website Information Sheets on Fescue Toxicosis. Available at: https://www.dechra-us.com/Files/Files/SupportMaterialDownloads/us/at_a_glance_fescue_toxicosis.pdf
https://www.dechra-us.com/Files/Files/SupportMaterialDownloads/us/fescue_factsheet.pdf (accessed February 21, 2020).

Suggested Reading

Brendemuehl JP, Boosinger TR, Pugh DG, Shelby RA. Influence of endophyte-infected tall fescue on cyclicity, pregnancy rate and early embryonic loss in the mare. Theriogenology 1994; 42(3):489–500.

Boosinger TR, Brendemuehl JP, Bransby DL, et al. Prolonged gestation, decreased triiodothyronine concentration, and thyroid gland histomorphologic features in newborn foals of mares grazing Acremonium *coenophialum*-infected fescue. Am J Vet Res 1995; 56:66–69.

Cross DL, Redmond LM, Strickland JR. Equine fescue toxicosis: signs and solutions. J Anim Sci 1995; 73(3):899–908.

Cross DL. Fescue toxicosis in horses. In: Bacon CW, Hill NS, eds. Neotyphodium/Grass Interactions. New York: Plenum Press, 1997; pp. 289–309.

Evans TJ. Endocrine disruptive effects of ergopeptine alkaloids on pregnant mares. Vet Clin North Am Equine Pract 2011; 27(1):165–173.

Evans TJ, Youngquist RS, Loch WE, Cross DL. A comparison of the relative efficacies of domperidone and reserpine in treating equine "fescue toxicosis". Proc Ann Convention AAEP, Albuquerque, NM 1999 (abstract, p. 207).

Klotz JL, McDowell KJ. Tall fescue ergot alkaloids are vasoactive in equine vasculature. J Anim Sci 2017; 95(11):5151–5160.

Authors: Tim J. Evans, DVM, MS, PhD, DACT, DABVT
Consulting Editors: Robert H. Poppenga, DVM, PhD, DABVT; Lynn R. Hovda, DPh, DVM, MS, DACVIM

Fumonisins

Chapter 44

DEFINITION/OVERVIEW

- Fumonisins are a group of mycotoxins produced by *Fusarium* species, including *F. verticilloides* and *F. proliferatum*, that can contaminate corn and occasionally other grains.
- Fumonisins B1 and B2 are clinically relevant.
- In horses, fumonisins can cause equine leukoencephalomalacia (ELEM), liver failure, and cardiac dysfunction.

ETIOLOGY/PATHOPHYSIOLOGY

Mechanism of Action

- Altered sphingolipid metabolism leads to accumulation of sphingolipid intermediates and depletion of complex sphingolipids critical for cellular metabolism.
- Target organs are the CNS, the liver, and the heart.

Toxicity

- Horses appear to be the most sensitive species.
- Toxic dose depends on duration of exposure.
- One study found ELEM associated with ingestion of feed containing > 10 ppm fumonisin B1.
- For equine rations, the FDA's recommended maximum level of total fumonisins is 1 ppm.

Systems Affected

- Nervous – altered mentation, depression, somnolence, head-pressing, circling, aimless wandering, excitation, frenzied behavior, compulsive walking, apparent blindness, tonic-clonic seizures, sudden death.
- Neuromuscular – ataxia, stumbling, falling, paresis, facial paralysis.
- Gastrointestinal – decreased appetite.
- Hepatobiliary – icterus.
- Hemic/lymphatic/immune – petechiae, ecchymoses, hemorrhage.
- Cardiovascular – bradycardia, decreased cardiac output.
- Respiratory – dyspnea.

Blackwell's Five-Minute Veterinary Consult Clinical Companion: Equine Toxicology, First Edition. Edited by Lynn R. Hovda, Dionne Benson, and Robert H. Poppenga.
© 2022 John Wiley & Sons, Inc. Published 2022 by John Wiley & Sons, Inc.
Companion website: www.wiley.com/go/hovda/equine

SIGNALMENT/HISTORY

Risk Factors

- Fumonisin production is increased when periods of insect damage, drought, or other plant stresses are followed by cool, wet weather during pollination.
- Corn or corn by-products in the diet. Corn screenings, broken kernels, and distiller's grain products carry highest risk of contamination.

Historical Findings

- Abrupt onset of neurological signs including aimless wandering, circling, depression, somnolence, head-pressing, compulsive walking, frenzied behavior, ataxia, seizures, and death.
- Early neurologic signs can be subtle, and can include decreased tongue tone, difficulty chewing, conscious proprioception deficits, and mild ataxia.
- May also have a history of decreased appetite.
- Multiple animals on a farm are usually affected if consuming the same diet.

CLINICAL FEATURES

- Can occur within 5–8 days of ingesting large amounts of fumonisin, or can be delayed for weeks with repeated lower dosages.
- Onset of signs can occur 12 days or more after removal of contaminated feed.
- Signs of ELEM include altered mentation, depression, somnolence, head-pressing, compulsive walking, frenzy, hyperexcitability, marked ataxia, muscle tremors, and recumbency.
- Hepatotoxicosis can cause icterus, depression, hemorrhage, and death.
- Cardiovascular effects include bradycardia and decreased cardiac output.

DIFFERENTIAL DIAGNOSIS

- Other causes of neurologic dysfunction:
    - Infectious – rabies, arboviral encephalitides (e.g., EEE, WNV), bacterial infection/abscess.
    - Trauma.
    - Toxic – lead, sodium, botulism, blue-green algae, mushrooms, plants (locoweeds).
    - Metabolic – hyperammonemia.
    - Neoplasia.
- Other causes of liver disease:
    - Toxic – pyrrolizidine alkaloid-containing plants, mushrooms, cocklebur (*Xanthium strumarium*), lantana (*Lantana camera*), alsike clover, aflatoxin, blue-green algae, phenolics, coal tar derivatives, and iron.
    - Infectious – viral (Theiler's disease), bacterial (leptospirosis).
    - Inflammatory – hepatitis, cholangitis, cholangiohepatitis.
    - Metabolic – hepatic lipidosis.
    - Cholelithiasis.
    - Neoplasia.

DIAGNOSTICS

- History and clinical signs.
- Corn or corn by-products in the diet.

CBC/Serum Chemistry/Urinalysis

- Chemistry – elevated liver enzymes with hepatotoxic syndrome.

Other Diagnostic Tests

- CSF – elevated albumin, total protein, and IgG.
- Fumonisin testing of feed is usually unrewarding due to delayed onset of clinical signs. Contaminated feed is often gone by the time clinical signs are apparent.
  - Methods include ELISA and HPLC.
  - See www.aavld.org for a list of accredited veterinary diagnostic laboratories.
- Currently no tests for fumonisin residues in biological samples.

Pathological Findings

- Softening and necrosis of cerebral and/or brainstem white matter. Often bilaterally asymmetrical, but can be unilateral. Lesions range from pinpoint necrosis to extensive cavitation and collapse of grey matter.
- Hepatomegaly, yellowish liver, and hepatocyte vacuolation and necrosis can be seen with hepatotoxic syndrome.

THERAPEUTICS

- Remove affected feeds and provide supportive care. Treatment unrewarding with ELEM. Animals with liver damage only can recover but might not regain normal liver function.

Detoxification

- Delayed onset of clinical signs precludes decontamination.

Appropriate Health Care

- Offer a high-quality diet.
- Maintain perfusion and electrolyte balance with crystalloid IV fluids.
- Supplement with dextrose and/or electrolytes as necessary.

Antidotes

- No antidote is available.

Drugs of Choice

- Hepatic support:
  - N-acetylcysteine.
  - SAM-e.
  - Silymarin (milk thistle).

Precautions/Interactions

- Avoid drugs metabolized by the liver in hepatotoxic syndrome.

COMMENTS

Patient Monitoring

- Liver enzymes in hepatotoxic syndrome

Prevention/Avoidance

- Do not feed corn screenings, broken kernels, distiller's grain products, or moldy feeds.
- Screen feeds periodically for mycotoxins.

Expected Course and Prognosis

- Prognosis is grave for ELEM. Most symptomatic animals die.
- Prognosis for hepatotoxic syndrome is guarded even with treatment.

Abbreviations

See Appendix 1 for a complete list.

Suggested Reading

Caloni F, Cortinovis C. Effects of fusariotoxins in the equine species. Vet J 2010; 186:1 7-1-1.
Mostrom MS. Fumonisin toxicosis. In: Wilson DA, ed. Clinical Veterinary Advisor: The Horse. St Louis: Elsevier, 2012.
Riet-Correa F, Rivero R, Odriozola E, et al. Mycotoxicoses of ruminants and horses. J Vet Diag Invest 2013; 25(6):692–708.
Smith GW, Constable PD. Fumonisin. In: Plumlee KH, ed. Clinical Veterinary Toxicology. St Louis: Elsevier, 2004.

Author: Megan C. Romano, DVM, DABVT
Consulting Editor: Robert H. Poppenga, DVM, PhD, DABVT

Fusaria

Chapter 45

DEFINITION/OVERVIEW

- The *Fusarium* spp. produce a number of mycotoxins, including the trichothecenes, zearalenone, and fumonisins (see Chapter 44).
- The trichothecene class is produced predominantly by *Fusarium sporotrichioides*, and consists of approximately 150 mycotoxins including deoxynivalenol (DON; Vomitoxin), T-2 toxin, diacetoxyscirpenol (DAS), and nivalenol.
- Zearalenone, a weak estrogen, is produced primarily *Fusarium roseum* (*Fusarium graminearum*) in corn, but has also been reported in wheat, barley, rice, and *Sorghum*.
- Zearalenone toxicosis is uncommon in horses.
- Feeds may be co-contaminated with multiple mycotoxins.
- Most commonly found in Canada and north-central USA and primarily in corn and wheat.
- Fungal infection of grain, with or without toxin production, reduces nutrient quality, leading to poor production and nutritional impairment of animals.
- Once produced, the trichothecenes and zearalenone are environmentally stable compounds.

ETIOLOGY/PATHOPHYSIOLOGY

Mechanism of Action

- Trichothecenes have multiple effects on cells including inhibition of protein, RNA, and DNA synthesis.
- The trichothecenes are potent inhibitors of protein synthesis and other effects could be secondary to decreased protein synthesis.

Toxicity

- Although trichothecenes are toxic to multiple species, few studies specific to horses have been published.
- Dietary tolerance concentration guidelines in the total ration dry matter for horses are suggested to be:
  - T-2 toxin: 0.7–1.5 ppm.
  - DON: 2.5–6 ppm.

- Zearalenone: 3.9–7 ppm.
- Higher concentrations are potentially harmful.

Systems Affected

- Gastrointestinal.
- Hemic/lymphatic/immune.
- Integument (dermal).
- Reproductive.

SIGNALMENT/HISTORY

- Neonatal animals are more susceptible to effects of the trichothecenes.
- Failure of implantation and early embryonic death were reported in swine administered zearalenone.

Risk Factors

- Ingestion of contaminated grain or processed feed, or inhalation via contaminated bedding.

Historical Findings

- Trichothecene mycotoxins and zearalenone are resistant to heat and pressure of food processing and are stable in the environment.
- Unusually cool weather conditions in late summer and early fall coupled with heavy rainfall can result in trichothecene production.
- High concentrations of zearalenone usually result from improper storage at high moisture concentrations (> 30–40%).

CLINICAL FEATURES

- Horses appear to be resistant to the effects of DON; feed refusal is reported in sensitive animals.
- Experimentally, T-2 and DAS can cause dermal irritation and necrosis, lymphoid depletion, gastroenteritis, cardiovascular failure and death at concentrations which are unlikely to occur in the field.
- In one case report, zearalenone was associated with edema and flaccidity of the equine genitals.

DIFFERENTIAL DIAGNOSIS

- For the GI effects of the trichothecenes:
  - Cantharidin toxicosis – detection of cantharidin in gastric contents or urine, evidence of insects in hay or GI contents, characteristic lesions.
  - *Ranunculus* spp. – blistering of skin and mouth, erythema and swelling of muzzle and lips, evidence of ingestion.
  - NSAIDs.
  - Arsenic – arsenic concentration in liver, kidney, urine, hair, feed, hemorrhagic gastroenteritis.

- Castor bean (*Ricinus communis*) and other toxic lectins – clinical signs, detection of ricin in tissues, evidence of beans in GI contents, histopathology.
- Gastroenteritis due to a number of infectious agents such as *Salmonella* serovars, *Clostridium* spp., *Aeromonas* spp., coronavirus, and cyathostomiasis.
■ For the reproductive effects of zearalenone:
- Fescue toxicosis

DIAGNOSTICS

CBC/Serum Chemistry/Urinalysis
■ No clinically significant changes.

Other Diagnostic Tests
■ Feed can be tested for mycotoxins.
■ Due to uneven distribution of mycotoxins in feeds it is critical to obtain a representative sample for testing.

Pathological Findings
■ No pathognomonic lesions for DON.
■ T-2 and DAS – dermal and mucosal irritation, necrosis, intestinal inflammation, lymphoid necrosis.
■ Zearalenone – swelling of vulva and uterus, ovarian atrophy.

THERAPEUTICS

Detoxification
■ Removal of contaminated feed and/or bedding. Animals should return to normal performance in weeks to months following removal from toxin.

Appropriate Health Care
■ There is no specific treatment for the trichothecenes or zearalenone.
■ Symptomatic and supportive treatment is recommended.

Antidotes
■ There are no antidotes.

COMMENTS

Prevention/Avoidance
■ Feed should be visually inspected and tested for the presence of mycotoxins.
■ Avoiding late harvests, removing overwintered stubble from fields, and avoiding a corn/wheat rotation that favors *Fusarium* growth in crop residue can reduce contamination of grains.

- Store grains at less than 13–14% moisture to prevent mycotoxin production.
- Various binders such as clay-based and yeast cell wall extracts for inclusion in mycotoxin-contaminated feeds have been suggested to prevent adverse effects. However, long-term effects of binding agents are unclear, and they should be used with caution.

Possible Complications

- Poor performance in exposed animals.

Expected Course and Prognosis

- The clinical effects are expected to resolve following removal of the toxin.

See Also

Fescue
Fumonisins

Abbreviations

See Appendix 1 for a complete list.

Internet Resources

Molds, Mycotoxins and their Effect on Horses. Available at: http://www.omafra.gov.on.ca/english/livestock/horses/facts/info_mycotoxin.htm#levels.

Suggested Reading

Caloni F, Cortinovis C. Effects of fusariotoxins in the equine species. Vet J 2010; 186:157–161.
Mostrom MS. Zearalenone. In: Gupta RC, ed. Veterinary Toxicology: Basic and Clinical Principles, 2nd edn. San Diego, CA: Elsevier, 2012; p. 1266.
Mostrom MS, Raisbeck MF. Trichothecenes. In: Gupta RC, ed. Veterinary Toxicology: Basic and Clinical Principles, 2nd edn. San Diego, CA: Elsevier, 2012; pp. 1239.
Osweiler GD. Mycotoxins. Vet Clin North Am Equine Pract 2001; 17:547–566.
Songsermsakul P, Bohm J, Aurich C, et al. The levels of zearalenone and its metabolites in plasma, urine and faeces of horses fed with naturally, Fusarium toxin-contaminated oats. J Anim Physiol Anim Nutr (Berl) 2013; 97:155–161.
Villar D, Carson TL. Trichothecene mycotoxins. In: Plumlee KH, ed. Clinical Veterinary Toxicology. St Louis, MO: Mosby, 2004; pp. 270.

Acknowledgement: The author and editors acknowledge the prior contribution of Petra Volmer.

Author: Robert H. Poppenga DVM, PhD, DABVT
Consulting Editor: Lynn R. Hovda, RPh, DVM, MS, DACVIM; Robert H. Poppenga DVM, PhD, DABVT

Chapter 46

Slaframine

DEFINITION/OVERVIEW

- Slaframine is a mycotoxin produced by *Rhizoctonia leguminicola*, the causative organism of black patch disease of red clover and other legumes. Slaframine causes the "slobbers" syndrome of livestock characterized by excessive salivation.

ETIOLOGY/PATHOPHYSIOLOGY

Mechanism of Action

- The active metabolite is a parasympathomimetic cholinergic agonist, with a structure similar to acetylcholine and a high affinity for M3 muscarinic receptors.
- Causes profound stimulation of exocrine glands, particularly salivary glands.

Toxicokinetics

- Rapidly absorbed from the GI tract.
- Activated by hepatic microsomal enzymes to active ketoimine metabolite.

Systems Affected

- Skin/exocrine – excessive salivation, lacrimation.
- Gastrointestinal – anorexia, bloat, colic, diarrhea.
- Renal/urologic – polyuria.
- Musculoskeletal – stiff joints.
- Nervous – lethargy, depression.

SIGNALMENT/HISTORY

Risk Factors

- Risk of slaframine toxicosis higher with increased amounts of red clover hay or other legume forage in the diet.
- Primary host of *R. leguminicola* is red clover. Infection of other legumes typically occurs when red clover is also present in the pasture.

Blackwell's Five-Minute Veterinary Consult Clinical Companion: Equine Toxicology, First Edition. Edited by Lynn R. Hovda, Dionne Benson, and Robert H. Poppenga. © 2022 John Wiley & Sons, Inc. Published 2022 by John Wiley & Sons, Inc. Companion website: www.wiley.com/go/hovda/equine

- Risk of fungal infection of legumes is highest in cool, wet weather.
- Affected hay may retain slaframine for as long as 2 years.

Historical Findings

- Profuse salivation.

CLINICAL FEATURES

- Ptyalism.
- Dehydration.
- Occasionally colic, bloat, or diarrhea.
- Rarely develop other clinical signs, including polyuria, stiff joints, depression, and very rarely death. Some of these signs may be due to swainsonine, another toxic alkaloid produced by *R. leguminicola*.

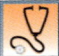

DIFFERENTIAL DIAGNOSIS

- Other causes of excessive salivation:
  - Rabies.
  - Oral, esophageal, GI, or other neurologic system infection.
  - Trauma – grass awns (foxtail, needlegrass), burs (cocklebur, burdock), insoluble oxalates (dumbcane), acid or alkali ingestion.
  - Toxic – cholinesterase inhibitors (organophosphates, carbamates), plants (azalea, horse nettle, milkweeds, spurge), blister beetles, bufo toads, phenols.
  - Inflammatory – gingivitis.
  - Neoplastic – oral, esophageal, GI, or neurologic system neoplasia.

DIAGNOSTICS

- Clinical signs.
- Legume forage in the diet.
- Examine forage for mold.
- Forage testing for slaframine is available, but not routinely pursued.
  - See www.aavld.org for a list of accredited veterinary diagnostic laboratories.

Pathological Findings

- Not described. Rarely fatal.

THERAPEUTICS

- Remove source and provide supportive care.

Appropriate Health Care

- Fluid support as needed.

Antidotes

- Atropine may help decrease salivation in severe cases, but is less effective at treating than preventing excessive salivation.
- Atropine can have serious adverse effects in equines, including potentially fatal ileus, and is not routinely used to treat slaframine toxicosis.

COMMENTS

Client Education

- Clinical signs may persist for several days after contaminated forage is removed.

Prevention/Avoidance

- Never feed moldy feeds or forages.
- Attempts at detoxifying slaframine in pastures or hay have been unsuccessful.
- Controlling fungal infection of legumes relies on selecting more resistant varieties and chemically treating seeds. Fungicide treatments applied to plants have been largely unsuccessful.

Expected Course and Prognosis

- Excellent once removed from source.

Abbreviations

See Appendix 1 for a complete list.

Suggested Reading

Imerman PM. Slaframine toxicosis. In: Wilson DA, ed. Clinical Veterinary Advisor: The Horse. St Louis: Elsevier, 2012.
Meerdink GL. Slaframine. In: Plumlee KH, ed. Clinical Veterinary Toxicology. St Louis: Elsevier, 2004.
Riet-Correa F, Rivero R, Odriozola E, et al. Mycotoxicoses of ruminants and horses. J Vet Diagn Invest 2013; 25(6):692–708.
Smith GW. Slaframine. In: Gupta RC, ed. Veterinary Toxicology. Cambridge: Elsevier, 2018.

Author: Megan C. Romano, DVM, DABVT
Consulting Editor: Robert H. Poppenga, DVM, PhD, DABVT

Chapter 47

Tremorgenic Mycotoxins

DEFINITION/OVERVIEW

- Tremorgenic mycotoxins include lolitrems and paspalitrems.
- Lolitrems (lolitrems A, B, C, and D) are produced by *Neotyphodium lolii* and cause perennial ryegrass (*Lolium perenne*) staggers.
    - *N. lolii* is an endophytic fungus of ryegrass and propagates via seed.
- Paspalitrems (paspalinine, paspalitrem A, B and C) are produced by *Claviceps paspali* and cause dallis grass or paspalum staggers [associated with dallis grass (*Paspalum dilatatum*) and bahia grass (*Bahia oppositifolia*)].
    - *C. paspali* is a soil fungus that invades dallis and bahia grass under favorable environmental conditions
- Annual ryegrass toxicosis, the clinical presentation of which is similar to that of tremorgenic mycotoxins, can result when the bacterium *Clavibacter toxicus* is carried into annual ryegrass seedheads by the nematode *Anguina funesta*.
    - *C. toxicus* produces the neurotoxin corynetoxin, a glycolipid that inhibits the synthesis of lipid-linked oligosaccharides and blocks protein glycosylation.
- The specific tremorgen associated with Bermuda grass (*Cynodon dactylon*) has not been isolated.

ETIOLOGY/PATHOPHYSIOLOGY

Mechanism of Action

- Some tremorgens competitively inhibit CNS postsynaptic GABA receptors and cause chloride influx; GABA receptor antagonism leads to increased nerve discharge and neurologic signs.
- Lolitrem B inhibits calcium-activated potassium channels, thereby perturbing motor function.

Toxicokinetics

- Signs typically occur within 5–10 days of being on affected highly toxic pastures.
- Recovery occurs in several weeks after being removed from pastures.

Blackwell's Five-Minute Veterinary Consult Clinical Companion: Equine Toxicology, First Edition. Edited by Lynn R. Hovda, Dionne Benson, and Robert H. Poppenga.
© 2022 John Wiley & Sons, Inc. Published 2022 by John Wiley & Sons, Inc.
Companion website: www.wiley.com/go/hovda/equine

Systems Affected
- Nervous.

SIGNALMENT/HISTORY

- No breed, sex, or age predispositions.

Risk Factors
- Perennial ryegrass staggers:
  - Incidence is greater during the late summer and fall and on ryegrass pastures that have been heavily grazed.
  - Environmental temperatures are generally > 23°C.
  - Frequency of intoxication is related to the degree of fungal infection of the ryegrass. Infection rates < 25% are associated with sporadic outbreaks, whereas rates > 90% are associated with large outbreaks.
- Paspalum staggers:
  - Toxin production is greatest during a warm and wet period following seedhead formation.
- Annual ryegrass staggers:
  - Toxin concentration increases in seedheads during the summer and is greatest as the plant dries and seeds ripen.
  - Annual ryegrass occurs in patches, and alterations in grazing patterns may predispose to ingestion.
  - Newly introduced animals may ingest more ryegrass.

Historical Findings – see "Risk factors."

Location and Circumstances of Poisoning – see "Risk factors."

CLINICAL FEATURES

- Ryegrass staggers (perennial and annual):
  - Signs occur 5–10 days after grazing highly toxic pastures.
  - Signs include head tremors and muscle fasciculations of the neck and legs, which progress to head nodding and swaying while standing.
  - Animals that are forced to move develop dysmetria and leg stiffening, leading to collapse and tetanic spasms; if left alone, animals recover in a few minutes and walk away with a relatively normal gait.
  - Affected animals rarely die unless they injure themselves during a tetanic spasm.
  - Affected animals may lose weight and are difficult to handle or move because of inducible spasms.
- Paspalum staggers:
  - Signs are identical to those above but often less severe.

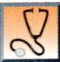
DIFFERENTIAL DIAGNOSIS

- Other plant intoxications such as locoism (*Astragalus* spp.) and white snakeroot (*Eupatorium rugosum*) – evidence of plant consumption, characteristic histopathologic lesions, detection of tremetol in white snakeroot toxicosis.
- Viral or bacterial encephalopathy.

DIAGNOSTICS

CBC/Serum Chemistry/Urinalysis
- No particular changes.

Other Diagnostic Tests
- Perennial ryegrass staggers:
  - Positive identification of perennial ryegrass.
  - Microscopic detection of fungus in ryegrass.
  - While testing for specific toxins is limited, some laboratories do offer testing (http://oregonstate.edu/endophyte-lab/) and should be consulted for costs and appropriate samples to submit:
    - Detection of lolitrems in ryegrass – concentrations of lolitrem B > 2 ppm is associated with effects in sheep and cattle.
    - ELISA for detection of lolitrem B.
- Paspalum staggers:
  - Positive identification of dallis or bahia grass and associated fungal sclerotia on grass seedheads.
  - Detection of tremorgen
- Annual ryegrass staggers:
  - Positive identification of annual ryegrass.
  - Identification of galls associated with nematode infestation.
  - ELISA for detection of corynetoxin.

Pathological Findings
- Gross lesions generally are absent
- Animals with chronic ryegrass staggers may have loss of Purkinje cells in the cerebellum, which is believed to be secondary to hypoxia and hypoglycemia.
- Histopathologic changes associated with annual ryegrass staggers include cerebellar, hepatic, and splenic hemorrhages that may be secondary to endothelial cell damage.

THERAPEUTICS

Detoxification
- As clinical signs develop over several days, decontamination is not effective.

Appropriate Health Care

- Remove animals from affected grass pastures.
- Attempt to prevent self-injury during tetanic spasms.
- Symptomatic and supportive care.

Antidotes

- There is no antidote.

Drugs of Choice

- Tremors:
    - Methocarbamol 4.4–22 mg/kg IV for moderate signs and 22–55 mg/kg IV for severe signs. Administer ½, pause until relaxation occurs, then administer remainder to effect. Do not exceed 330 mg/kg/day.
- Sedation:
    - Detomidine 0.02–0.04 mg/kg IV.
    - Romifidine 0.04–0.12 mg/kg IV.
    - Xylazine 1.1mg/kg IV; 2.2 mg/kg IM.
- Sedation/seizures:
    - Diazepam 25–50 mg IV (adults); 0.1–0.4 mg/kg IV (foals).

Precautions/Interactions

- Care should be taken for people dealing with a neurological horse.

COMMENTS

Prevention/Avoidance

- Perennial ryegrass staggers:
    - Reduce overgrazing of pastures.
    - Remove animals from pastures during critical periods – late summer and fall for endophyte-infested ryegrass pastures.
    - Use endophyte-free ryegrass seed.
    - Use fungicides – reduces seed viability.
- Paspalum staggers:
    - Inspect pastures for ergotized seedheads.
    - Mow pastures to remove toxic seedheads.
- Annual ryegrass staggers:
    - Break nematode life cycle by killing ryegrass for two or three growing seasons.
    - Integrated control measures – herbicide use in the spring, seeding pastures with legumes, burning infested pastures in the early fall, applying herbicides to selectively kill ryegrass during the summer, and heavy winter grazing.

Possible Complications

- Traumatic injury.
- Bloating or drowning during tetanic spasm.

Expected Course and Prognosis

- Once removed from affected pastures, animals generally recover within several weeks without treatment.
- Degenerative CNS lesions associated with chronic perennial ryegrass staggers is likely prevent full recovery.

Abbreviations

See Appendix 1 for a complete list.

Suggested Reading

Cawdell-Smith AJ, Scrivener CJ, Bryden WL. Staggers in horses grazing paspalum infected with *Claviceps paspali*. Aust Vet J 2010; 88(10):393–395.

Plumlee KH, Galey FD. Neurotoxic mycotoxins: a review of fungal toxins that cause neurologic disease in large animals. J Vet Intern Med 1994; 8:49–54.

Authors: Arya Sobhakumari, DVM, PhD, ERT, DABT, DABVT; Robert H. Poppenga, DVM, PhD, DABVT

Consulting Editors: Lynn R. Hovda, RPh, DVM, MS, DACVIM; Robert H. Poppenga, DVM, PhD, DABVT

Other Toxins

Chapter 48

Clostridium botulinum Toxin

DEFINITION/OVERVIEW

- Anerobic, spore-forming, rod-shaped Gram-positive bacterium.
- Botulism neurotoxin (BoNT) is the potent neurotoxin responsible for clinical signs:
  - Eight serotypes types (A, B, C1, C2, D, E, F, G).
  - Types A, B, C1, and D have been reported to cause disease in domestic animals.
- The spores can be found in the soil in most regions around the world:
  - In the United States, botulism of soil origin affecting horses is caused by BoNT types A and B (occasionally type C).
  - Animals may also ingest feed contaminated with animal carcasses. This source usually contains BoNT types C and D.

ETIOLOGY/PATHOPHYSIOLOGY

Mechanism of Action

- Tissue proteases activate the BoNT by cleavage into light and heavy chains connected by a disulfide bridge.
- Toxins are taken up into endosomes and translocated into the cytosol of the cell where they cleave with SNARE (soluble n-ethylmaleimide sensitive factor attachment protein receptor) proteins.
  - SNARE proteins are required for neurotransmitter release.
- When BoNT combines with a SNARE protein, it destabilizes or prevents the formation of a SNARE complex which does not allow for acetylcholine release.
- This action occurs at the level of the neuromuscular junction.

Toxicokinetics

- There are three sources of intoxication:
  - Ingestion of toxin:
    - Contaminated forage.
    - Round bales that are tightly wrapped in plastic film are often a source of intoxication.
  - Wound infection:
    - Sporulation within a wound and subsequent systemic absorption.

Blackwell's Five-Minute Veterinary Consult Clinical Companion: Equine Toxicology,
First Edition. Edited by Lynn R. Hovda, Dionne Benson, and Robert H. Poppenga.
© 2022 John Wiley & Sons, Inc. Published 2022 by John Wiley & Sons, Inc.
Companion website: www.wiley.com/go/hovda/equine

- Toxicoinfectious botulism:
  - Ingestion of spores which then germinate within the gastrointestinal tract where the toxin is absorbed systemically.
- Once the toxin has bound the motor end plate, new axon and new motor end plate formation must occur for resolution of clinical signs. This could take weeks to months.

Toxicity

- Ingestion of contaminated feed material is the most common route of infection.
- Shaker foal syndrome:
  - Toxicoinfectious botulism (caused by type B).

Systems Affected

- Musculoskeletal system – flaccid paralysis:
  - Skeletal muscle.
  - Can also affect smooth muscle.
- Respiratory system – hypoventilation, aspiration pneumonia:
  - Seen in more severe cases where the muscles of respiration become weak.
  - Pneumonia may be seen in cases where regurgitation has occurred.

SIGNALMENT/HISTORY

- Can affect horses of all ages and breeds.

Risk Factors

- Round bales that are tightly wrapped in plastic film are often a source of intoxication.
- Occasionally, carcasses of small rodents can be incorporated into round bales or grain augers.
- Spore germination and toxin formation occurs in conditions of high pH, low oxygen, and high-water content.

Historical Findings

- Horses who have access to round bales may be at an increased risk of ingesting spores or the toxin.
- A horse displaying clinical signs of botulism that is also being treated for an infected wound could have botulism spores within the wound.
- Shaker foal syndrome. Typically seen in foals aged 2–6 weeks.

Location and Circumstances of Poisoning

- United States distribution:
  - BoNT type A is most commonly seen in Western states, particularly in Idaho and Oregon.
  - BoNT type B is endemic in Kentucky and the mid-Atlantic states.
  - BoNT type C cases are seen occasionally throughout the country.
  - BoNt type D cases are rare in horses.

CLINICAL FEATURES

- The severity and progression of disease are dose-dependent.
- Low toxin dose:
    - The only clinical sign may be mild dysphagia, which presents as a slow-eating horse that is clumsy about chewing and drops feed.
    - These cases typically progress over the course of 5–7 days and resolve with minimal treatment.
- High toxin dose:
    - Horses who are affected by a high toxin load will become recumbent within 8–12 hours and often die within 48 hours of the first clinical signs.
- Subtle signs of muscle weakness:
    - Tongue weakness.
        - This is an important and consistent early sign of intoxication.
        - Tongue strength can be tested by gently pulling on the tongue and observing the horse's ability to retract it.
    - Food may be retained in the cheeks.
        - As the disease progresses in severity, water may run out of the nostrils when the horse attempts to drink.
    - Sluggish pupillary light reflex.
    - Horses may walk with a shuffling gait and low head carriage.

DIFFERENTIAL DIAGNOSIS

- Diseases that cause infectious encephalomyelitis:
    - Equine protozoal myeloencephalitis.
    - Eastern equine encephalitis.
    - Western equine encephalitis.
    - Venezuelan equine encephalitis.
    - Equine herpesvirus myeloencephalopathy.
    - West Nile encephalitis.
- Diseases associated with generalized myopathy.
- Polysaccharide storage myopathy.
- Equine motor neuron disease.
- Grass sickness.
- Hyperkalemic periodic paralysis.
- Heavy metal toxicity.

DIAGNOSTICS

CBC/Serum Chemistry/Urinalysis

- Complete blood count and serum chemistry panels tend to be unhelpful and abnormalities are non-specific.

Other Diagnostic Tests

- In order for a definitive diagnosis to be made, spores must be present.
- The toxin may be found in blood serum, gastrointestinal material or infected wounds.
- Antibodies may be seen in the serum.
- If contaminated feed is the suspected source, spores may be found within that feed material.

 THERAPEUTICS

Detoxification

- Removal of suspected contaminated food source.
- Cleaning of open wound with antibacterial solution.

Appropriate Health Care

- Dysphagic horses should be administered water and food slurries via nasogastric tube.
  - Feedings should only be performed with horses in sternal recumbency.
- Recumbent horses need to be kept on deep, clean bedding with bony prominences padded with pillows or inflatable, circular tubes to prevent the formation of decubital ulcers
  - Horses unable to maintain sternal recumbency should have their recumbency changes several times per day by manually rolling.
  - These horses are at greater risk for colic.
- Horses who are not recumbent but have weak neck muscles will hang their heads:
  - These horses are at an increased risk of developing facial and upper respiratory tract edema.
  - The head needs to be supported such that it is maintained at the level of, or above the heart.
- Frequent blood work:
  - Packed cell volume and total protein can be monitored daily to evaluate hydration status.
  - Total CO_2:
    - A value < 18 mEq/L indicates metabolic acidosis.
    - A value > 35 mEq/L indicates metabolic alkalosis. This finding suggests that the body is compensating for respiratory acidosis that may be secondary to hypoventilation due to respiratory muscle paralysis or aspiration pneumonia
  - Arterial blood gas:
    - PaO_2 < 65 mmHg indicates that the horse or foal should be administered humidified oxygen via nasal cannula insufflation.
    - Patients who develop respiratory acidosis secondary to hypoventilation may require mechanical ventilation if $PaCO_2$ > 60 mmHg. This is realistically only feasible in foals.

Antidotes

- A trivalent antitoxin is commercially available in the United States:
  - Adult horses – 50,000 IU.
  - Foals – 20,000 IU.

- A single dose is usually sufficient due to the long half-life.
▪ Minimal efficacy if administered after the onset of recumbency in adult horses.

Drugs of Choice

▪ Antibiotic therapy is indicated in the case of wound botulism or if secondary aspiration pneumonia develops.
▪ These patients may also require gastroprotection therapy with proton pump inhibitors and H_2 blockers:
  - Omeprazole 4 mg/kg q24h.
  - Ranitidine 6.6–10 mg/kg q8h.

Precautions/Interactions

▪ Aminoglycosides, tetracycline, procaine penicillin and metronidazole are contraindicated.
  - Aminoglycosides block neurotransmission and will potentiate the effects of the toxin on the neuromuscular junction.
  - Tetracycline, procaine penicillin, and metronidazole will damage the cell walls of the bacteria which will release more toxin.

COMMENTS

Prevention/Avoidance

▪ Remove plastic wrap from around bales and allow bales to dry.
▪ Clean wounds daily.

Possible Complications

▪ Metabolic acidosis – can be treated with IV fluid therapy.

Expected Course and Prognosis

▪ Administration of antitoxin before clinical signs become severe greatly increases survival rate.
▪ Rate of recovery is dependent on the toxin type and dose.
▪ Dysphagic horses who are able to stand should gradually regain the ability to swallow over the course of 1–14 days.

Abbreviations

See Appendix 1 for a complete list.

Suggested Reading

Coffield JA, Whelchel DD. Botulinum neurotoxin. In: Veterinary Toxicology. St Louis, MO: Elsevier Saunders, 2007; pp. 755–770.
Galey FD. Botulism in the horse. Vet Clin North Am: Equine Practice 2001; 17(3):579–588.
Diseases of the nervous system: motor unit and cauda equina diseases - botulism. In: Smith B, ed. Large Animal Internal Medicine, 5th edn. St Louis, MO: Elsevier Saunders, 2015; pp. 1000–1002.

Author: Sarah Jarosinski, DVM
Consulting Editor: Lynn R. Hovda, RPh, DVM, MS, DACVIM

Chapter 49

Cyanide

DEFINITION/OVERVIEW

- Cyanide toxicosis can occur through the ingestion of plants containing cyanogenic glycosides (CG) resulting in acute death. Over 3,000 species of plants are known to contain varying concentrations of the 75 known CG.
- Common plant sources for animals include species from the genera *Prunus* (almond, apricot, chokecherry, peaches, wild black cherry), *Sorghum* (Johnson grass, milo sorghum, sudan grass), *Suckleya suckleyana* (poison suckleya), *Sambucus nigre* (elderberry), and *Mannihot esculentum* (cassava).
- Seeds of plants contain the highest concentration of CG followed by the leaves, bark, and fruit.
- Intoxication in equine species is rare but has been reported.

ETIOLOGY/PATHOPHYSIOLOGY

Mechanism of Action

- Damage to the plant through various means, including but not limited to freezing, cutting, crushing, and mastication releases intrinsic enzymes that degrade CGs, resulting in the release of cyanide.
- Cyanide binds the ferric (Fe^{3+}) heme moiety of cytochrome *c* oxidase, resulting in impairment of the mitochondrial ETC.
- Oxygen is still carried by the blood, but it cannot be utilized, resulting in anoxia and death.

Toxicokinetics

- Absorption – cyanide is rapidly absorbed from the GI tract.
- Excretion – cyanide is excreted in the urine as thiocyanate after combining with endogenous thiosulfate.

Toxicity

- LD = 4.4 mg/kg.

Blackwell's Five-Minute Veterinary Consult Clinical Companion: Equine Toxicology, First Edition. Edited by Lynn R. Hovda, Dionne Benson, and Robert H. Poppenga.
© 2022 John Wiley & Sons, Inc. Published 2022 by John Wiley & Sons, Inc.
Companion website: www.wiley.com/go/hovda/equine

Systems Affected

- As a result of the inability to utilize oxygen and cellular hypoxia, all body systems are affected.
- Cardiovascular – arrhythmias and hypotension.
- Respiratory – respiratory distress and difficulty breathing.
- Nervous – ataxia and tremors can be observed.

SIGNALMENT/HISTORY

- There are no breed, sex, or age predilections.

Risk Factors

- Young plants < 60 cm tall contain higher concentrations of CG.
- Events that damage plants resulting in the release of hydrolytic enzymes and free cyanide.
- Poisoning occurs following the consumption of fresh leaves that have fallen as a result of freezing or wind.
- Intoxication has been reported in individuals consuming bark from cherry trees.

Historical Findings

- Onset of clinical signs is rapid and can occur within 15–20 minutes. Animals are likely to be found dead.
- Staggering.
- Weakness.
- Respiratory difficulty/acute dyspnea.
- Tremoring.
- Convulsions.
- Death.

Location and Circumstances of Poisoning

- Plants located in arid regions tend to have greater concentrations of hydrogen cyanide.

CLINICAL FEATURES

- Cherry red blood may be observed.

DIFFERENTIAL DIAGNOSIS

- CO – measurement of carboxyhemoglobin in the blood.
- Yew (*Taxus*) – identification of plant material or detection of taxine alkaloids in the stomach contents.

- Cyanobacteria – exposure to algal blooms, identification of toxin-producing algal species, or detection of cyanotoxins in tissue or GI tract.
- Ionophores – myocardial or skeletal muscle necrosis, detection of ionophores in feed GI contents or tissues.

DIAGNOSTICS

- Cyanide analysis of whole blood, liver, GI contents, and suspect material.
- Samples should be collected in an air-tight container and frozen immediately.

Pathological Findings

- Gross and histological lesions are not commonly observed.
- Bright cherry red blood.
- Ingesta may possess a bitter almond odor.
- Cystitis and degeneration of nerve fibers may be observed with chronic intoxications.

THERAPEUTICS

Detoxification

- AC may help bind cyanide within the GI tract.
- Sodium thiosulfate at 20 g in solution may be used orally to detoxify cyanide in the GI tract.

Appropriate Health Care

- Treatment and supportive care should be provided immediately to be effective.
- The goal of treatment is to re-establish the mitochondrial ETC by breaking the bond between cyanide and cytochrome *c* oxidase.
- Supportive care includes supplemental oxygen.

Drugs of Choice

- Sodium nitrite and sodium thiosulfate may be used in conjunction with each other.
- Initial administration of sodium nitrite induces a methemoglobinemia that draws cyanide from cytochrome *c* oxidase to form cyanomethemoglobin.
- Administration of sodium thiosulfate converts cyanomethemoglobin to thiocyanate to be excreted in the urine.
    - Sodium nitrite 10–20 mg/kg as a 20% solution.
    - Sodium thiosulfate 30–40 mg/kg as a 20% solution.
    - Can be administered IV as a mixture of 1 mL of 20% sodium nitrite and 3mL of 20% sodium thiosulfate at 4 mL per 45 kg of body weight.
- Sodium thiosulfate may be used alone in unconfirmed cases but should ideally be used in sequence with sodium nitrite.
- Rapid onset of clinical signs and potentially rapid recovery often preclude therapeutic intervention.

Precautions/Interactions

- Sodium nitrite should be used with caution in unconfirmed cyanide intoxication, and if repeat dosing is necessary, 10 mg/kg every 2–4 hours can be given IV to reduce potential for nitrite intoxication and severe methemoglobinemia.
- Vomiting and hypotension can occur with sodium thiosulfate.

Alternative Drugs

- 1% methylene blue at 4–22 mg/kg IV can be used to induce methemoglobinemia but is not as effective as sodium nitrite.
- Hydroxycobalamin (vitamin B_{12}) may be used to attract cyanide from cytochrome c oxidase but may cause injection site reactions, GI upset, pruritus, and dysphagia.

COMMENTS

Client Education

- Be aware of potential sources of cyanide that horses may be exposed to, including vegetation and cyanide salts.

Prevention/Avoidance

- Avoid exposure to and consumption of cyanogenic plants.
- Avoid grazing *Sorghum* species when < 60 cm.
- Avoid turning out animals that have had been withheld from feed into high-risk environments.
- Allow forages and vegetation to dry prior to feeding.

Expected Course and Prognosis

- Death or recovery occurs rapidly.

Abbreviations

See Appendix 1 for a complete list.

Suggested Reading

Cheeke PR. Natural Toxicants in Feeds, Forages, and Poisonous Plants, 2nd edn. Danville, IL: Interstate Publishers, 1998.
Cope R. Overview of cyanide poisoning. In: Aiello SE, Moses MA, eds. Merck Veterinary Manual, 11th edn. Kenilworth, NJ: Merck Sharp & Dohme Corp., 2016
Jackson T. Cyanide poisoning in two donkeys. Vet Hum Toxicol; 37:567–568.
Osweiler GD, Carson TL, Buck WB, Van Gelder GA. Clinical and Diagnostic Veterinary Toxicology, 3rd edn. Dubuque, IA: Kendall/Hunt Publishing Company, 1985.
Thompson, LJ. Cyanide toxicosis. In: Blackwell's Five-Minute Veterinary Consultant Equine, 3rd edn. Hoboken, NJ: John Wiley and Sons Inc., 2020.

Acknowledgement: The editors acknowledge the prior contribution of Larry J. Thompson.

Author: Scott L. Radke, DVM, MS
Consulting Editor: Robert H. Poppenga, DVM, PhD, DABVT

Chapter 50

Sodium Chloride (Salt)

DEFINITION/OVERVIEW

- Sodium is the major extracellular cation in the body, and is therefore critical for maintenance of the extracellular space
- Serum sodium concentration reflects the ratio of whole-body sodium to whole-body water; knowledge of the hydration state is important for accurate interpretation of serum sodium concentrations
- The "normal" serum sodium concentration is generally < 144 mEq/L. There is no true "cut-off", but serum sodium concentrations > 155 mEq/L require some treatment.
- Salt toxicity is rare in horses and usually occurs from chronic ingestion of improperly mixed or formulated feeds, owners over-supplementing in cold winter months, or an overzealous horse consuming several large salt blocks.
- Alternatively, iatrogenic administration of excessive amounts of sodium bicarbonate or hypertonic saline can result in toxicity, particularly in foals.
- Rarely, road salt contaminates a pasture or field, but as a general rule not enough is left to cause any issues.
- Hypernatremia from water loss may occur when a horse has a limited water supply, primarily in the winter when stock tanks and waterers have frozen.

ETIOLOGY/PATHOPHYSIOLOGY

Mechanism of Action

- Two mechanisms affect the brain:
  - Sudden increases in serum sodium and osmolality cause water to shift out of the cells, resulting in cellular dehydration.
  - Brain mass shrinks from cerebral tissue dehydration. Tearing of small meningeal vessels and secondary hemorrhage or hematoma formation occur.
- Rapid increases in serum sodium may cause hypervolemia as fluid shifts from the intracellular compartment into the vasculature.

Blackwell's Five-Minute Veterinary Consult Clinical Companion: Equine Toxicology,
First Edition. Edited by Lynn R. Hovda, Dionne Benson, and Robert H. Poppenga.
© 2022 John Wiley & Sons, Inc. Published 2022 by John Wiley & Sons, Inc.
Companion website: www.wiley.com/go/hovda/equine

Toxicity

- While there is no true "cut-off" for horses, serum concentrations > 155 mEq/L are generally associated with hypernatremia.
- Different forms of hypernatremia:
  - High whole-body sodium – excessive sodium chloride intake (i.e., salt poisoning) with water restriction; IV or oral administration of hypertonic saline or sodium bicarbonate solutions.
  - Normal whole-body sodium with pure water loss – water deprivation because of unavailable water source or physical abnormality causing decreased ingestion (e.g., botulism or dysphagia); prolonged hyperventilation; central and nephrogenic diabetes insipidus; evaporative loss from extensive burns; exhausted horse syndrome.
  - Low whole-body sodium with hypotonic fluid loss – urinary loss (osmotic diuresis, e.g., osmotic diuretic administration such as mannitol); gastrointestinal loss (early stages of diarrhea, before the point of compensatory water intake occurs).

Systems Affected

- Nervous – lethargy, depression, ataxia, seizures.
- Cardiovascular – tachycardia.
- Endocrine – hypernatremia, hyperchloremia, metabolic acidosis, hyperthermia.
- Renal – PU/PD.
- Respiratory – changes secondary to hypervolemia.
- Gastrointestinal – anorexia, diarrhea.
- Musculoskeletal – tremors.

SIGNALMENT/HISTORY

- No true age, breed, or sex predilection, although foals, in particular ill foals, are more likely to have iatrogenic-induced hypernatremia.

Risk Factors

- Access to large amounts of salt or limited access to fresh water.

CLINICAL FEATURES

- Severity of clinical signs depends on the duration and degree of hypernatremia.
- Lethargy.
- Weakness.
- Hyperthermia.
- Tachycardia.
- Tremors.

- Seizures.
- Coma.
- Death.
- Other signs depend on the underlying cause.

DIFFERENTIAL DIAGNOSIS

- Pure water loss – heat stroke, hyperthermia, severe burns, lack of water supply or decreased intake; other medical conditions (diabetes insipidus).
- Hypotonic fluid losses – excess diuretic administration; GI disease, renal failure.

DIAGNOSTICS

CBC/Serum Chemistry/Urinalysis

- High serum sodium concentration.
- ± high chloride concentration.
- Plasma osmolality – should be high with hypernatremia.
- Hyposthenuria – consider diabetes insipidus.

Other Diagnostic Tests

- Urinary FE_{Na} (fractional excretion of sodium) – a single urine sample can be used for sodium and creatinine measurements, which are compared with serum sodium and creatinine concentrations determined at the same time ($[Na^+_u/Na^+_s]/[Cr_u/Cr_s]$; normal < 1%); suspect extrarenal water loss if urine volume with $FE_{Na} < 1\%$ and clinical signs of dehydration; suspect osmotic diuresis if urine volume is increased with an $FE_{Na} = 1\%$ and clinical signs of dehydration.

THERAPEUTICS

Detoxification

- Reflux with large-bore tube for witnessed acute ingestions, otherwise no other decontamination.

Appropriate Health Care

- Hospitalize as needed and monitor electrolytes, acid–base status, urine output, water intake, and body weight.
- Treatment depends on whether the intoxication is acute or chronic, the severity of hypernatremia, and whether there is an underlying disorder.
- If increases in sodium and chloride are proportional, administer IV fluids such that decreases in serum sodium concentration do not exceed 0.5 mEq/L/hour.

- IV crystalloids to correct dehydration in acute intoxications. If chronic ensure that crystalloids are iso-osmotic with patient (i.e., match the serum sodium).
- Free water replacement to correct the water deficit – either orally or IV. If giving IV, 5% dextrose in water is recommended.
- If chloride is increased disproportionately compared with sodium, evaluate and treat the acid–base imbalance.

Antidotes

- There is no antidote.

Drugs of Choice

- Anticonvulsants as needed:
  - Diazepam 25–50 mg IV (adults); 0.1–0.4 mg/kg IV (foals).
  - Phenobarbital 16–20 mg/kg IV × one dose.
- Methocarbamol if tremors are severe:
  - 4.4–22 mg/kg IV (moderate signs); 22–55 mg/kg (severe signs). Administer ½ of the dose, pause until relaxation occurs, then administer remainder to effect. Do not exceed 330 mg/kg/day.

Precautions/Interactions

- The combination of hypernatremia and dehydration is a therapeutic dilemma because rapid reduction of serum sodium concentrations can lead to cerebral and pulmonary edema.
- The use of furosemide to aid in sodium excretion in hypervolemic animals (only) must be carefully balanced against dehydration.

COMMENTS

Client Education

- Prevent ingestion of salt sources.
- Provide access to water.

Possible Complications

- Seizures, convulsions, and probable permanent neurologic damage in severe, longstanding cases, or with rapid correction of serum sodium concentrations.

Expected Course and Prognosis

- Prognosis for acute exposure with mild signs is excellent with signs typically resolving in 12–24 hours.
- Prognosis for chronic exposures with more severe signs or an underlying condition is guarded to poor.

Abbreviations

See Appendix 1 for a complete list.

Suggested Reading

George JW, Zabolotzky SM. Water, electrolytes, and acid base. In: Latimer KS, ed. Duncan & Prasse's Veterinary Laboratory Medicine Clinical Pathology, 5th edn. Hoboken, NJ: Wiley Blackwell 2011; pp. 146–147.

Jose-Cunilleras E. Abnormalities of body fluids and electrolytes in athletic horses. In: Hinchcliff KW, Kaneps AJ, Geor RJ, eds. Equine Sports Medicine and Surgery, 2nd edn. Philadelphia, PA: Saunders, 2013; pp. 881–885.

Acknowledgment: The author acknowledges the prior contributions of Wendy S. Sprague and Martin David.

Author: Lynn R. Hovda, RPh, DVM, MS, DACVIM
Consulting Editor: Lynn R. Hovda, RPh, DVM, MS, DACVIM

Plants and Biotoxins

Alsike Clover (*Trifolium hybridum*)

Chapter 51

DEFINITION/OVERVIEW

- *Trifolium hybridum* (alsike clover) has been implicated as the cause of equine hepatic failure and neurologic impairment but evidence is limited.
  - Not reported in other species.
- Occurrence of the two syndromes is associated with ingestion of alsike clover, but a specific toxin has not been identified.
- Clinical manifestations of intoxication are acute and neurologic or chronic and cachectic.
- Postmortem histopathologic lesions are consistently found in the liver and include biliary fibrosis and marked bile duct proliferation.
- Photosensitization can occur in conjunction with both syndromes but is uncommon
- A reversible, alsike clover-induced photosensitization has been described and is considered by some to be unrelated to the other two syndromes.

ETIOLOGY/PATHOPHYSIOLOGY

Mechanism of Action
- Unknown since toxin(s) have not been identified.

Toxicokinetics
- Unknown.

Toxicity
- Ingestion of a diet of 20% alsike clover for a minimum of 2 weeks can cause signs of liver disease although much longer exposure times might occur.

Systems Affected
- Hepatobiliary – secondary to hepatic failure.
- Nervous – secondary to hepatic encephalopathy.
- Skin/Exocrine – secondary to photosensitization.

Blackwell's Five-Minute Veterinary Consult Clinical Companion: Equine Toxicology, First Edition. Edited by Lynn R. Hovda, Dionne Benson, and Robert H. Poppenga.
© 2022 John Wiley & Sons, Inc. Published 2022 by John Wiley & Sons, Inc.
Companion website: www.wiley.com/go/hovda/equine

SIGNALMENT/HISTORY

Risk Factors

- When both syndromes are considered together, there are no apparent breed, age or sex predispositions; however, a retrospective study of alsike clover-associated disease suggested the nervous form occurs more commonly in old, female horses.
- The disease is associated with ingestion of alsike clover-containing pasture or hay.
- Alsike clover is believed to be less palatable than other forages and horses on pasture may eat less if alternative plants are available.
  - Individual palatability differences might account for sporadic nature of affected horses in an exposed group.
- The ability of horses to avoid alsike clover in hay is less than on pasture; thus, horses fed alsike clover-containing hay may ingest more of the plant.

Historical Findings

- Feeding alsike clover hay or access to pasture containing alsike clover.

Location and Circumstances of Poisoning

- Some evidence for geographic distribution of cases in Canada.
- Environmental factors that might contribute to disease occurrence are unknown.

CLINICAL FEATURES

- Acute and neurologic – alternating depression and excitement, head pressing, aimless walking, incoordination, yawning and bruxism, coma, and death.
- Chronic and cachectic – variable appetite, progressive loss of body condition, weakness, sluggishness, dry and rough haircoat, icterus, yawning, head pressing, and periodic excitement preceding sudden death.
- Photosensitization – skin erythema and swelling, pruritus, exudation of serum, hair matting, skin exfoliation, lacrimation, conjunctivitis, photophobia, and keratitis.

DIFFERENTIAL DIAGNOSIS

- Ingestion of plants containing pyrrolizidine alkaloids.
- Locoism (*Astragalus* spp.).
- *Equisetum arvense* (horsetail) or *Pteridium aquilinum* (bracken fern).
- Fumonisin mycotoxins.
- Rabies.
- Equine protozoal myelitis.
- Viral encephalitis.
- Brain abscesses or meningitis.
- Narcolepsy.

- Other causes of liver disease such as cholangiohepatitis of infectious (Gram-negative bacteria such as *Salmonella* spp. *Escherichia coli*, *Pseudomonas* spp., and *Actinobacillus* spp.) or other etiology (e.g., cholelithiasis, duodenitis, intestinal obstruction, neoplasia, and parasitism), with or without hepatoencephalopathy.

DIAGNOSTICS

CBC/Serum Chemistry/Urinalysis
- Hyperbilirubinemia.
- Increases in liver enzymes (GGT, SDH and other less specific for hepatic damage).
- Increases in bile acids.
- Increased blood ammonia in horses with hepatic encephalopathy.

Other Diagnostic Tests
- Liver biopsy can be useful in differentiating alsike clover toxicosis from other liver diseases.

Imaging
- Ultrasonography – enlarge and irregular liver.

Pathological Findings
- Gross
  - Enlarged and irregular liver.
  - Some fibrosis may be evident.
  - Icterus is variable.
- Histopathologic:
  - Biliary hyperplasia.
  - Hepatic lesions include fibrosis of portal triads and around proliferating biliary epithelium.
  - Typically no inflammation and minimal parenchymal damage.

THERAPEUTICS

Detoxification
- Decontamination is not useful given the delay in onset of signs after exposure begins.

Appropriate Health Care
- Treat photosensitivity by preventing sun exposure.
- Remove animal from the source of the plant.
- Treatment of the hepatic and nervous syndromes commonly is unrewarding.
- Supportive care including sedation for nervous syndrome, balanced electrolyte fluid administration, correction of hypoglycemia if present, and treatment of liver failure and hyperammonemia.

- Small meals given frequently are suggested.
- Diet should provide adequate energy and limited protein, primarily as branched-chain amino acids.

Antidotes

- None.

Drugs of Choice

- Treatment for liver dysfunction is largely supportive.
- Crystalloid fluids (50 mL/kg/day) with supplemental 5% dextrose and potassium can be beneficial in some cases and is indicated in animals with hepatic encephalopathy.
- Branched-chain amino acid treatment might decrease severity of neurologic signs.
- Lactulose (0.3 mL/kg q6–12h) or neomycin (10 mg/kg q6h) PO in animals with hepatic encephalopathy to decrease ammonia production.
- Antibiotics, if infectious cholangiohepatitis is an initial differential diagnosis.

Precautions/Interactions

- Potential to alter hepatic drug metabolism or biliary excretion due to liver dysfunction.

COMMENTS

Patient Monitoring

- Monitor hepatic function.

Prevention/Avoidance

- Because the conditions under which animals are intoxicated are poorly defined, the best specific recommendation is to prevent horses from ingesting alsike clover.

Expected Course and Prognosis

- Recovery from hepatic and neurologic syndromes is unlikely.
- Recovery from uncomplicated photosensitization is expected with appropriate treatment.

Abbreviations

See Appendix 1 for a complete list.

Suggested Reading

Elfenbein, JR, House, AM. Review of pasture-associated liver disease. AAEP Proc 2011; 57:206–210.
Nation, PN. Alsike clover poisoning: a review. Can Vet J 1989; 30:410–415.
Nation PN. Hepatic disease in Alberta horses: a retrospective study of "alsike clover poisoning" (1973–1988). Can Vet J 1991; 32:602–607.

Authors: Robert H. Poppenga, DVM, PhD, DABVT; Arya Sobhakumari, DVM, PhD, DABT, DABVT
Consulting Editor: Robert H. Poppenga, DVM, PhD, DABVT

Blue-green Algae (Cyanobacteria)

Chapter 52

DEFINITION/OVERVIEW

- Blue-green algae are also called cyanobacteria, and toxin-producing blooms (i.e., rapid multiplication) occur worldwide in a variety of fresh and brackish bodies of water.
- Algal blooms can be made of a single or multiple species of algae and each species can produce more than one toxin.
- Cyanotoxins are generally grouped into hepatotoxins and neurotoxins:
  - Microcystins are potent hepatotoxins and the most common in North America.
  - There are multiple microcystin congeners that vary in their toxicity.
  - Anatoxin-a and Anatoxin-a(s) are the most common neurotoxins.
- Poisonings by cyanotoxins have occurred in pets, livestock, and humans, and suspected in a horse given a blue-green algae dietary supplement.
- The following discussion focuses on the main toxins encountered in North America (i.e., microcystins and anatoxins.)

ETIOLOGY/PATHOPHYSIOLOGY

Mechanism of Action

- Microcystins:
  - Microcystins inhibit serine and threonine protein phosphatases in hepatocytes, which leads to reorganization of cytoskeletal infrastructure and eventual apoptosis.
- Anatoxin-a:
  - Anatoxin-a is a potent acetylcholine-receptor agonist and exhibits greater affinity for nicotinic over muscarinic receptors.
- Anatoxin-a(s):
  - Anatoxin-a(s) is a naturally occurring organophosphorus compound and is a potent inhibitor of acetylcholinesterase.

Toxicokinetics

- Pharmacokinetic and bioavailability data are lacking for horses.
- Microcystins:

Blackwell's Five-Minute Veterinary Consult Clinical Companion: Equine Toxicology, First Edition. Edited by Lynn R. Hovda, Dionne Benson, and Robert H. Poppenga. © 2022 John Wiley & Sons, Inc. Published 2022 by John Wiley & Sons, Inc. Companion website: www.wiley.com/go/hovda/equine

- Microcystins are readily hydrophilic compounds that are actively absorbed from the small intestines and are preferentially taken up by hepatocytes via the organic anion transporting protein.
- Inhalation may present another route of exposure.
- Radiolabeled experiments have identified the kidney as the main excretory organ in rats.
- Metabolism is poorly defined, but glutathione and cysteine conjugation have been proposed.
- Anatoxins:
    - Based on the rapid onset of clinical signs, anatoxins are rapidly absorbed after ingestion.
    - Anatoxin-a has been detected in the urine and bile of a dog suggesting at least some renal and biliary excretion.

Toxicity

- Microcystins:
    - Reported LD_{50} values range from 50 µg/kg to 11 mg/kg dependent upon the microcystin congener, species, and route of administration and is undefined in horses.
- Anatoxins:
    - Toxicity data are based mostly on IV and IP administration to mice.
        - IP LD_{50} for anatoxin-a(s) in mice is approximately 50 µg/kg.
        - The data suggest wide species variation.
    - Calves dosed orally with a bloom containing anatoxin-a developed clinical disease, suggesting natural blooms can contain enough toxin to produce disease after oral consumption.

Systems Affected

- Microcystins:
    - Hepatobiliary.
    - Hematopoietic.
    - Gastrointestinal.
- Anatoxins:
    - Nervous.
    - Musculoskeletal.
    - Respiratory.

 # SIGNALMENT/HISTORY

- There are no known species, breed, age, or sex predilections.
- Morbidity and mortality are high in exposed animals.

Risk Factors

- Risk factors associated with harmful algal blooms are focused on environmental conditions.

- Warm (> 70°F), stagnant, nutrient-rich waters are most at risk.
- Nitrogen and phosphorus are the main nutrients of concern.
- Often, the waters receive runoff from residential, commercial, or agricultural areas contributing to nutrient loading.

Historical Findings
- Animals are often found dead.
- Accessible water sources often have obvious algal blooms present.

Microcystins
- Death due to microcystin occurs within hours to days.
- Anorexia, depression, colic, diarrhea, weakness, pale mucous membranes, and hypovolemic shock may be observed prior to death.
- Animals that survive the initial hepatic insult can have secondary photosensitivity and chronic hepatic insufficiency.

Anatoxin-a
- Death due to anatoxin-a exposure is often within minutes to hours.
- Clinical signs may include muscle tremors, paralysis, coma, and cyanosis.
- Death is due to respiratory paralysis.

Anatoxin-a(s)
- Death due to anatoxin-a(s) exposure is often within minutes to hours.
- Clinical signs will mirror anatoxin-a but with the addition of salivation, lacrimation, urination, and defecation as a result of significant action on muscarinic receptors.
- Death is due to respiratory paralysis.

Location and Circumstances of Poisoning
- Animals must have access to a water source capable of supporting a bloom.
- Blooms do not occur in automatic watering systems due to water movement and no avenue of nutrient loading.
- Animals will often be found near the water source, especially after consuming one of the anatoxins.
- Blooms generally occur in the late summer months when temperatures rise and rainfall tapers off.

CLINICAL FEATURES

- Physical exam findings will vary based on the amount and type of toxin encountered.
- Microcystins:
  - Weakness, lethargy, colic, diarrhea, and pale mucous membranes.
  - Photosensitization can occur with sub-lethal intoxication
- Anatoxins:
  - Anatoxins are so potent that animals generally die prior to veterinary intervention.

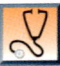
DIFFERENTIAL DIAGNOSIS

- Microcystins:
    - Theiler's disease, Tyzzer's disease, iron, pyrrolizidine alkaloids (*Senecio* spp. *Amsinckia* spp.; more chronic liver disease), Kleingrass (*Panicum coloratum*), alsike clover (*Trifolium hybridum*), cocklebur (*Xanthium* spp.).
- Anatoxin-a:
    - Numerous plants including poison hemlock (*Conium maculatum*), oleander (*Nerium oleander*), yew (*Taxus* spp.), cyanide producers, insecticides, ionophores, and other causes of acute death (e.g., lightning, trauma, intestinal torsion).
- Anatoxin-a(s):
    - OP/carbamate insecticides, slaframine.

DIAGNOSTICS

- Identification of algae and/or their toxins in a suspect water source is suggestive.
- Detection of algal toxins in gastric content is considered confirmatory.
- There are new assays using antemortem urine samples, but these need more development to be useful in a point-of-care situation.

CBC/Serum Chemistry/Urinalysis

- Microcystin – elevations in liver enzymes (AST, SDH, and bile acids), hyperammonemia, hyperkalemia, hypoglycemia, hyperbilirubinemia.
- Anatoxins – no significant laboratory abnormalities.

Other Diagnostic Tests

- Anatoxin-a(s) will depress acetylcholinesterase activity in the circulation but cannot cross the blood–brain barrier so brain acetylcholinesterase activity will remain normal.

Pathological Findings

- Microcystins:
    - Severe, massive hepatocellular degeneration and necrosis with intrahepatic hemorrhage
    - Potentially – acute renal tubular necrosis with granular casts
- Anatoxins – no known associated histopathological lesions.

THERAPEUTICS

- Therapy is often unsuccessful due to the rapid onset and progression of clinical signs.

Decontamination

- GI decontamination is likely of little use once clinical signs are observed.

Appropriate Health Care

- Microcystins:
    - Mainly supportive care, fluid therapy to combat hypovolemic shock and electrolyte disturbances.
    - Blood transfusions may be necessary in severe cases.
- Anatoxin-a:
    - General supportive care and seizure control.
- Anatoxin-a(s):
    - A test dose of atropine can be given to assess efficacy.

Antidotes

- There are no known specific antidotes for cyanotoxins.
- For anatoxin-a(s), atropine might be considered an antidote.

Drugs of Choice

- Microcystins:
    - Activated charcoal – 1–4 g/kg in a water slurry PO.
        - Questionable efficacy after clinical signs observed.
    - Lactulose (0.5 mL/kg via nasogastric tube every 6 hours).
- Anatoxin-a:
    - Diazepam to control seizures:
        - Adults – 25–50 mg IV every 30 minutes as necessary.
        - Foals – 0.05–0.4 mg/kg IV every 30 minutes as necessary.
- Anatoxin-a(s):
    - Atropine IV to effect.

Precautions/Interactions

- Atropine can cause severe GI stasis and colic.

COMMENTS

Client Education

- Clients should be made aware of the potential issues associated with blue-green algae blooms.
- Surface waters used for drinking water should be monitored.

Patient Monitoring

- Microcystins:
    - Animals that survive the acute poisoning should have liver enzymes and coagulation capabilities monitored and clients should be warned about the potential for photosensitivity to develop.

- Anatoxins:
  - Not much is known about long-term effects associated with anatoxin exposure.

Prevention/Avoidance

- Water sources should be monitored.
- Horses should not be allowed access to waters with visible algal blooms.
- There are many theories about preventing blooms in a given water source. Much research is needed in order to develop effective and economic prevention strategies.

Expected Course and Prognosis

- Animals poisoning by blue-green algae are often found dead.
- Animals that survive acute microcystin exposure may suffer from photosensitivity and chronic hepatic insufficiency.
- Animals generally do not survive anatoxin exposure.

Abbreviations

See Appendix 1 for a complete list.

Suggested Reading

Carmichael WW. The cyanotoxins. In: Callow JA, ed. Advances in Botanical Research, Vol 27. San Diego, CA: Academic Press, 1997; pp. 211–256.

McLellan NL, Manderville RA. Toxic mechanisms of microcystins in mammals. Toxicol Res (Camb). 2017; 6(4):391–405.

Puschner B. Cyanobacterial (blue-green algae) toxins. In: Gupta RC, ed. Veterinary Toxicology: Basic and Clinical Principles, 3rd edn. San Diego, CA: Elsevier, 2018; pp. 763–777.

Authors: Scott Fritz, DVM; Steve Ensley, DVM, PhD
Consulting Editor: Robert H. Poppenga, DVM, PhD, DABVT

Chapter 53

Cardiotoxic Plants

DEFINITION/OVERVIEW

- Cardiac glycosides, the major cardiac toxins, are found in a number of unrelated plants, e.g., oleander (*Nerium oleander*), summer pheasant's eye (*Adonis aestivalis*), foxglove (*Digitalis purpurea*), lily of the valley (*Convallaria majalis*), dogbane (*Apocynum* spp.), and some species of milkweed (*Asclepias* spp.).
- Other cardiotoxic plants that have poisoned horses include yew (*Taxus* spp.), grayanotoxin-containing plants (*Rhododendron* spp., *Kalmia* spp., and *Pieris japonica*), avocado (*Persea* spp.), death camas (*Zigadenus* spp.), and cheeseweed mallow (*Malva parviflora*).
- Milkweed (*Asclepias* spp.), oleander (*Nerium oleander*), rhododendron (*Rhododendron* spp.), yew (*Taxus* spp.), and death camas (*Zigadenus* spp.) are highly toxic to horses and each have a separate chapter in this book.

ETIOLOGY/PATHOPHYSIOLOGY

Mechanism of Action

- Digitalis cardiac glycosides work at the cellular level by interfering with action of the Na^+/K^+-ATPase pump on cardiac and other tissues, resulting in decreased intracellular potassium, increased serum potassium, increased sodium in the myocytes, and increased intracellular Ca^{2+}. This elevated intracellular Ca^{2+} causes a positive inotropic effect with increased cardiac contractions and bradycardia. They also have direct effects on the sympathetic nervous system.
- Taxine alkaloids, the toxin in yews, increases cytoplasmic calcium, resulting in the depression of cardiac depolarization and conduction. Yews also contain nitriles (cyanogenic glycoside esters), ephedrine, and irritant oils that may cause colic and diarrhea.
- Grayanotoxins are diterpenes that exert toxicity by maintaining cells in a state of depolarization. The membrane effects caused by grayanotoxins account for the observed responses of skeletal and myocardial muscle, nerves, and the central nervous system.
- The toxic compound in avocado is persin, but the exact mechanism of action remains unclear.

Blackwell's Five-Minute Veterinary Consult Clinical Companion: Equine Toxicology,
First Edition. Edited by Lynn R. Hovda, Dionne Benson, and Robert H. Poppenga.
© 2022 John Wiley & Sons, Inc. Published 2022 by John Wiley & Sons, Inc.
Companion website: www.wiley.com/go/hovda/equine

- Death camas contains steroidal alkaloids such as zygacine and zygadenine. The alkaloids decrease blood pressure, slow the heart rate, and lead to respiratory depression.
- Cyclopropene fatty acids present in cheeseweed mallow are suspected to impair beta-oxidation, leading to acute myopathy and cardiomyopathy.

Toxicokinetics

- Rapidly absorbed from the GI tract.
- Yews contain taxine alkaloids (major alkaloids are taxine A and taxine B) that are rapidly absorbed, metabolized, conjugated in the liver, and eliminated in urine as conjugated benzoic acid (hippuric acid).

Toxicity

- Most of these are high toxic with the majority of horses dying acutely.
- Yew, death camas, and avocado poisoning are relatively uncommon in horses.
- Grayanotoxin and cheeseweed mallow poisonings are uncommon in horses.

Systems Affected

- Cardiovascular.
- Gastrointestinal.

SIGNALMENT/HISTORY

- No breed, age, or sex predilection.

Risk Factors

- Fresh plant material is often considered to be of low palatability, so animals are most likely to ingest dried plant material.
- Contamination of hay or hay cubes with oleander is a significant risk.
- The Guatemalan "race" of avocados and its hybrid ("Fuerte") are reportedly toxic, while the Mexican "race" has low toxicity.

Historical Findings

- Ingestion of dried oleander clippings or oleander-contaminated hay is a common cause of toxicity.

Location and Circumstances of Poisoning

- Cardiotoxic plants have specific distributions in the USA.
- Oleander grows throughout southwest and southern USA.
- Summer pheasant's eye is limited to northern California.
- Grayanotoxins are widely distributed in the USA.
- Avocado is extensively cultivated in California and Florida.
- Death camas species are most abundant in the spring.
- Cheeseweed mallow is a common weed found in pastures in the USA.

CLINICAL FEATURES

- Digitalis cardiac glycosides – abdominal pain, colic, diarrhea, dehydration, weakness, bradycardia (rarely tachycardia), cardiac arrhythmias, heart block.
- Summer pheasant's eye – GI stasis, anorexia, dyspnea, and cardiac arrhythmias.
- Avocado – subcutaneous edema of the head and chest, submandibular edema, respiratory dyspnea, and cardiac arrhythmias.
- Yew – incoordination, nervousness, difficulty in breathing, bradycardia, diarrhea, and convulsions, but sudden death is often all that is seen.
- Grayanotoxins – depression, severe salivation, and abdominal pain. In severe cases, the animals may become laterally recumbent and develop seizures, tachycardia, tachypnea, and pyrexia.
- Cheeseweed mallow – diffuse sweating, muscle tremors, and tachycardia.

DIFFERENTIAL DIAGNOSIS

- Ionophore antibiotics – detection in the feed, histologic lesions.
- Cyanide poisoning – mucous membranes are initially bright cherry red; evidence of exposure to cyanogenic plants, chemical analysis for cyanide in GI contents, liver, or muscle.
- Organophosphorus or carbamate insecticide exposure – commonly associated with GI and neurologic signs, evaluation of cholinesterase activity, detection in GI contents.
- Neurotoxic plants such as poison hemlock, water hemlock, tree tobacco, lupine – chemical analysis for plant toxins in GI contents, history of presence of plants in the environment.
- Myocarditis – murmurs are usually present; differentiate echocardiographically.
- Endocarditis – fever; differentiate echocardiographically.
- Intestinal compromise – physical examination.

DIAGNOSTICS

CBC/Serum Chemistry/Urinalysis

- Serum chemistry changes are limited. Hyperkalemia may occur especially in digitalis cardiac glycoside intoxications.
- Myocardial damage may result in hyperkalemia, elevated LDH, CK, and AST activities, and elevated cTnI.

Other Diagnostic Tests

- Analytic detection of cardiotoxins in serum, stomach, cecal, or colon contents, and liver.
- Visual and microscopic examination of stomach or intestinal contents for plant fragments.

- Acyl carnitine profiles are altered after cheeseweed mallow exposure.
- ECG disturbances are supportive – AV conduction blocks and ventricular arrhythmias.

Pathological Findings

- No lesions in peracute cases.
- Oleander poisoning – fluid in the pericardium and body cavities, endocardial hemorrhages, and multifocal myocardial degeneration and necrosis. Mural thrombi and subepicardial hemorrhage can be seen.
- Yew poisoning – mild-to-moderate endocardial hemorrhages in both ventricles. Histologically, acute multifocal contraction band necrosis of the ventricular wall and the papillary muscles and occasional neutrophilic and lymphocytic infiltrates in the interstitium of the myocardium are noted.
- Grayantoxin and death camas – no or very few lesions.
- Avocado poisoning – fluid accumulation in the pericardial sac and in the thoracic and abdominal cavities.
- Cheeseweed mallow poisoning results in myocardial necrosis in atrial and ventricular walls. Skeletal muscle necrosis may also be seen.

THERAPEUTICS

Detoxification

- The use of activated charcoal (1–3 g/kg) in a watery slurry may be helpful in early or smaller ingestions, but many of these horses are found dead or die acutely. Multidose activated charcoal may be beneficial in oleander intoxications.

Appropriate Health Care

- Immediate removal of the toxic plant material to prevent further exposure. Provide the animals with high-quality diet.
- Treatment of animals is primarily supportive and symptomatic.
- Keep the animal quiet and avoid stress.
- IV crystalloids as needed; fluid choice should be based on serum electrolytes.
- Hyperkalemia may be present in digitalis cardiac glycoside intoxications.
- Monitor progression of clinical signs and evaluate ECG.
- Temporary pacemakers have been used experimentally for bradycardia unresponsive to medical management

Antidotes

- There is no specific antidote, although in humans, small animals, and a limited number of horses, digoxin specific Fab antibody fragments (Digibind, DigiFab) have been used successfully for yew, oleander, and some of the cardiac glycoside intoxications.

Drugs of Choice

- Bradycardia:
    - Atropine 0.01–0.02 mg/kg IV.
    - Glycopyrrolate 5–10 mcg/kg IV prn.

- Antiarrhythmics (guided by ECG monitoring):
  - Lidocaine 0.25–0.5 mg/kg IV slowly, repeat in 5–10 minutes if needed. Do not exceed 2 mg/kg total doses as boluses. If multiple doses are required, consider CRI.
- GI protectants:
  - Sucralfate 10–20 mg/kg PO q6–8h.
  - Omeprazole 4 mg/kg PO q24h.
- Edema is present in avocado poisoning:
  - Furosemide 250–500 mg IV or IM q6–8h.

Precautions/Interactions

- Do not administer potassium in fluids if hyperkalemia is present.
- Avoid calcium-containing solutions and quinidine.

Alternative Drugs

- Digoxin specific Fab antibodies have been used successfully in humans, small animals, and some equine oleander intoxications. Their efficacy for other cardiotoxic plant intoxications in horses is unknown.

COMMENTS

Client Education

- Recognize cardiotoxic plants of concern in the geographic location and prevent access by the horse.
- Provide adequate forage to limit ingestion of toxic plants.
- Clippings from cardiotoxic landscaped plants such as yew and rhododendron and holiday wreaths made of yew are toxic to horses if discarded in their pasture or paddock or displayed where horses have ready access.

Prevention/Avoidance

- Horses should be denied access to landscaped yards.
- Clippings should *not* be discarded in pastures, paddocks, or turnout areas.
- Suspect forage should be inspected for the presence of cardiotoxic plants before allowing access.
- Hay should be inspected carefully for weeds, as many cardiotoxic plants remain toxic when dried (oleander, death camas, yew).

Possible Complications

- Horses that survive the acute poisoning may suffer from myocardial damage and may be more prone to stress.

Expected Course and Prognosis

- Animals poisoned with cardiotoxic plants are often found dead.

- Cardiotoxic plant exposure progresses so rapidly that treatment is often too late; however, if treatment is initiated promptly after the onset of clinical signs, the prognosis is fair.
- In oleander and yew intoxications, the prognosis is poor.

Abbreviations

See Appendix 1 for a complete list.

Suggested Reading

Bauquier J, Stent A, Gibney J, et al. Evidence for marsh mallow (*Malva parviflora*) toxicosis causing myocardial disease and myopathy in four horses. Equine Vet J 2017; 49(3):307–313

Clark RF, Selden BS, Curry SC. Digoxin-specific Fab fragments in the treatment of oleander toxicity in a canine model. Annals Emerg Med 1991; 20(10):1073–1077.

Galey FG. Cardiac glycosides. In: Plumlee KH, ed. Clinical Veterinary Toxicology. St Louis, MO: Mosby, 2004; pp. 386–388.

Puschner B. Grayanotoxins. In: Plumlee KH, ed. Clinical Veterinary Toxicology. St Louis MO: Mosby, 2004; pp. 412–415.

Tiwary AK, Puschner B, Kinde H, et al. Diagnosis of *Taxus* (yew) poisoning in a horse. J Vet Diagn Invest 2005; 17:252–255.

Acknowledgment: The author and editor acknowledge the prior contribution of Birgit Puchner.

Author: Lynn R. Hovda, RPh, DVM, MS, DACVIM
Consulting Editor: Lynn R. Hovda, RPh, DVM, MS, DACVIM

Day Blooming Jessamine (*Cestrum diurnum*)

DEFINITION/OVERVIEW

- *Cestrum diurnum* (day blooming jessamine or jasmine) is a large shrub with alternate, simple leaves having smooth margins and are lanceolate or elliptic in shape.
- The fragrant and showy blooms are *c.* 2.5 cm in length and are five-part flowers appearing in the axillary clusters. The flowers are white and sweet-scented in the day.
- The fruit is a small spheric berry tuning black when mature.
- Toxins concentrate in the leaves so ingestion occurs from grazing on shrubs or leaves in hay.
- Ingestion results in hypercalcemia with mineralization of the aorta, pulmonary arteries, heart and lungs, consistent with enzootic calcinosis.

ETIOLOGY/PATHOPHYSIOLOGY

Mechanism of Action

- Chronic ingestion results in increased absorption of calcium and phosphorous from the intestine, ultimately resulting metastatic tissue calcification.

Toxicokinetics

- Slow onset; signs increase over a 2- to 6-month period.

Toxicity

- The plant is a member of the Solanaceae family and contains several toxins. The unripe berry contains solanine, a GI irritant, and a cholinesterase-inhibiting glycoalkaloid. The ripe berry contains tropane alkaloids. Traces of saponins and nicotine are found as well.
- The agent of greatest concern is 1,25-dihydroxycholecalciferol. The glycoside is hydrolyzed to yield the active vitamin D_3 (calcitriol). There are about 30 000 IU of D_3 equivalents/kg of plant.

Blackwell's Five-Minute Veterinary Consult Clinical Companion: Equine Toxicology,
First Edition. Edited by Lynn R. Hovda, Dionne Benson, and Robert H. Poppenga.
© 2022 John Wiley & Sons, Inc. Published 2022 by John Wiley & Sons, Inc.
Companion website: www.wiley.com/go/hovda/equine

Systems Affected

- Cardiovascular – metastatic tissue calcification.
- Respiratory – metastatic tissue calcification.
- Musculoskeletal – metastatic tissue calcification.
- Renal – metastatic tissue calcification.

SIGNALMENT/HISTORY

- There is no breed, sex, or age predilection.

Risk Factors

- Consumption of *C. diurnum*, most often from boredom, curiosity or hunger.

Historical Findings

- Horses generally will not graze on these plants unless there is no other forage available.

Location and Circumstances of Poisoning

- The plant, introduced into the USA from the West Indies, prefers warmer areas, and is used ornamentally in the south. It also may be found wild in the Florida Keys and in south Texas.

CLINICAL FEATURES

- Progressive weight loss and lameness, increasing in severity during a 2- to 6-month period.
- Affected horses become stiff, are reluctant to move, and develop a short, choppy gait.
- Flexor and suspensory ligaments sensitive to palpation.
- Slight to moderate kyphosis.
- Elevated pulse and respiratory rates.
- Polyuria.

DIFFERENTIAL DIAGNOSIS

- Vitamin D intoxication from other sources – vitamin D supplement overdose; other plants associated with enzootic calcinosis (*Solanum malacoxylon* – South America; *Solanum sodemauim* – Hawaii; *Trisetum flavescens* – Germany); cholecalciferol rodenticides.
- Primary thyroid/parathyroid tumors, although rare in equines, can cause hypercalcemia.

DIAGNOSTICS

CBC/Serum Chemistry/Urinalysis

- Hypercalcemia.
- Hyperphosphatemia.
- Increased BUN and creatinine as disease progress.

Other Diagnostic Tests

- Ionized calcium.

Imaging

- Evidence of tissue calcification is visible on radiology or ultrasound.

Pathological Findings

- Gross:
  - Hypervitaminosis D results in widespread soft tissue mineralization (i.e., calcification.) Grossly, mineralization is seen as gritty white deposits in kidneys, intestines, stomach, heart, lungs, arteries, bones, tendons, and ligament.
  - Forelimb flexor tendons are more severely affected than those of the pelvic limb; however, all suspensory ligaments are calcified.
  - Calcification occurs in the kidneys, lungs, large blood vessels, and GI tract but is not a consistent finding.
  - Heart calcification can occur, with the most severely calcified portion of the heart being the left atrium.
  - Generalized osteoporosis and emaciation.
  - In response to chronic hypercalcemia, the thyroid cells often become hyperplastic and the parathyroid will become atrophic.
- Histopathology:
  - Hyperplasia of the parathyroid chief cells (i.e., C cells).

THERAPEUTICS

Detoxification

- This is a chronic disease, so no detoxification is recommended.

Appropriate Health Care

- No documented efficacious treatment once hypercalcemia has become chronic.
- Remove the animal from the plant or the plant from the horse's environment and feed a good-quality, low-calcium diet (i.e., check supplements).
- Promote diuresis and calciuresis with IV normal saline.
- Monitor serum calcium and phosphorous concentrations.
- Provide pain relief.

Antidote

- There is no specific antidote. Bisphosphonate drugs have been used successfully in humans and small animals for the treatment of hypercalcemia-related intoxications. There are no reports as yet in horses.

Drugs of Choice

- Diuresis and calciuresis:
  - 0.9% sodium chloride IV at 1.5–2× normal

- Furosemide 1 mg/kg IV initial dose; if no increase in urine output is noted within 1 hour, increase dose to 2–4 mg/kg IV or IM. However, care should be taken to ensure the horse does not become dehydrated.
- Decrease bone release, intestinal absorption of calcium and promote calciuresis:
  - Prednisolone has been used successfully in small animal medicine.
- NSAIDS for inflammation and pain control:
  - Phenylbutazone 2.2 –4.4 mg/kg IV or PO q12–24h.
  - Flunixin meglumine 1.1 mg/kg IV q12–24h.
- Butorphanol for severe pain:
  - 0.05–0.1 mg/kg IV q3–4h.

Precautions/Interactions

- Use NSAIDs very cautiously and monitor BUN and creatinine.
- Avoid the use of calcium-containing IV fluids.

Alternative Drugs

- Salmon calcitonin prevents mobilization of calcium from bones but is rarely used any more in human or veterinary medicine.
- Pamidronate disodium (pamidronic acid) and other bisphosphonate drugs may be useful but must be used early and will not reverse mineralization

 COMMENTS

Client Education

- Learn to identify this plant and remove it from the pasture, paddock or turnout area.

Prevention/Avoidance

- Do not plant as an ornamental shrub along fence lines or buildings.
- Provide adequate forage so horses will not graze on wild plants in pastures.

Possible Complications

- Heart failure, renal failure, recumbency.

Expected Course and Prognosis

- Once clinical signs develop the prognosis is very poor and most horses are humanely euthanized.

Abbreviations

See Appendix 1 for a complete list.

Suggested Reading

Burrow GE, Tyrl RJ. Toxic Plants of North America. Ames, IA: Iowa State University Press, 2001; pp. 1111–1113.
Krook L, Wasserman RH, Shively JN, et al. Hypercalcemia and calcinosis in Florida horses: implication of the shrub, *Cestrum diurnum*, as the causative agent. Cornell Vet 1975; 65:26–56.

Odriozola ER, Rodríguez AM, Micheloud JF, et al. Enzootic calcinosis in horses grazing *Solanum glaucophyllum* in Argentina. J Vet Diagn Invest 2018; 30(2):286–289.

Villagrán CC, Frank N, Schumacher J, et al. Case report persistent hypercalcemia and hyperparathyroidism in a horse. Hindawi Publishing Corporation Case Reports in Veterinary Medicine Vol 2014, Article ID 465425, http://dx.doi.org/10.1155/2014/465425

Author: Tam Garland, DVM, PhD, DABVT
Consulting Editor: Lynn R. Hovda, RPh, DVM, MS, DACVIM

Chapter 55

Death camas (*Zigadenus* spp.)

DEFINITION/OVERVIEW

- Death camas (*Zigadenus* spp.) are so called due to their resemblance to edible Camassia species.
- *Zigadenus* spp. are members of the lily family (Liliaceae).
- Over 20 species exist, most of which are indigenous to North and Central America.
- Horses generally encounter the plant in hay.
- Clinical signs can include salivation, depression, colic, trembling and ataxia.

ETIOLOGY/PATHOPHYSIOLOGY

- Horses rarely consume this plant due to bitterness; actual incidence of toxicity is unknown.
- *Zigadenus* spp. are found throughout north and central America but are rare in other regions of the world.

Mechanism of Action

- The toxic principles in *Zigadenus* are a variety of cevanine-type ester alkaloids similar to those found in *Veratrum* spp. One of these esters is zygadene, but several others are uncharacterized.
- The alkaloids in the plant increase reflex activity and sensitize afferent pathway receptors in the absence of stimuli.
- Clinically this means they are neurotoxicants and hypotensive agents.
- The alkaloids bind to open sodium channels and interfere with closure of the channels thus allowing increased movement of Na^+, Ca^{2+}, and K^+ through the cell membrane.
- Channel closure delay lasts several seconds; repolarization delay results in increased repetitive activity, with a single stimulus producing multiple discharges.
- The most sensitive neurons appear to be vagal afferent fibers.
- Clinical effects include bradycardia, peripheral vasodilation, and hypotension as well as organophosphate-like effects (salivation, urination, defecation).

Blackwell's Five-Minute Veterinary Consult Clinical Companion: Equine Toxicology,
First Edition. Edited by Lynn R. Hovda, Dionne Benson, and Robert H. Poppenga.
© 2022 John Wiley & Sons, Inc. Published 2022 by John Wiley & Sons, Inc.
Companion website: www.wiley.com/go/hovda/equine

Toxicity

- Seeds and fruit contain the highest levels of toxins, but early-growth leaves also contain high concentrations and represent the greatest risk to grazing animals.
- The plant is seldom grazed by horses due to extreme bitterness.
- Most intoxications in horses are due to consumption in hay.
- Number and variety of toxins vary by species.
- No specific toxic dose has been established for horses; lethal dose for sheep and cattle is estimated at 0.6–0.7% body weight of dry matter.
- Clinical signs may be seen several hours to a day following ingestion.
- Disease course is typically 1–2 days.
- Death is believed to occur due to central respiratory depression.
- Death is rare in horses.

Systems Affected

- Neurological – depression, trembling, pelvic limb ataxia and weakness, hypothermia, coma in terminal cases.
- Gastrointestinal – hypersalivation (often the first sign noted), colic, retching, bruxism, frequent defecation.
- Cardiovascular – bradycardia, hypotension.
- Respiratory – labored respiration in terminal cases.
- Renal/urologic – frequent urination.

SIGNALMENT/HISTORY

- No breed or sex predilection has been reported.
- Grazing equids of any age may be affected.
- No information is available describing risk for suckling foals; it is unknown if the toxins are present in the milk of lactating animals that consume the plant.

Risk Factors

- The time of highest risk for pasture-kept animals is early spring, before ample grass is available for grazing.
- *Zigadenus* spp. withers by early summer and is unlikely to be grazed, but withered foliage may be incorporated into hay.
- Any hay has the potential to be contaminated with death camas.
- The most toxic species (*Z. nuttallii*, *Z. venenosus*, and *Z. paniculatus*) occur in the western half of the US.

CLINICAL FEATURES

- Horses first present with hypersalivation and depression.
- Signs of abdominal pain may be present: bruxism, hunched back, typical colic signs and frequent defecation.

- Later in the disease course the horse may tremble, demonstrate ataxia more prominent in the pelvic limbs and weakness.
- Frequent urination may be seen.
- Auscultation may reveal increased borborygmi and bradycardia.
- Hypotension may be present.
- Hypothermia may be present.

DIFFERENTIAL DIAGNOSIS

- Slaframine (red clover) intoxication.
- Organophosphate toxicity.
- Carbamate insecticide toxicity.
- Botulism.
- Fumonisin.
- Ivermectin toxicity.
- Locoweed (swainsonine).
- Cannabis toxicity.
- Phosphide salts.
- Ryegrass staggers.
- Selenium toxicosis.
- Sudan grass.
- White snakeroot.

DIAGNOSTICS

Other Diagnostic Tests

- No specific antemortem diagnostics have been described.
- Examination of gastric lavage specimens for plant parts.
- Extraction of gut content or ocular fluid for identification of the alkaloids.
- Inspection of pasture or hay for the plant.

Pathological Findings

- Horses seldom die from *Zigadenus* consumption.
- Gross pathology is subtle.
- Pulmonary congestion and edema with scattered small hemorrhages.
- Reddening of the gastric mucosa.
- Plant parts may be found in ingesta.
- No specific histopathologic lesions have been described.

THERAPEUTICS

Detoxification

- No specific detoxification process has been described for *Zigadenus* spp.

Appropriate Health Care

- Gastric lavage.
- Activated charcoal 1–2 g/kg administered via NG tube in a slurry (1g charcoal to 5 mL water).
- Cathartics (not evaluated in *Zigadenus* toxicity): sodium or magnesium sulfate, 250–500 mg/kg slurry via NG tube.
- Atropine.
- Sympathomimetics if needed.
- Fluid support if indicated.

Antidotes

- No specific antidote exists. Atropine may be helpful.

Drugs of Choice

- Atropine up to 1 mg/kg IV; may be repeated subcutaneously OR glycopyrrolate 0.01 mg/kg IV (not approved in horses).
- For hypotension: dobutamine, 2–15 µg/kg/min diluted in saline solution or dopamine 2–15 µg/kg/min diluted in saline.

Precautions/Interactions

- Note: pralidoxime hydrochloride (2-PAM) is specific to organophosphates and will be ineffective in death camas toxicity.

Alternative Drugs

- Picrotoxin (a CNS stimulant) plus atropine have been historically used in sheep (8 mg picrotoxin per 100 lb BW), but no literature describes the combination in horses.
- Picrotoxin is a GABA antagonist. It is no longer available as a therapeutic but is still used in research.

COMMENTS

Client Education

- Inspect pastures in spring for *Zigadenus* spp. and uproot if found.
- Consultation with a forage extension agent may be helpful.

Prevention/Avoidance

- Inspect pastures and hay for the presence of the plants.

Expected Course and Prognosis

- Most horses recover fully within 48 hours of ingestion.

Abbreviations

See Appendix 1 for a complete list.

Suggested Reading

Burrows GE, Tyrl RJ. *Zigadenus Michx*. In: Burrows GE, Tyrl RJ, eds. Toxic Plants of North America, 2nd edn. Ames, IA: John Wiley and Sons, 2013; pp. 789–794.

Divers TJ. Nervous system treatment and procedures. In: Equine Emergencies, 4th edn. St. Louis, MO: Saunders, 2014; pp. 339–378.

Panter KE, James LF. Death camas: early grazing can be dangerous. Rangelands 1989 11(4)147–149.

Author: Tamara Gull, DVM, PhD, DACVIM (LAIM), DACVPM, DACVM
Consulting Editor: Lynn R. Hovda, RPh, DVM, MS, DACVIM

Hemlock (Poison Hemlock – *Conium maculatum*; Water Hemlock – *Cicuta* spp.)

Chapter 56

DEFINITION/OVERVIEW

- Poison hemlock (*Conium maculatum*) and water hemlock (*Cicuta* spp.) are two very different poisonous plants with unique plant habits, growth patterns, toxins, mechanisms of toxicity, clinical disease, and potential treatments.
- Both contain neurotoxins that fatally poison horses, humans, livestock, and wildlife.
- Human poisoning of both poison hemlock and water hemlock occur when they are confused with wild carrot or parsnip and are mistakenly eaten.
- Neither produces consistent gross or microscopic lesions so diagnosis is made by documenting exposure, chemical identification of plant toxin in biologic samples, and the lack of gross and histologic lesions with correlation with consistent clinical course and signs.

ETIOLOGY/PATHOPHYSIOLOGY

- Poison hemlock (*C. maculatum*) (Figs 56.1 and 56.2):
  - Native to Europe and North Africa, has become naturalized in North and South America, Asia and Australia.
  - It is highly invasive and expansive as it often dominates pastures and marginal areas.
  - It is the first plant to sprout in the spring and grows to several meters tall, allowing it to dominate many plant communities.
- Water hemlock (*Cicuta* spp.):
  - Native to North America and Europe where it grows in temperate regions in wet meadows and along canals and stream banks.
  - It is highly toxic, producing violent grand mal seizures and death.
  - Poisoning occurs when horses eat the tubers, green sprouts in the spring or the seed heads later in the season.

Mechanism of Action

- Poison hemlock (*C. maculatum*) (Fig. 56.3):
  - Coniine, the poison hemlock toxin, is a nicotinic antagonist that activates and then blocks nicotinic acetylcholine receptors.

Blackwell's Five-Minute Veterinary Consult Clinical Companion: Equine Toxicology, First Edition. Edited by Lynn R. Hovda, Dionne Benson, and Robert H. Poppenga.
© 2022 John Wiley & Sons, Inc. Published 2022 by John Wiley & Sons, Inc.
Companion website: www.wiley.com/go/hovda/equine

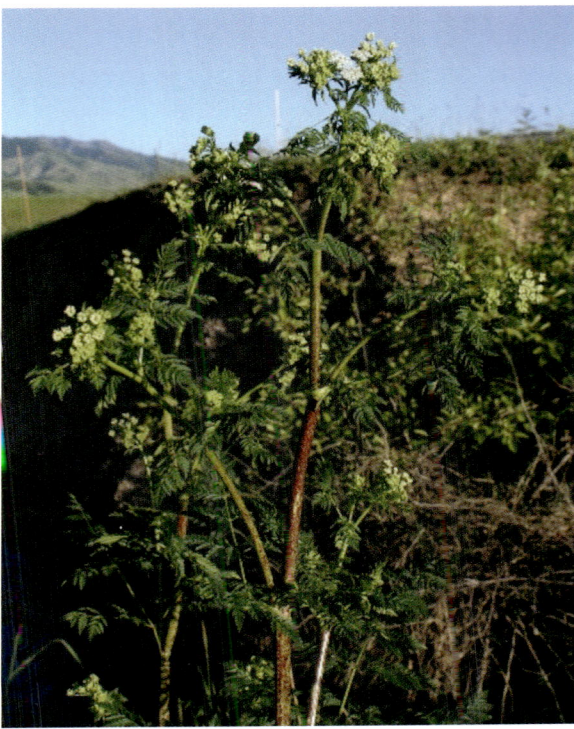

■ **Fig. 56.1.** *Conium maculatum* (poison hemlock) is a biennial that grows up to 2.5 m tall. It has a smooth glabrous, hollow stem that often has purple spots or streaks. The carrot-like leaves have two to four pinnate finely divided sections that can be 50 cm long. The small five-petaled flowers form umbral-like clusters. *Source:* Bryan Steiglemeier/USDA.

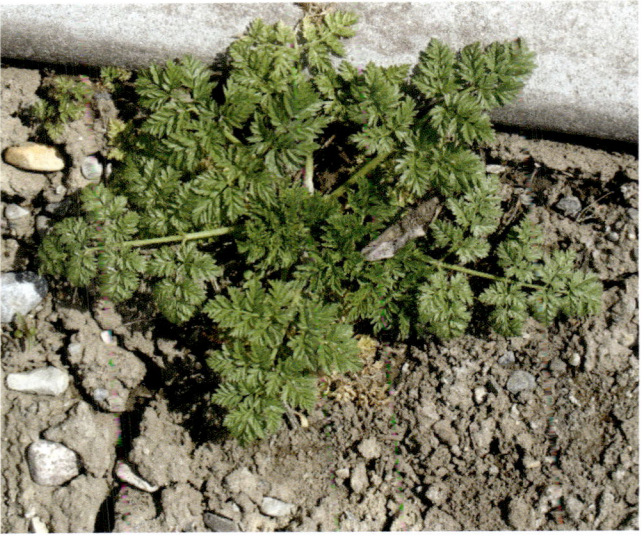

■ **Fig. 56.2.** *Conium maculatum* (poison hemlock) grows in the spring. This small carrot-like growth is cold-tolerant and is often the only feed available other than the woody shells and stems that remain from the previous season. If the only feed available, horses may become poisoned by eating these sprouts. *Source:* Bryan Steiglemeier/USDA.

CHAPTER 56 HEMLOCK (POISON HEMLOCK – *CONIUM MACULATUM*; WATER HEMLOCK – *CICUTA* SPP.)

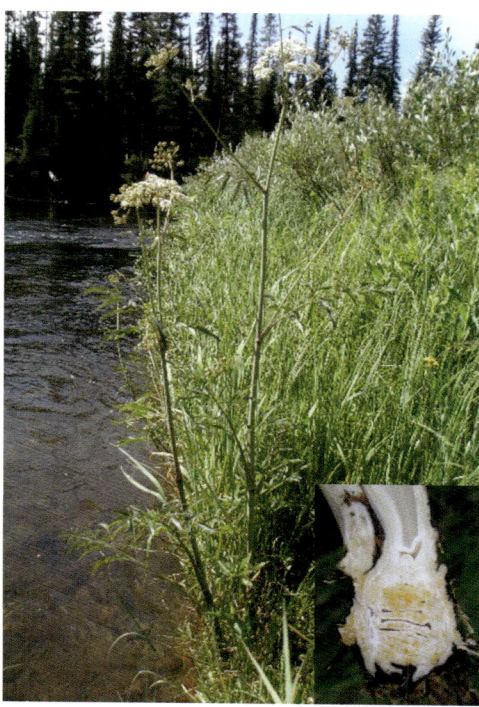

■ **Fig. 56.3.** *Cicuta douglasii* (Western water hemlock) is an erect perennial that, depending on conditions, grows between 0.5 and 2.5 m tall. It also has hollow, glabrous stems and the tubers are compartmentalized and often filled with yellow thick fluid (inset). The tubers are highly toxic. The leaves are alternate with three to four pinnate and toothed edges. The flowers are white and form distinct umbrels. Later the flowers develop into flat oval fruits. *Source.* Bryan Steiglemeier/USDA.

- Similar to nicotine, poison hemlock poisoning produces nausea, vomiting (in animals that can vomit), tremors, muscular weakness, incoordination, tachycardia, tachypnea, increased salivation and lacrimation, coma, and death.
■ Water hemlock (*Cicuta* spp.):
  - Water hemlock toxins (cicutoxin is generally used as an indicator) act as a GABA antagonist that results in massive neuronal depolarization.
  - This results in severe clonic seizures that can impair respiration, producing asphyxia and death.

Toxicokinetics

■ Poison hemlock (*C. maculatum*):
  - Onset of action 30 minutes to 2 hours.
  - Poisoning in horses often results in recumbency that resolves as the toxin is cleared. Clearance may take 1–2 days.
  - With larger ingestions, death may occur in 5–10 hours.
  - Both coniine and γ-coniceine are present in fresh poison hemlock.
  - It seems that most the γ-coniceine breaks down into coniine. *in vivo* conversion is rapid, as nearly all excreted in the urine as coniine. It has been suggested that this

conversion occurs quickly in the bovine rumen and this might account for the apparent susceptibility of cattle to poison hemlock poisoning.
- The toxic dose in horses is 15.5 mg/kg BW, while that of cattle is 3.3 mg coniine/kg BW and sheep 44 mg/kg.
- Water hemlock (*Cicuta* spp.):
  - Onset minutes; rapid death (1–2 hours; rarely up to 8 hours).
  - There is little toxicity data for cicutoxin or the other *Cicuta* C17 polyacetylenes in horses.
  - The tubers are highly toxic.
  - Additional metabolism and excretion are largely unknown, but it is speculated that it is slow as clinical signs often persist for days after ingestion.
  - Fatal seizure-related deaths generally occur quickly within 8 hours of exposure, suggesting that a least part of its metabolism occurs within several hours. All species appear to be susceptible to poisoning, including fatal human intoxication, which generally occurs a result of plant misidentification.

Toxicity

- Poison hemlock (*C. maculatum*):
  - Horses are likely to eat young plants that emerge in the early spring before other green forages. The doses thus tend to be lower, resulting in less severe poisoning seen as weakness and recumbency. If they remain calm in sternal recumbency to allow toxin clearance, most will recover.
  - Older plants are unpalatable for most livestock. Highly susceptible cattle may be fatally poisoned if they are fed contaminated green chopped forages.
- Water hemlock (*Cicuta* spp.:)
  - All parts of water hemlock are toxic, but the roots are highly toxic and generally associated with poisoning.
  - Animals show signs (nervousness and excessive salivation) within minutes. These are followed by seizures and fatal asphyxia within 1–2 hours.

Systems Affected

- Nervous – primarily.
- Respiratory – secondary to convulsions and hypoxia.
- Musculoskeletal – secondary to convulsions and hypoxia.
- Cardiovascular.

SIGNALMENT/HISTORY

- All species appear to be susceptible and human poisoning generally occurs when it is mistaken for an edible plant.

Risk Factors

- Poison hemlock (*C. maculatum*):
  - The plant appears during the early spring when other forages are unavailable, resulting in poisoning.

- Older plants are not palatable for most species; however, it can poison livestock if they are fed contaminated green chopped forages.
- Contaminated dry hay and forages rarely contain toxic coniine concentrations and some have suggested that the coniine degrades during the drying and storage process.
■ Water hemlock (*Cicuta* spp.):
- Water hemlock grows in marginal areas along streams and canals, so it rarely contaminates feeds and most poisoning occur when animals graze free-standing plants or pull up and eat the tubers.

Location and Circumstances of Poisoning

■ See "Risk Factors".

CLINICAL FEATURES

■ Poison hemlock (*C. maculatum*):
- Initial signs include mydriasis, salivation, lacrimation, depression, colic, and diarrhea.
- Neurologic signs develop rapidly and include apprehension, muscle tremors, muscular weakness, incoordination, recumbency, paralysis, and coma.
- Cardiovascular depression is seen as a weak pulse and cold extremities.
- Horses may become recumbent and comatose and remain that way for hours to days before either recovering or dying from respiratory depression.
- Death results from respiratory failure.
■ Water hemlock (*Cicuta* spp.):
- Initial signs include excessive salivation, vigorous chewing movement, and grinding teeth.
- Neurologic signs include tremors and severe convulsions.
- With severe seizures, respiration becomes labored and finally fails. Death usually occurs within 2–3 hours of ingestion.

DIFFERENTIAL DIAGNOSIS

■ Other plants that cause similar clinical signs – death camas, *Veratrum californium*, and acute lupine poisoning.
■ Tetanus.
■ Epileptic-like seizures.
■ Other causes of sudden death in horses – ionophore toxicosis, cardiac dysfunction/arrhythmia, aortic aneurysm/rupture, blister beetle toxicosis.

DIAGNOSTICS

CBC/Serum Chemistry/Urinalysis

■ Elevated CK and cTnI concentration, especially if the clinical course is prolonged.

Other Diagnostic Tests

- Chemical identification of coniine or other *Conium* alkaloids.
- Chemical identification of *Cicuta* C17 polyacetylenes

Pathological Findings

- Plant material in stomach; stomach contents, urine, and exhaled air may have a characteristic mousy odor.
- Lack of specific gross and microscopic findings. Nonspecific lesions at necropsy include diffuse congestion of the lungs, liver, and myocardium.

THERAPEUTICS

Detoxification

- AC (1–4 g/kg PO in water slurry, 1 g of AC in 5 mL of water). Give with one dose of cathartic PO if no diarrhea or ileus – 70% sorbitol (3 mL/kg) or sodium or magnesium sulfate (250–500 mg/kg).

Appropriate Health Care

- Hospitalize if able and provide general supportive treatment.
- Early GI decontamination may be useful if it can be safely achieved.
- Maintain body fluid and electrolyte balance.
- Adequate nursing care of recumbent animals.
- Respiratory support by mechanical ventilation has been suggested.

Antidotes

- There is no specific antidote.

Drugs of Choice

- Convulsions:
  - Diazepam 25–50 mg slow IV (adults); 0.1–0.4 mg/kg IV (foals).
  - Phenobarbital 16–20 mg/kg IV.

Precautions/Interactions

- Use excessive care when dealing with horses poisoned with water hemlock as seizures may be very violent, making any therapy difficult and dangerous.

COMMENTS

Client Education

- Poison hemlock (*C. maculatum*):
  - Older plants are unpalatable for nearly all species. Mature plants can be several meters tall and are untouched as animals graze around them.

- Herbicide treatment of such mature plants should be done with care to exclude animals until the plants have died and dried up, as some reports suggest sprayed plants become more palatable.
- Water hemlock (*Cicuta* spp.):
  - This plant grows along controlled drainage ditches, canals and stream banks and these areas should be fenced to avoid exposure.
  - Be very cautious when working around these plants as human exposure and death have occurred.

Prevention/Avoidance

- See "Client Education".

Possible Complications

- Poison hemlock – in pregnant cattle and sheep, non-fatal doses can cause contracture-type birth defects. It is unknown if this is a problem in horses.

Expected Course and Prognosis

- Poison hemlock (*C. maculatum*):
  - Very guarded early prognosis.
  - Because both the quantity of alkaloid in the plant and the quantity of plant consumed vary, not all horses that eat poison hemlock die.
  - Onset of signs within 2 hours and may last several hours up to 1–2 days.
  - Not reported in horses, but cattle fed poison hemlock-contaminated green chopped forage can be fatally poisoned. Depending on the amount of contamination, mortality can be high as numerous animals are affected.
- Water hemlock (*Cicuta* spp.):
  - Extremely poor to no prognosis.
  - Onset of signs within minutes and death within a few hours.

Abbreviations

See Appendix 1 for a complete list.

Suggested Reading

Burrows GM, Tyrl RJ. Toxic Plants of North America, 2n edn. Ames, IA: Wiley Blackwell, 2013; pp. 66–70.

Green BT, Goulart KD, Welch JA, et al. The non-competitive blockade of GABA A receptors by an aqueous extract of water hemlock (*Cicuta douglasii*) tubers. Toxicon 2015; 108:11–14.

Karakasi MVS, Tologkos V, Papadatou N, et al. *Conium maculatum* intoxication: literature review and case report on hemlock poisoning. Forensic Sci Rev 2019; 31:23–36.

Keeler RF, Balls LD, Shupe JL, et al. Teratogenicity and toxicity of coniine in cows, ewes, and mares. Cornell Vet 1980; 70:19–26.

Lopez TA, Cid MS, Bianchini ML. Biochemistry of hemlock (*Conium maculatum* L.) alkaloids and their acute and chronic toxicity in livestock. A review. Toxicon 1999; 37:841–865.

Acknowledgment: The author and editors acknowledge the prior contribution of Sharon Gwaltney-Brant.

Author: Bryan L. Stegelmeier, DVM, PhD, DACVP
Consulting Editor: Lynn R. Hovda, RPh, DVM, MS, DACVIM

Chapter 57

Hoary Alyssum (*Berteroa incana*)

DEFINITION/OVERVIEW

- Hoary alyssum (*Berteroa incana*) is a weed that grows well in climates with cold winters and hot, dry summers.
- It grows in sandy, gravelly, and disturbed soil along roads, ditches, trails and vacant lots as well as pastures and hayfields in the northeastern and north central United States and Canada.
- The small, white flower has four deeply divided petals (see Fig. 57.1). Several flowers are found in clusters around each stem.
- The tall, erect stem (about 0.6 m) is branched with small alternating, lance-shaped, downy leaves (see Fig 57.2).
- Difficult to distinguish hoary alyssum stems from alfalfa stems in baled hay.
- Toxic as fresh plant on pasture and when baled into hay (toxic for up to 9 months).
- Edema and swelling of the distal limbs, fever, and laminitis occur 12–24 hours following ingestion.
- Not all horses will develop clinical signs; it depends on the specific horse, amount ingested, concentration of toxin, and other factors.

ETIOLOGY/PATHOPHYSIOLOGY

Mechanism of Action

- The exact mechanism is unknown.
- Distal limb edema may be due to the leakage of plasma constituents at vascular beds.

Toxicokinetics

- Onset of action – 12–24 hours after ingestion of toxic amount.
- Duration of action – 2–4 days after treatment or removal from source.

Toxicity

- Unknown toxin.
- Active in fresh plants on pasture and in hay up to 9 months after it is cut and stored.
- Hay containing more than 30% is considered toxic.
- Only about 50% of exposed horses will develop clinical signs.

Blackwell's Five-Minute Veterinary Consult Clinical Companion: Equine Toxicology, First Edition. Edited by Lynn R. Hovda, Dionne Benson, and Robert H. Poppenga.
© 2022 John Wiley & Sons, Inc. Published 2022 by John Wiley & Sons, Inc.
Companion website: www.wiley.com/go/hovda/equine

CHAPTER 57 HOARY ALYSSUM (*BERTEROA INCANA*)

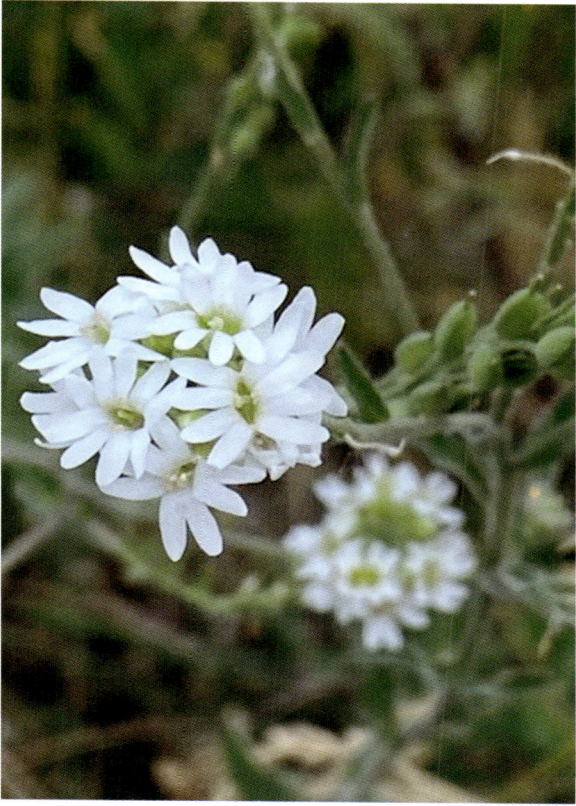

■ **Fig. 57.1.** Small, white flower of *Berteroa incana* (hoary alyssum). Note the four deeply divided petals. *Source:* Photo courtesy of Lynn Hovda.

Systems Affected

- Musculoskeletal – warm edematous distal limbs.
- Endocrine – increased body temperature.
- Cardiovascular – tachycardia.
- Respiratory.
- Gastrointestinal.
- Reproductive – less often.

 SIGNALMENT/HISTORY

- There is no specific age, breed, or sex distinction for generalized signs.

Risk Factors

- Overgrazed pastures, stressed meadows, ditch hay.
- Housed horses fed only baled hay may be affected more frequently.
- Due to housing and feeding practices, racehorses may be more susceptible.

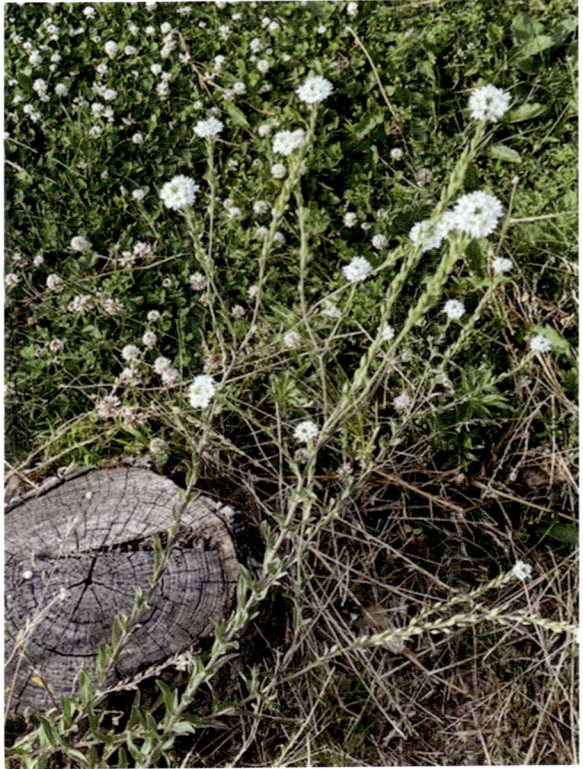

■ Fig. 57.2. *Berteroa incana* (hoary alyssum) plant. *Source*: Photo courtesy of Lynn Hovda.

Historical Findings

- Most cases occur in the summer after recently cut hay.
- Few cases in the winter.

Location and Circumstances of Poisoning

- Northeastern and north central United States and Canada.
- Less often, Washington, Oregon, Montana.

 CLINICAL FEATURES

- Distal limb edema (generally pitting edema).
- Warm hoof walls, digital pulses, reluctant to move.
- Elevated body temperature.
- Tachycardia.
- Tachypnea.
- Dehydration, hypovolemia.
- RBC destruction.
- +/- diarrhea.
- Abortion – less often.

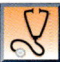
DIFFERENTIAL DIAGNOSIS

- Infectious diseases including *Salmonella*, *Purpura hemorrhagica*, Potomac horse fever (*Neorickettsia risticii*), anaplasmosis (*Anaplasma phagocytophilum*, formerly *Ehrlichia equi*), Lyme's (*Borrelia burgdorferi*a), and equine viral arteritis.
- Black walnut shavings (*Acer negundo*).
- Other causes of laminitis.

DIAGNOSTICS

CBC/Serum Chemistry/Urinalysis

- Varies depending on individual horse:
  - Elevated PCV consistent with dehydration and hypovolemia.
  - Decreased PCV consistent with RBC destruction and anemia.
  - Neutropenia ± left shift.
  - Elevated BUN and creatinine consistent with dehydration and hypovolemia.
  - Hematuria.

Imaging

- Radiographs of feet for evidence of distal phalanx rotation.

Pathological Findings

- Gross – subcutaneous edema of limbs. Perirenal hemorrhage, hemoperitoneum, hemothorax, diffuse serosal petechiae and ecchymoses.
- Histopathology – pulmonary and intestinal congestion and edema, intratubular renal casts.

THERAPEUTICS

Detoxification

- Activated charcoal (1–3 g/kg) in a watery slurry × one dose may be helpful for very early cases but is not indicated once clinical signs have developed.

Appropriate Health Care

- Most cases can be managed conservatively on the property with anti-inflammatory medications to control the body temperature and pain, leg wraps to assist with edema, and attention to feet.
- Some horses with need to be hospitalized for supportive care:
  - IV fluids for dehydration and hypovolemia.
  - Anti-inflammatory drugs.
  - Pain medications as needed.

Antidotes

- There is no specific antidote.

Drugs of Choice

- NSAIDs – use judiciously and monitor BUN and creatinine:
  - Flunixin 1.1 mg/kg IV or PO q12–24h.
  - Phenylbutazone 2.2–4.4 mg/kg IV or PO q12–24h.
  - Ketoprofen 2.2 mg/kg IV q24h.
- Butorphanol for severe pain:
  - 0.05–0.1 mg/kg IV q3–4h.

Precautions/Interactions

- DMSO should be used cautiously as RBC destruction may occur in some horses with hoary alyssum toxicosis, and rapid IV administration of DMSO may result in intravascular hemolysis.

Alternative Drugs

- Most racetrack trainers use a "tightening" poultice and leg wraps in an attempt to counteract the edema.

COMMENTS

Client Education

- Learn to identify and remove hoary alyssum in pastures and paddocks. Hoary alyssum in fields and ditches is easy to identify, but difficult in cut and baled hay as it is looks very similar to alfalfa.
- Purchase hay from a reputable source that is knowledgeable about hoary alyssum.
- Do not feed hoary alyssum-contaminated hay to horses.
- Move horses that are on contaminated pastures to other areas.

Prevention/Avoidance

- Don't overgraze pastures – healthy pastures can prevent the growth of hoary alyssum
- Small areas can safely be removed by pulling or digging the weed out of the soil.
- Mowing pastures and contaminated areas before the weed flowers or goes to seed will help to decrease the presence.
- Some herbicides are effective on hoary alyssum but should be applied by a professional and all restrictions followed closely.

Possible Complications

- Abortion in pregnant mares.
- Complete rotation of the coffin bone through the sole of the foot or "sinking" at the coronary band with sloughing of the hoof wall are known sequela.

Expected Course and Prognosis

- The prognosis for most horses is good once the horse has been removed from the contaminated hay or pasture and received treatment.
- Death from complications of hoary alyssum toxicosis, although rare, has occurred even in those most well-managed cases.

Abbreviations

See Appendix 1 for a complete list.

Internet Resources

Hoary alyssum Available at: https://extension.umn.edu/horse-pastures-and-facilities/hoary-alyssum-most-common-poisonous-plant-horses-minnesota (accessed 12 April, 2021).

Suggested Reading

Geor RJ, Becker RL, Kanara EW, et al. Toxicosis in horses after ingestion of hoary alyssum. J Am Vet MedAssoc; 201(1):63–67.

Hovda LF, Rose ML. Hoary alyssum (*Berteroa incana*) toxicity in a herd of broodmare horses. Vet Hum Toxicol 1993;35(1):39–40.

Author: Lynn R. Hovda, RPh, DVM, MS, DACVIM
Consulting Editor: Lynn R. Hovda, RPh, DVM, MS, DACVIM

Chapter 58

Jimsonweed (Datura stramonium)

DEFINITION/OVERVIEW

- *Datura stramonium*, an annual herb commonly known as Jimsonweed is a member of the Solanaceae (potato and nightshade) family that grows extensively over North America.
- Alternate names include devil's trumpet and thorn apple.
- The plant is readily identifiable under field conditions growing to 0.9–1.52 m (3–5 ft) in height supported by a green or rhubarb-colored stem. The leaves are large with multiple irregular pointed lobes. The trumpet-shaped white or purple flowers bloom at night and typically remain closed during the day. However, flowers may open during the day under overcast conditions. (see Fig. 58.1) Spiny ovate seed pods, ~ 38 mm (1½ in) in length and diameter, are initially green but dry and turn brown before releasing dark-colored, pitted, irregularly shaped seeds. (see Fig. 58.2).
- The live plant has a strong, noxious odor and is bitter-tasting. It is unlikely to be voluntarily consumed by horses unless other feed is unavailable. Exposure is more likely from seed pods, seeds or plant material incorporated into hay or straw during harvesting and baling, processes that neutralize the plant's odor and taste to the extent that horses will consume it.
- Presumptive diagnosis of datura intoxication should be made, until ruled out, when seed pods (± seeds) are identified in hay or bedding.
- Inappetence, colic, abdominal distension, and mydriasis are the most commonly observed clinical signs observed in horses experiencing toxicity.
- Jimsonweed is recognized as a human substance of abuse for its hallucinogenic properties. It has traditional use in some religious rituals and has also been used in folkloric medicine for treating a range of maladies, including asthma, epilepsy, hemorrhoids, and schizophrenia. Scopolamine is available as a prescription medication as a transdermal patch for the control of nausea or motion sickness.

ETIOLOGY/PATHOPHYSIOLOGY

Mechanism of Action

Competitive inhibition of post-ganglionic muscarinic receptors in the parasympathetic nervous system.

Blackwell's Five-Minute Veterinary Consult Clinical Companion: Equine Toxicology, First Edition. Edited by Lynn R. Hovda, Dionne Benson, and Robert H. Poppenga.
© 2022 John Wiley & Sons, Inc. Published 2022 by John Wiley & Sons, Inc.
Companion website: www.wiley.com/go/hovda/equine

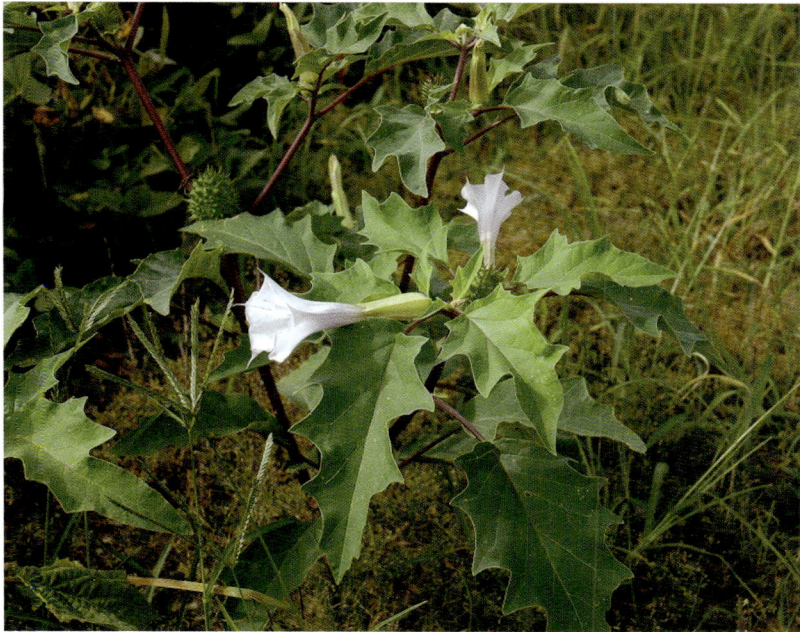

■ **Fig. 58.1.** Jimsonweed is readily identified under field conditions by its height, distinctive trumpet-shaped flowers, and thorny seed pods. Jimsonweed in Prince George's Co., Maryland (September 20, 2008). *Source*: Photo courtesy of Jim Brighton.

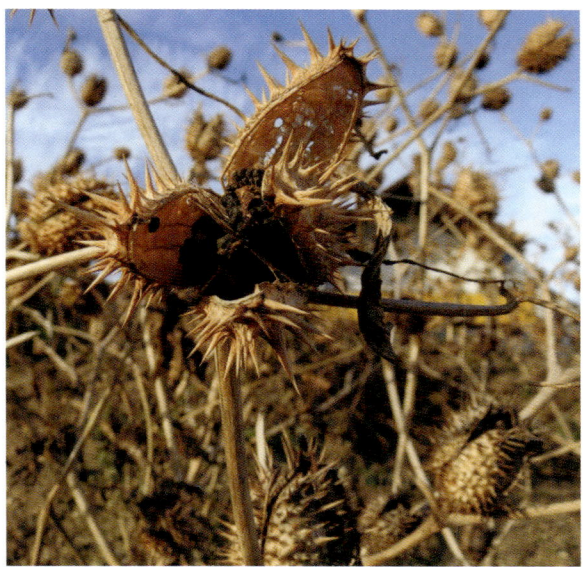

■ **Fig. 58.2.** Dried seed pods. The small black seeds may be difficult to observe in hay if released from the seed pod. Exposure should be presumed if entire seed pods or their fragments are identified in hay or straw. *Source*: Mary Scollay (https://upload.wikimedia.org/wikipedia/commons/4/48/20150113Datura_stramonium3.jpg).

Toxicokinetics

- This is based primarily on human literature:
  - Oral bioavailability is believed to be poor, potentially due to a high first-pass effect.
  - Peak plasma concentrations are achieved approximately 30 minutes post-ingestion.
  - Scopolamine crosses the blood–brain barrier, thus explaining its psychoactive effects when compared with the similar antimuscarinic alkaloid atropine.
  - Fecal elimination is the primary route of excretion.
  - Scopolamine is excreted in the urine as a glucuronide conjugate; < 3% of scopolamine is excreted as parent drug.

Toxicity

- Jimsonweed contains multiple plant alkaloids, including atropine and scopolamine (L-hyoscine), which, when consumed, result in dose-dependent clinical signs consistent with anticholinergic toxicity. While all parts of the plant contain these alkaloids, the highest concentration is found in the seeds.
- In horses administered an experimental dose of 6.5 g of *Datura* plant material, the peak urine concentration of free and conjugated scopolamine was 100 ng/mL. These horses did not demonstrate clinical signs of toxicity.

Systems Affected

- Gastrointestinal – colic; diminished or absent borborygmus; ileus.
- Nervous – mydriasis, photosensitivity, agitation, hyperactivity, ataxia, tremors, seizures.
- Cardiovascular – tachycardia.
- Respiratory – tachypnea.
- Endocrine/metabolic – fever.
- Genitourinary – bladder stasis/urine retention.

SIGNALMENT/HISTORY

Horses of all ages, genders, and breeds can be affected, although in one case study foals nursing from affected mares did not develop clinical signs.

Historical Findings

Cases of *Datura* intoxication tend to occur in clusters as multiple horses may share a pasture, whereas stabled horses typically have shared exposure to the same feed/bedding source.

CLINICAL FEATURES

- Clinical signs and history of exposure or evidence of jimsonweed in the environment can establish a presumptive diagnosis.
- Clinical signs are dose-dependent and can range from spontaneously resolving mild inappetence to convulsions and death.
- Most commonly observed signs are mydriasis, inappetence, colic, decreased or absent borborygmus.

- Other clinical signs reported include fever (101–102°F); tacky, hyperemic mucous membranes; decreased thirst; abdominal distension, often more prominent on the left side; tachycardia; tachypnea; anhidrosis; anuria and failure to defecate. CNS signs range from agitation to seizures.
- On rectal examination, typical findings include distended bladder; gas distended cecum and colon; and dry, mucus-coated fecal balls.

DIFFERENTIAL DIAGNOSIS

- *Atropa belladonna* (deadly nightshade) intoxication.
- Misadministration of antimuscarinic drugs.

DIAGNOSTICS

CBC/Serum Chemistry/Urinalysis

- Hematologic changes in affected horses included neutrophilia with a left shift and eosinopenia.
- Serum chemistry profiles in affected horses showed statistically significant elevations in blood glucose, total bilirubin, and AST.

Other Diagnostic Tests

- Detection of scopolamine ± atropine in a urine sample:
  - While atropine is contained in jimsonweed, it is not routinely detected in samples collected from affected horses. Atropine is eliminated more rapidly than scopolamine; its absence from a sample may be reflective the timing of sample collection post-exposure.
  - Detection of atropine without scopolamine is *not* indicative of *Datura* intoxication. (Note: This analysis should be conducted at an equine analytical chemistry laboratory that has validated methods and relevant sensitivity. Veterinarians are advised to make inquiries with respect to laboratory proficiency before submitting samples.)
  - The International Federation of Horseracing Authorities and the ARCI recognize a threshold of 60 ng/mL of free and conjugated scopolamine in the urine as acknowledgement of the potential for exposure through consumption of conventional feedstuffs.
  - The collection of serial samples may be more informative about *Datura* exposure than a single sample collected at one time point only.
- Identification of seeds or seed pods in gastric or intestinal contents on necropsy.

Pathological Findings

- On necropsy, necrotic or lytic changes were noted in liver, kidney, intestinal mucosa, and myocardium. However, none of these lesions, alone or in combination, is pathognomonic for scopolamine intoxication.
- Several cases were diagnosed at necropsy with gastric rupture.

THERAPEUTICS

Detoxification

- Activated charcoal is administered in cases of human intoxication and was described in one report of an equine case cluster.
- The potential benefit of administration in the horse should be weighed against the extent and severity of the GI signs, particularly when there is evidence of ileus or gut stasis.

Appropriate Health Care

- Eliminate source of exposure.
- Hospitalization is indicated for horses demonstrating clinical signs that warrant intervention.
- Supportive nursing care directed at clinical signs.
- Withhold feed and maintain hydration via parenteral fluids until GI signs resolve.
- Gastric decompression via nasogastric intubation with refluxing.

Antidotes

There is no specific antidote.

Drugs of Choice

- In one case report pilocarpine (5% solution) was administered SC at 100 mg q2–6h to severely affected horses and resulted in transient improvement in clinical signs.
- NSAIDS for inflammation and pain control:
    - Flunixin meglumine 1.1 mg/kg IV or PO q12–24h.
    - Phenylbutazone 2.2–4.4 mg/kg IV or PO q12 – 24h.
- Sedation for agitation:
    - Diazepam 0.02–0.1 mg/kg slow IV.
    - Xylazine 1.1 mg/kg IV or 2.2 mg/kg IM prn.

Precautions/Interactions

- Avoid medications with antimuscarinic effects.
- *Datura* exposure should be investigated if a horse develops signs of toxicity following a conventional dose of an antimuscarinic medication.
- Horses ingesting subclinical doses of Datura may be at risk of toxicity if administered antimuscarinic drugs, including:
    - Antihistamines.
    - Atropine.
    - Dextromethorphan.
    - N-butylscopolamine (Buscopan™).
    - Tramadol or other opioids.

Alternative Drugs

Physostigmine is used to treat human intoxications but there are no descriptions of its use in horses.

COMMENTS

Prevention/Avoidance

- Pasture management including weed control and forage quality monitoring.
- Plants are readily identifiable and can be manually removed from pastures or paddocks.
- Avoidance can be achieved by ensuring adequate access to conventional forages
- Inspection of hay may be unreliable in preventing exposure; there can be high variability in jimsonweed distribution within an individual field and so with the hay harvested from it. Further, while seed pods may not be observed, seeds may remain entrapped in the cured plant material.

Possible Complications

Mydriasis may result in impaired vision and/or physical discomfort when affected horses are exposed to sunlight. Providing a secure, shaded or darkened environment is recommended until mydriasis resolves, typically 2–3 days following cessation of *Datura* exposure, but mydriasis has been reported to persist for up to 7 days.

Expected Course and Prognosis

- Clinical signs and prognosis are dose-dependent.
- Improved prognosis is associated with the development of polydipsia and polyuria during the recovery interval after source of exposure is withdrawn.
- While some exposures have resulted in fatalities due to GI stasis or gastric rupture, most cases spontaneously recover in 48–168 hours with appropriate nursing care and with no lasting adverse effects.

Abbreviations

See Appendix 1 for a complete list.

Suggested Reading

Binev R, Valchev I, Nikolov J. Clinical and pathological studies on intoxication in horses from freshly cut Jimson weed (*Datura stramonium*) contaminated maize intended for ensiling. J S Afr Vet Ass 2006; 77(4):215–219.

Brewer K, Dirikolu L, Hughes CG, Tobin T. Scopolamine in racing horses: Trace identifications associated with dietary or environmental exposure. Vet Journal 2014; 199:324–331.

Gerber R, Naudé TW, de Kock SS. Confirmed *Datura* poisoning in a horse most probably due to *D. ferox* in contaminated tef hay. J S Afr Vet Assoc 2006; 77(2):86–89.

Author: Mary Scollay, DVM
Consulting Editor: Lynn R. Hovda, RPh, DVM, MS, DACVIM

Kleingrass (Panicum coloratum)

DEFINITION/OVERVIEW

- *Panicum coloratum* (kleingrass, kleingrass 75) is a tufted, perennial grass with stems usually 60–135 cm in height from a firm, knotty base. The blades are elongate, 2–8 mm in width, smooth or stiff, with bristly hairs on one or both surfaces.
- Loosely branched, pyramidal flower clusters are mostly 8–25 cm in length, with spikelets on spreading branches; the spikelets are 2.8–3.2 mm in length and smooth.
- The rootstock is hearty and easily develops rhizomes.
- *Panicum* spp. grow in Australia, New Zealand, South Africa, South America, Afghanistan, India, and Texas. In Texas, they reach from the high plains to Edward's Plateau and the Trans-Pecos area. Some native species found outside the USA generally are not toxic.
- Horses have developed liver disease while grazing kleingrass or eating kleingrass hay but hepatic-related photosensitization has not been reported with *Panicum coloratum*.
- *Panicum dichotomiflorum* (fall panicum) hay, found in the eastern USA has been associated with an outbreak in horses. In this instance, the onset was much more rapid (days to weeks) and liver disease with photosensitization occurred.

ETIOLOGY/PATHOPHYSIOLOGY

Mechanism of Action

- The exact mechanism of action has not been fully described.
- Cattle are not affected by the toxin; sheep, goats and horses are susceptible.
- The suspected toxin is a saponin (saponins are composed of sapogenins and a sugar moiety), probably the same as that found in *Tribulus*, *Nolina*, and *Agave* spp.

Toxicokinetics

- The onset of action is variable, but generally several months.

Toxicity

- Variable and may depend on the specific strain of kleingrass, stage of growth, or the concentration of saponin.

Blackwell's Five-Minute Veterinary Consult Clinical Companion: Equine Toxicology, First Edition. Edited by Lynn R. Hovda, Dionne Benson, and Robert H. Poppenga.
© 2022 John Wiley & Sons, Inc. Published 2022 by John Wiley & Sons, Inc.
Companion website: www.wiley.com/go/hovda/equine

Systems Affected

- Hepatobiliary.
- Integument – ± photosensitization.

 ## SIGNALMENT/HISTORY

- No known breed, sex, or age predispositions.

Risk Factors

- Consumption of *P. coloratum* (kleingrass) either on pasture or in hay.
- Lack of knowledge about the effects on horses. Cattle are not affected, and horses turned out on kleingrass pasture with them or receiving kleingrass hay may develop signs.

Historical Findings

- *Panicum* spp. were introduced into the USA from South Africa during the 1950s; *P. coloratum* was developed by Texas A&M University during the early 1970s and prefers improved pastures.

Location and Circumstances of Poisoning

- Areas where kleingrass is grown as pasture grass or baled into hay.

 ## CLINICAL FEATURES

- Anorexia and weight loss.
- Icterus.
- Hepatoencephalopathy with head pressing and violent behavior.
- Horses tend not to develop secondary or hepatogenous photosensitization.
- Intermittent colic.

 ## DIFFERENTIAL DIAGNOSIS

- History of being on kleingrass pasture or fed kleingrass hay; compatible clinical signs.
- Other hepatotoxins – aflatoxin (detection in feed and histopathology), pyrrolizidine alkaloids (ingestion of alkaloid-containing plants and histopathology), and iron toxicosis (tissue iron concentrations and histopathology).
- Exposure to other hepatotoxic plants – *Nolina texana*, *Agave lechuguilla*, *Panicum* spp., and *Trifolium hybridum* (identification in animal's environment, evidence of consumption).
- Theiler's disease (history, histopathology).

DIAGNOSTICS

CBC/Serum Chemistry/Urinalysis

- Markedly elevated serum GGT, total and direct bilirubin, blood ammonia
- Variable elevations in SDH, AST and SAP.

Other Diagnostic Tests

- Sulfobromophthalein (or bromsulphalein) clearance times are slowed several-fold.

Imaging

- Hepatic ultrasound may show areas of fibrosis. Ultrasound may be used to guide liver biopsy.

Pathological Findings

- Histopathologically, chronic hepatitis with varying degrees of fibrosis, which is dependent on the length of exposure.
- Characteristic microscopic lesions – bridging hepatic fibrosis, cholangitis, and hepatocellular regeneration.

THERAPEUTICS

Detoxification

- None suggested as this is a chronic disease.

Appropriate Health Care

- Remove horse(s) from kleingrass.
- Provide access to high-quality feeds and hay.
- Protect from sunlight if needed.
- Monitor liver enzymes.
- Consider liver biopsy to determine amount of fibrosis and other hepatic damage.
- IV crystalloids as needed for dehydration.

Antidotes

- None.

Drugs of Choice

- No specific therapeutic interventions.
- Sedation for those horses with behavior issues secondary to hepatic encephalopathy.

Precautions/Interactions

- Impaired hepatic function may prolong clearance of drugs metabolized by the liver.
- Handle carefully if horse shows any signs of hepatic encephalopathy.

Alternative Drugs

- SAM-e or NAC for hepatic support.

COMMENTS

Client Education

- Be knowledgeable about pasture grasses and grasses in baled hay. This is especially important if horses are grazed and fed with cattle.

Prevention/Avoidance

- Do not allow horses to graze *Panicum* spp. or ingest hays containing the grass.

Possible Complications

- The occurrence of photosensitization in horses is questionable. Photosensitization has been noted in other *Panicum* spp., but not *P. coloratum*.

Expected Course and Prognosis

- Onset of clinical signs is associated with significant hepatic fibrosis, making the long-term prognosis guarded to very poor.
- If medical attention is provided prior to the onset of clinical signs, the prognosis is better, but some residual liver damage may be present.

Abbreviations

See Appendix 1 for a complete list.

Internet Resources

Kleingrass (*Panicum coloratum* L.). Available at: http://plants.usda.gov/factsheet/pdf/fs_paco2.pdf (accessed April 14, 2021).

Suggested Reading

Burrows GE, Tyrl RJ. Toxic Plants of North America. Ames, IA: Iowa State University Press, 2001; pp. 913–915.

Cornick JL, Carter GK, Bridges CH. Kleingrass-associated hepatotoxicosis in horses. J Am Vet Med Assoc 1988; 193:932–935.

Hart CR, Garland T, Barr AC, et al. Toxic Plants of Texas. College Station, TX, Texas Agrilife Extension Service, 2003; p. 144.

Johnson AL, Divers TJ, Freckleton ML, et al. Fall *Panicum* (*Panicum dichotomiflorum*) hepatotoxicosis in horses and sheep. J Vet Intern Med 2006; 20:1414–1421.

Author Tam Garland, DVM, PhD, DABVT
Consulting Editor: Lynn R. Hovda, RPh, DVM, MS, DACVIM

Chapter 60

Lantana (*Lantana camara*)

DEFINITION/OVERVIEW

- *Lantana camara* (lantana or red sage) is an herbaceous, perennial, ornamental shrub. It is erect or sprawling, clumped, stout, hairy and grows to 210 cm tall, with several stems arising out of the base. It has square twigs or stems having small, scattered spines. The branches have an opposite arrangement which is characteristic even in the dormant phase (see Fig. 60.1).
- The leaves are simple, opposite or whorled, and are oval-shaped, with a petiole up to 1.5 cm long. The net-veined leaf blade is aromatic when crushed; the blades are broadly lanceolate and 5–11 cm long and 2.5–6 cm wide, with a wedge-shaped base and regularly spaced, toothed margins.
- The flowers most often consist of two colors, ranging from white, yellow, or orange to red, blue, or even dark violet; the flowers are small and tubular in flat-topped clusters (see Fig. 60.2).
- A green, immature, berry-like fruit is also found, with hard seeds turning blue to black at maturity.
- The green berry apparently is the most toxic, although the entire plant is toxic.
- The plant is regarded as ornamental, but some varieties have escaped cultivation over most of the USA and Canada. It also grows widely in tropical and subtropical countries around the world.
- Lantana toxins cause intrahepatic cholestasis, characterized by inhibition of bile secretion without extensive hepatocyte necrosis and may cause kidney failure as well.
- Horses display hepatic dysfunction with severe and intense icterus but may not develop photosensitization that occurs in ruminants. This may be due to a difference in metabolism or which toxin is involved.

ETIOLOGY/PATHOPHYSIOLOGY

Mechanism of Action

- Toxins cause intrahepatic cholestasis by inhibiting bile secretion.
- Hepatic metabolism differences between species may account for the variable susceptibility to lantana toxins

---

Blackwell's Five-Minute Veterinary Consult Clinical Companion: Equine Toxicology, First Edition. Edited by Lynn R. Hovda, Dionne Benson, and Robert H. Poppenga.
© 2022 John Wiley & Sons, Inc. Published 2022 by John Wiley & Sons, Inc.
Companion website: www.wiley.com/go/hovda/equine

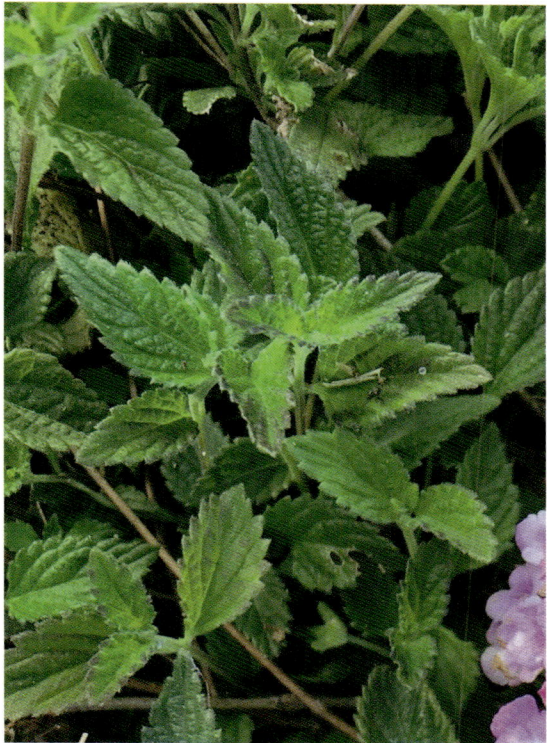

■ **Fig. 60 1.** Lantana (*Lantana camara*) leaves. *Source:* Photo courtesy of Robert Poppenga.

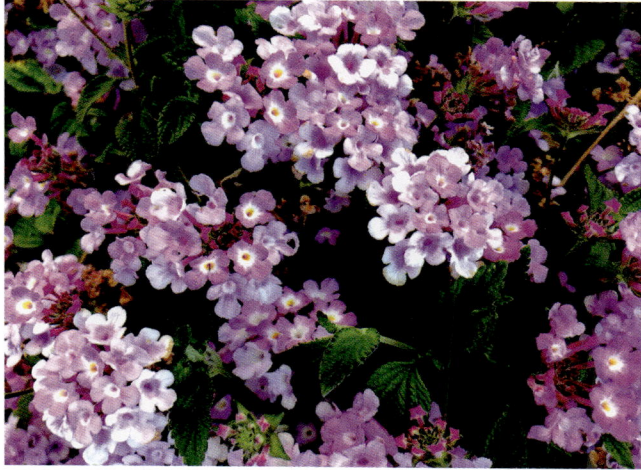

■ **Fig. 60.2.** Lantana (*Lantana camara*) leaves and flowers. *Source:* Photo courtesy of Robert Poppenga.

Toxicokinetics

- Inappetence and anorexia within 2 hours followed by lethargy, sedation, swelling of the eyelids and dermatitis within 24–48 hours. Colitis and severe jaundice follow in a few days.
- Death within 1–4 weeks if exposure continues.
- Injury to the liver cells could result from the action of the metabolite rather than the parent compound.
- There is no information in horses about transfer to milk or placenta or to offspring.

Toxicity

- The toxins are polycyclic triterpenoids – lantadene A and lantadene B.
- Sheep dosed with 60 mg/kg lantadene A developed hepatitis.
- There are numerous cultivars and hybrids, and toxicity seems to vary considerably among them. Common pink-flowered types are low in lantadene A and B, while the red-flowered type is high is lantadene A and B. Nevertheless, caution is warranted not to rely only on flower color as judge of toxicity.

Systems Affected

- Hepatic.
- Gastrointestinal.
- Renal.
- Integument.

SIGNALMENT/HISTORY

Risk Factors

- Hungry horses or those unfamiliar with the plants are more likely to consume L. camara.

Historical Findings

- The incidence of lantana poisoning in horses is generally low but may occur more frequently after a prolonged drought when there is little alternate forage available for food.

Location and Circumstances of Poisoning

- Pastures in the southern USA.

CLINICAL FEATURES

- Anorexia, lethargy, icterus (may be severe), constipation, PU/PD.
- Horses are not believed to develop photosensitization with lantana intoxication, but one report described associated crusty, contact-type lesions around the muzzles and light-skinned areas.

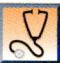
DIFFERENTIAL DIAGNOSIS

- Other hepatotoxins – aflatoxin (detection in feed and histopathology), PAs (ingestion of alkaloid-containing plants and histopathology), and iron toxicosis (tissue iron concentrations and histopathology).
- Exposure to other hepatotoxic plants – *Nolina texana*, *Agave lechuguilla*, *Panicum* spp., and *Trifolium hybridum*.
- Theiler's disease (history and histopathology).

DIAGNOSTICS

CBC/Serum Chemistry/Urinalysis

- Hyperbilirubinemia (conjugated) is the most consistent finding.
- Elevation in liver enzymes.
- ± increases in BUN and creatinine.

Other Laboratory Tests

- Lantadenes may be detected in stomach contents if death occurs close to the time of consumption.
- Portions of the plant may be identified in the stomach contents by a competent microscopist.

Imaging

- Ultrastructural studies have observed obstructive cholangitis.

Pathological Findings

- Liver lesions – cholestasis, pigmentation and degeneration of hepatocytes, and fibrosis.
- Kidney lesions – vacuolation and degeneration of convoluted tubule epithelium and presence of various casts. Occasionally, multifocal, interstitial, mononuclear cell infiltration, and fibrosis may be evident.

THERAPEUTICS

Detoxification

- Activated charcoal 2–4 g/kg PO in a water slurry (1 g of AC per 5 mL of water) if recent ingestion.
- Sodium thiosulfate 0.5 g/kg IV.

Appropriate Health Care

- Primarily supportive care.
- IV crystalloid fluids as needed for dehydration and diuresis.

Antidotes

- There is no specific antidote.

Alternative Drugs

- NAC or SAM-e for hepatic support.

COMMENTS

Client Education

- Become familiar with this plant and remove from pastures. Do not plant it as an ornamental shrub in pastures or along fence lines when horses have access

Prevention/Avoidance

- Preventing access to the plant is the best solution for avoiding toxicosis.
- Herbicides can be used to control the plant. It is quite susceptible to the herbicide 2,4-dichlorophenoxyacetic acid.

Possible Complications

- Chronic hepatic or renal failure in horses that survive.
- ± crusting skin lesions.

Expected Course and Prognosis

- The prognosis is good for horses that are removed from pasture and treated within the first 24 hours of exposure.
- Continued exposure results in a very poor prognosis.

Abbreviations

See Appendix 1 for a complete list.

Suggested Reading

Burrow GE, Tyrl RJ. Toxic Plants of North America. Ames, IA: Iowa State University Press, 2001; pp. 1170–1174.

Morton JF. Lantana, or red sage (Lantana camara L., [Verbenaceae]), notorious weed and popular garden flower; some cases of poisoning in Florida. Economic Botany. 1994 Jul 1;48(3):259.

Pass MA. Poisoning of livestock by lantana plants. In: Keeler RF, Tu AT, eds. Toxicology of Plant and Fungal Compounds: Handbook of Natural Toxins. New York, NY: Marcel Dekker, 1991; pp. 297–311.

Sharma OP, Sharma S, Pattabhi V, et al. A review of the hepatotoxic plant Lantana camara. Critical reviews in toxicology. 2007; 37(4):313–352.

Author: Tam Garland, DVM, PhD, DABVT
Consulting Editor: Lynn R. Hovda, RPh, DVM, MS, DACVIM

Locoweed (*Astragalus* and *Oxytropis*) Poisoning in Horses

Chapter 61

DEFINITION/OVERVIEW

- Locoweed poisoning is caused by about 20 species of the *Astragalus* and *Oxytropis* genera that contain the indolizidine alkaloid, swainsonine (see Table 61.1 and Fig. 61.1).
- Prolonged swainsonine ingestion produces cellular storage disease and abnormal glycosylation of many different glycoproteins, resulting in vacuoles in cells that disrupt normal cellular function.
- All locoweed plant parts, including dry hulls or stems, contain swainsonine.
- Horses are uniquely susceptible, and they readily eat locoweed and they often become poisoned regardless of the accessibility of alternative forages.
- Most susceptible animals require several weeks of poisoning to develop mild neurologic disease.
- Poisoning affects nearly all body systems and poisoning becomes more severe with prolonged and repeated poisoning.
- Clinical poisoning includes depression, reluctance to move, proprioceptive deficits, tremors, weakness, loss of body condition, wasting and dull rough coat that fails to shed properly. When exposure is discontinued, most lesions quickly resolve and many animals are useful if they do not have severe neurologic damage.

ETIOLOGY/PATHOPHYSIOLOGY

Mechanism of Action

- Essentially a plant-induced lysosomal storage disease.
- Swainsonine is not directly cytotoxic; rather it inhibits cellular α-mannosidase and mannosidase II. These enzymes hydrolyze mannose-rich polysaccharides, glycoproteins and oligosaccharides.
  - Prolonged swainsonine ingestion produces cellular storage disease and abnormal glycosylation of many different glycoproteins.
  - Without these enzymes, oligosaccharides and abnormally glycosylated proteins accumulate in the cell, lysosomal numbers increase, vacuoles form, and normal cellular function is disrupted.
- Clinical disease requires extended enzyme inhibition.

Blackwell's Five-Minute Veterinary Consult Clinical Companion: Equine Toxicology,
First Edition. Edited by Lynn R. Hovda, Dionne Benson, and Robert H. Poppenga.
© 2022 John Wiley & Sons, Inc. Published 2022 by John Wiley & Sons, Inc.
Companion website: www.wiley.com/go/hovda/equine

TABLE 61.1 Common locoweeds present in the United States.

Locoweeds		
Scientific name	Common name	Location
Astragalus allochrous	Halfmoon milkvetch	California, Arizona
A. amphioxys	Crescent milkvetch	Southwest North America
A. assymetricus	San Joaquin milkvetch	California
A. flavus	Yellow milkvetch	Colorado plateau, canyonlands
A. lentiginosus	Spotted locoweed	Western North America
A. mollissimus	Woolly locoweed	Colorado plateau, canyonlands
A. missouriensis	Missouri milkvetch	Central North America
A. nothoxys	Sheep milkvetch	Southwest North America
A. oxyphysus	Diablo milkvetch	California
A. pubentissimus	Green river milkvetch	Utah, Wyoming, Colorado
A. purshii	Woollypod milkvetch	Western and northwestern North America
A. pycnostachyus	Marsh milkvetch	California
A. thurberi	Thurber's milkvetch	Arizona, New Mexico
A. wootoni	Half moon milkvetch, Garboncillo	Texas, southwest north America
Oxytropis besseyi	Bessey's locoweed	Mountain western United States
O. campestris	Field locoweed	Northern North America
O. lambertii	Purple or Lambert's locoweed	Northern North America
O. sericea	White locoweed	Western North America

Source: USDA/ARS Poisonous Plant Research Laboratory.

Toxicokinetics

- Swainsonine is highly soluble, and this is seen *in vivo* as rapid absorption and excretion in urine and milk.
- There is little information about the toxicokinetics in horses. The half-life in sheep associated with a natural poisoning research model was about 18 hours. This indicates that serum swainsonine concentrations at just over 2 days post-exposure will be below current detection concentrations and limits the use of swainsonine as an indicator of locoweed poisoning if sampling is delayed.

Toxicity

- There is marked species difference in susceptibility to poisoning:
  - Horses and goats seem to be the most susceptible (about 0.25 mg swainsonine/kg BW for 30 days).
  - Sheep and cattle are a little less (about 0.4 mg swainsonine/kg BW for 30 days).
  - Mule deer, rats, hamsters, mice, and guinea pigs are more resistant (about 1.5 mg/kg BW for 30 days).

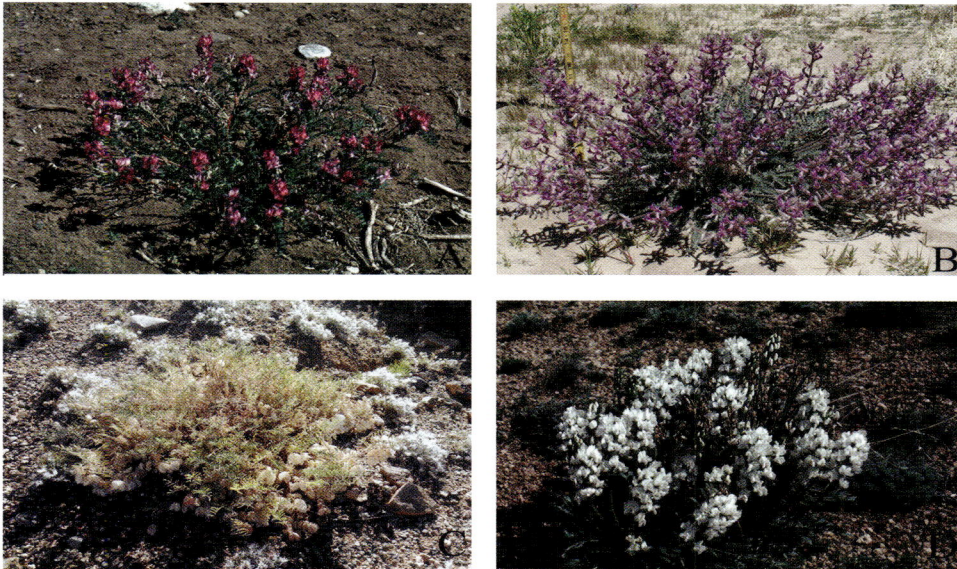

■ **Fig. 61.1.** Locoweeds that commonly poison horses and livestock in North America. (A) *Astragalus lentiginosus* (spotted locoweed) is a perennial or annual common to the western North American Great Basin area. It has 12- to 15-cm leaves that are divided pairs of small leaflets. The pea-like flowers may be purple to white that mature into a grooved pod that has red mottling (spotted). (B) *Astragalus mollissimus* (wooly locoweed) is a perennial of desert western North America. It is similar to *A. lentiginosus*, but the leaves and stems are covered with small fine hairs. The flowers form on a slightly taller stalk than spotted locoweed and they also can be purple, white or bicolored. The pods are egg-shaped and are covered with small hairs. (C) *Astragalus wootonii* (garboncillo, rattleweed, or half-moon milkvetch) is found in the trans-pecos region (Texas, New Mexico and Arizona). It is also multi-branched with erect hair stems 6–15 cm long. The leaves have 19 pea-like leaflets that are hairy underneath. The flowers are white to purple the mature into inflated pods that when dry easily break off and rattle. (D) *Oxytropis sericea* (white point locoweed) is a perennial with a wide distribution that can be found from the great plains through the western mountain states of North America. It grows to about 30 cm tall and may have several flowering stalks. The flowers are usually white and they mature into 2.5-cm pods that contain hairy, kidney-shaped seeds. *Source*: Bryan Steiglemeier/USDA.

- Birds seem to be completely resistant to poisoning, although only pigeons and chickens have been evaluated.
■ The duration of exposure is critical:
  - In sheep, frequent intermittent exposures allowing 7-day withdrawal periods do not produce disease or lesions.
  - Long chronic exposures result in neurologic lesions including neuronal cell death.
  - Repeated poisoning, as often occurs with the use of contaminated pastures and ranges each year, results in progressive disease until neuronal damage is extensive, and animals are unable to function or be productive.

Systems Affected

■ Nearly all body systems can be affected. As neurologic disease is often irreversible and more permanent, it is the system more closely studied and characterized. The lesions in other systems generally resolve if exposure is discontinued.
■ Nervous – primarily; abnormal behavior and neurological deficits.
■ Cardiovascular/circulatory.
■ Endocrine.

- Gastrointestinal – malnutrition, weight loss.
- Integument – dull, dry hair coat.
- Musculoskeletal.
- Ophthalmic.
- Reproductive – infertility, fetal death, teratogenicity, weak neonates.

SIGNALMENT/HISTORY

- Transplacental and transmammary poisoning occurs; neonates and foals can be poisoned and develop neurologic disease and neurovisceral vacuolation similar to adults.

Risk Factors
- Locoweed-contaminated pasture.

History
- As extended mannosidase inhibition is required to produce disease, exposures of weeks and months are required to poison animals.

Location and Circumstances of Poisoning
- Access to locoweed.

CLINICAL FEATURES

- The clinical presentation of poisoning is generally depression, reluctance to move, and intention tremors when the horse moves, especially when navigating over obstacles or backing.
- With prolonged poisoning, the coat becomes rough and dull, and the winter coat is often incompletely shed.
- Malnutrition, weight loss, and muscle atrophy.
- Decreased tear production and dull appearing eyes.
- With extended poisoning, neurologic disease may become more severe as animals lose proprioception and the ability to step over and around obstacles. This often causes anxiety, and erratic behavior that may result in dangerous aggression.
- Reproductive function is altered as female estrus cycle is disrupted and arrested. Poisoning has also been associated with fetal death and resorption, mild teratogenesis and weak neonates that cannot stand and nurse without assistance.
- If exposure is discontinued before permanent neurologic damage, most of these signs quickly resolve within a matter of weeks.

DIFFERENTIAL DIAGNOSIS

- Equine herpes myeloencephalitis (EHM).
- EPM.
- Cholesterol granulomas.

- Rabies.
- Other toxins – methyl bromide.
- Trauma.

DIAGNOSTICS

CBC/Serum Chemistry/Urinalysis

- Mild non-regenerative anemia.
- Increased AST.

Other Diagnostic Tests

- Locoweed toxin, swainsonine in serum, liver or other tissues. Samples must be taken during locoweed exposure and ingestion as rapid swainsonine clearance will result in undetectable concentrations within 2 days of discontinuing exposure.
- Similarly, serum α-D-mannosidase activities will be depressed in the presence of serum swainsonine. This will also quickly return to normal as swainsonine concentrations rapidly decrease when locoweed ingestion is discontinued.
- Supporting clinical findings include increased serum AST activities, decreased thyroid hormones, and alterations in micronutrient metabolism.

Pathological Findings

- Swainsonine-induced vacuolation is most prominent and characteristic in the cerebellar Purkinje cells and granular layer neurons. The vacuoles are small and often displace the nucleus to the cell margins.
  - Affected neurons are enlarged and swollen and they lose many axonal connections.
  - Secondary axonal changes include axonal hillock formation with swelling and spheroids.
  - With extended poisoning, affected neurons become degenerative and necrotic, inciting mild gliosis. Prolonged intoxication causes lesions in neurons of both the central and peripheral nervous system.
  - Combinations of vacuolation of intestinal ganglionic neurons and exocrine pancreas damage contribute to loss of condition, wasting and emaciation that characterizes locoweed poisoning.
  - If locoweed exposure is discontinued, much of the vacuolation resolves. However, some neuron lesions are permanent. These include reduced numbers of Purkinje cells and axonal spheroids in the cerebellar peduncles and medullary white tracts.
- Visceral and endocrine vacuolation is most prominent in thyroid follicular epithelium, exocrine pancreas, adrenal medulla, uroepithelium, renal proximal convoluted tubule epithelium, testes, ovary and macrophages in lymph nodes, splenic lymphoid follicles and interstitium of the heart, lung and liver.

THERAPEUTICS

Detoxification
- Historically various binding agents and mineral supplements have been suggested; however, none has proven to be effective.
- Swainsonine is not cytotoxic so activated charcoal and/or cathartics are not helpful.

Appropriate Health Care
- Affected horses should be removed from locoweed-contaminated pasture and provided a good nutritional source.
- Anxious animals with severe trembling may be treated with tranquilizers such as valium.
- Additional care is supportive as accidents and trauma are common in severely damaged animals.

Antidotes
- There is no antidote.

Drugs of Choice
- Diazepam 25–50 mg (adult dose) slow IV prn for seizures; 0.1–0.4 mg/kg IV (foals).

Precautions/Interactions
- Horses should be handled with caution as behavior may unpredictable and they may suddenly move from quiet to violent.

Alternative Drugs
- Many supplements and minerals have been suggested as preventative, but none has shown any positive effects.

COMMENTS

- Locoweed poisoning is a chronic disease that develops in horses grazing locoweeds over extended periods. A diagnosis of poisoning is made by documenting exposure to the plant, identifying the neurologic signs of poisoning, and analyzing serum for swainsonine.

Client Education
- As most horses on contaminated pasture will eat locoweed regardless of the accessibility of alternative forages, avoiding exposure is essential.

Prevention/Avoidance
- Monitor pastures and paddocks for locoweed and move horses to other pastures prior to the onset of disease.

Possible Complications

- Some of the neurologic changes are irreversible and permanent. If neuronal damage is severe, affected animals may not be able to breed or take care of neonates.
- Poisoning has also been associated with fetal death and resorption, mild teratogenesis usually seen as small and short-legged fetuses, placental dysplasia such as hydrops amnii and weak neonates that cannot stand and nurse without assistance.
- Prolonged and repeated exposures tend to result in severe disease that may not recover or be suitable for work or breeding.

Expected Course and Prognosis

- Locoweed poisoning severely compromises both male and female reproduction.
  - With 45 days of ingestion, mares become anestrus and most develop cystic ovaries.
  - With slightly longer exposures, males have abnormal spermatogenesis, resulting in abnormal and dysfunctional spermatozoa.
  - If poisoning is discontinued both males and females recover within a couple of estrus cycles and animals may be reproductively functional if neurologic damage is not severe enough to alter libido and breeding behavior.
- Residual neurologic deficits make the prognosis poor for animals used for draft, riding or competition as they are potentially hazardous to people who use them.

Abbreviations

See Appendix 1 for a complete list.

Internet Resources

Locoweed Poisoning in Horses. Available at: https://aces.nmsu.edu/pubs/_b/B713/welcome.html (accessed April 14, 2021).

Suggested Reading

Burrows GM, Tyrl RJ. Toxic Plants of North America, 2nd edn. Ames, IA: Wiley Blackwell, 2013; pp. 505–515.
Cook D, Gardner DR, Lee ST, et al. A swainsonine survey of North American *Astragalus* and *Oxytropis* taxa implicated as locoweeds. Toxicon 2016; 118:104–111.
Nollet H, Paater, Vanschandevijl K, et al. Suspected swainsonine poisoning in a Belgian horse. Eq Vet Educ 2008; 20(2):62–65.
Stegelmeier BL, Davis TZ, Clayton MJ. Neurotoxic plants that poison livestock. Vet Clin North Am Food Anim Pract 2020; 36(3):673–688.

Author: Bryan L. Stegelmeier, DVM, PhD, DACVP
Consulting Editor: Lynn R. Hovda, RPh, DVM, MS, DACVIM

Chapter 62

Narrowleaf Milkweed (Asclepias fascicularis)

DEFINITION/OVERVIEW

- Narrowleaf milkweed (*Asclepias fascicularis*, also known as Mexican milkweed or Mexican whorled milkweed) is one of the most toxic of the ~150 species of milkweeds.
- *A. fascicularis* is found in the western United States, including Utah, Nevada, Idaho, Arizona, California, Oregon, and Washington.
- The plant is perennial and may grow in a variety of habitats.
- Neurologic signs predominate.

ETIOLOGY/PATHOPHYSIOLOGY

Mechanism of Action

- Milkweeds contain both cardiotoxins and neurotoxins; the narrowleaf milkweed contains primarily neurotoxins.
- The toxic principle of *A. fascicularis* is unknown; other *Asclepias* species have been found to contain a variety of cinnamic ester pregnane glycoside neurotoxins.
- The mechanism of neurotoxicity is unknown, as is its metabolism.

Toxicity

- Clinical signs may appear following ingestion of as little as 0.22% body weight.
- Death may occur following ingestion of 0.5–1% body weight.
- Signs may be seen from 1–24 hours following ingestion of a toxic dose.
- Neurotoxic effects are cumulative.

Systems Affected

- Nervous – the primary system affected. Horses may show anxiety, depression, trembling, ataxia, weakness, recumbency, mydriasis, seizures with flexed thoracic limbs, and paddling leg movements.
- Respiratory – death occurs due to respiratory failure following seizure activity.
- Musculoskeletal – significant self-trauma often occurs during seizure activity.
- Cardiovascular – cardiac arrhythmias may be ausculted in some cases.
- Gastrointestinal – colic signs may be seen in the early stages of intoxication.

Blackwell's Five-Minute Veterinary Consult Clinical Companion: Equine Toxicology,
First Edition. Edited by Lynn R. Hovda, Dionne Benson, and Robert H. Poppenga.
© 2022 John Wiley & Sons, Inc. Published 2022 by John Wiley & Sons, Inc.
Companion website: www.wiley.com/go/hovda/equine

SIGNALMENT/HISTORY

Risk Factors

- Animals grazing pastures in the western United States may be at risk.
- No breed, sex, or age predilection is known.
- Narrowleaf milkweed often grows in dense localized patches.
- Narrowleaf milkweed is difficult to distinguish in hay but retains its toxicity when dried.

Location and Circumstances of Poisoning

- Affected animals will either be grazing pasture in the western United States or be fed hay originating from that area.

CLINICAL FEATURES

- Depression, weakness, trembling, ataxia, falling, recumbency.
- Sweating.
- Colic signs.
- Mydriasis.
- Pelvic limb paresis.
- Paddling, seizures with thoracic limbs flexed.
- Terminal dyspnea.
- Animals may be found dead.

DIFFERENTIAL DIAGNOSIS

- Other poisonous plants – *Astragalus/Oxytropis* (locoism), white snakeroot, bracken fern toxicosis.
- Mushroom intoxication.
- Tremorgenic mycotoxins (ryegrass or *Paspalum* staggers).
- Phosphide salts.
- Ivermectin toxicosis.
- Metals – arsenic, lead (acute).
- Cannabis toxicity.
- Brain abscess or neoplasia.
- Encephalitis/meningitis, EPM, hepatic encephalopathy.
- Hyperkalemic periodic paralysis.
- Propylene glycol toxicosis.
- Organophosphate intoxication.
- Strychnine poisoning.
- Hypocalcemia, hypomagnesemia.

DIAGNOSTICS

- No specific diagnostics are available for clinical disease.
- Pastures and hay should be carefully examined for the presence of narrowleaf *Asclepias* spp.
- A forage extension service may be helpful in this regard.

Pathological Findings

- Few gross pathologic changes are seen.
- GI content may be examined for *Asclepias*.
- There may be hemorrhages in the trachea, lungs and epicardium.
- Significant surface trauma may be seen.
- No characteristic histopathologic changes have been reported for neurotoxic *Asclepias*.

THERAPEUTICS

- Treatment objectives include removal of the plant from the digestive tract and supportive care through seizure activity.

Detoxification

- No specific detoxification.

Appropriate Health Care

- Gastric lavage if possible.
- Sedatives for control of seizure activity.
- IV fluids to maintain hydration and electrolyte balance.
- Padded stall or soft ground; limb or head padding as appropriate.

Antidotes

- No specific antidote is available.

Drugs of Choice

- Seizure control:
  - Diazepam 0.1–0.4 mg/kg IV (foal); 25–50 mg IV (horse).
  - Phenobarbital 5–15 mg/kg IV slowly to effect.
- Sedation:
  - Xylazine 0.2–1 mg/kg IV.

COMMENTS

Client Education

- Educate clients on appearance of narrowleaf milkweed and have them inspect pastures and hay.
- Avoidance or elimination of the plant is the only prevention.

Prevention/Avoidance

- Prevention of consumption or elimination of the plant is the only viable preventive measure.

Expected Course and Prognosis

- Survivors of acute intoxication may show residual neurologic signs for several days, but generally return to normal within 1–2 weeks.
- Prognosis depends on the amount of plant ingested and the level of supportive care available.

Abbreviations

See Appendix 1 for a complete list.

Internet Resources

Locoweed Poisoning in Horses. Available at: https://aces.nmsu.edu/pubs/_b/B713/welcome.html
USDA. *Asclepias fascicularis*. Available at: https://plants.sc.egov.usda.gov/core/profile?symbol=ASFA

Suggested Reading

Burrows GE, Tyrl RJ (eds). Asclepias L. in Toxic Plants of North America, 2nd edn. Ames, IA: John Wiley & Sons, 2013; pp. 85–94.
Divers TJ. Nervous system treatment and procedures. In: Equine Emergencies, 4th edn. St Louis, MO: Saunders, 2014; pp. 339–378.

Author: Tamara Gull, DVM, PhD, DACVIM (LAIM), DACVPM, DACVM
Consulting Editor: Lynn R. Hovda, RPh, DVM, MS, DACVIM

Chapter 63

Nightshades (*Solanum* spp.)

DEFINITION/OVERVIEW

- Numerous *Solanum* spp. (nightshade family) are potentially toxic to animals – *S. nigrum* (black nightshade), *S. dulcamera* (bittersweet nightshade), *S. carolinense* (horse nettle), *S. rostratum* (buffalo burr), *S. tuberosum* (potato), *S. elaeagnifolium* (Silverleaf nightshade) and *S. dimidiatum* (Western horse nettle), and others.
- Plants in this genus are widely distributed.
- Documented cases of equine intoxication are rare, and those in the literature do not provide significant information concerning pathophysiologic effects.
- Plants contain a variety of steroidal glycoalkaloids in varying concentrations of glycosides (attached sugars) and aglycones (no sugars attached).
- Reports of increased sensitivity to ivermectin (and presumably other macrolide endectocides as well) if horses are concurrently ingesting a *Solanum* spp.

ETIOLOGY/PATHOPHYSIOLOGY

Mechanism of Action

- Anticholinergic, muscarinic, and GI irritant effects have been described in intoxicated animals.
- Muscarinic effects may result from cholinesterase inhibition, but this has not been verified clinically.
- GI irritation is believed to result from a saponin-like effect of the steroidal glycoalkaloids.
- Increased sensitivity to macrolide endectocides is hypothesized to be due to *Solanum* toxins interfering with p-glycoprotein function, resulting in increased brain concentrations of the drug.

Toxicokinetics

- Limited information based upon human studies.
- Glycoalkaloids appear to be poorly absorbed from the GI tract.

Toxicity

- Toxicity is attributed primarily to tropane alkaloids and steroidal glycoalkaloids (e.g., solanine), but few equine data are available.
- Toxicity varies with environment, plant part ingested, and time of year.
- Unripe berries contain the highest glycoalkaloid concentration, which declines with maturity.
- Green portions of potato contain the highest toxin concentration.

Systems Affected

- Cardiovascular – arrhythmias.
- Gastrointestinal – irritation, increased or decreased motility.
- Nervous – CNS stimulation or depression described in some species and with ingestion of some *Solanum* spp.; mydriasis is a commonly reported effect across species

SIGNALMENT/HISTORY

Risk Factors

- No known breed, age, or sex predispositions.
- Contamination of hay with *Solanum* spp.
- Unavailability of alternative desirable forage.
- Access to cld potatoes or potato refuse.

CLINICAL FEATURES

- GI signs predominate – anorexia, nausea, salivation, colic, and diarrhea with or without blood.
- Nervous system signs – apathy, drowsiness, trembling, progressive weakness or paralysis, recumbency, and coma.

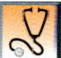
DIFFERENTIAL DIAGNOSIS

- Other causes of colic – physical examination, lack of exposure to *Solanum* spp.

DIAGNOSTICS

- Establishing the diagnosis relies on evidence of consumption of *Solanum* spp.

Other Diagnostic Tests

- Detection of alkaloids in GI contents is possible but not commonly performed.

Pathological Findings

- Gross findings:
  - Evidence of plant in the stomach.
  - Grossly, there may be evidence of GI irritation and diarrhea with or without hemorrhage.
- Histopathology:
  - Histopathologically, there is congestion, inflammation, hemorrhage, and ulceration of the GI mucosa.

THERAPEUTICS

Detoxification

- Remove animal from source of exposure.
- If soon after ingestion, consider GI decontamination.
- AC (1–4 g/kg PO in water slurry [1 g of AC in 5 mL or water]).
- One dose of cathartic (70% sorbitol at 3 mL/kg PO or sodium or magnesium sulfate at 250 mg/kg PO, the latter two being administered in a water slurry, with AC if no diarrhea or ileus.

Appropriate Health Care

- Symptomatic and supportive.

Drugs of Choice

- NSAIDs – flunixin meglumine (1.1 mg/kg IV q12h or as necessary) for abdominal pain.

Precautions/Interactions

- Use of NSAIDs in dehydrated animals.
- Potential for increased sensitivity to macrolide endectocides.

Alternative Drugs

- Many alternatives for pain control.

COMMENTS

Client Education

- Make sure clients are aware of the toxicity of *Solanum* spp.

Prevention/Avoidance

- Limit or prevent access to *Solanum* spp.
- Do not feed potatoes or potato waste.

Possible Complications

- Congenital craniofacial malformations have been induced in fetuses of pregnant laboratory animals fed *Solanum* spp. glycoalkaloids. The significance of this finding for horses is unknown, but pregnant mares should be prevented from ingesting any *Solanum* spp.

Expected Course and Prognosis

- With early intervention and appropriate symptomatic and supportive care, prospects for recovery are good.
- With severe clinical signs, prognosis is more guarded, but experience is limited.

Abbreviations

See Appendix 1 for a complete list.

Suggested Reading

Dalvi RR, Bowie WC. Toxicology of solanine: an overview. Vet Hum Toxicol 1983; 25:13–15.
Burrows GE, Tyrl RJ. Toxic Plants of North America, 2nd edn. Ames: Iowa State University Press, 2013.
Norman TE, Chaffin MK, Norton PL, Coleman MC, Stoughton WB, Mays T. Concurrent ivermectin and *Solanum* spp. toxicosis in a herd of horses. J Vet Intern Med 2012; 26:1439–1442.

Author: Robert H. Poppenga DVM, PhD, DABVT
Consulting Editor: Lynn R. Hovda, RPh, DVM, MS, DACVIM

Chapter 64

Oleander (*Nerium oleander* and *Cascabela thevetia*)

DEFINITION/OVERVIEW

- *Nerium oleander* (common oleander) is an evergreen shrub (family Apocynaceae) with leathery, dark, gray-green, sharply pointed leaves 10–30 cm (4–12 in) long with a prominent midrib and parallel secondary veins. Flowers are white, pink, red, peach, and salmon (see Figs 64.1 and 64.2)
- *Cascabela thevetia* (yellow oleander) is an evergreen tropical shrub (family Apocynaceae) with linear-lanceolate, glossy green leaves and fragrant, long, bell or funnel-shaped yellow flowers (see Fig. 64.3).
- *Thevetia peruviana* is the former and alternate name for yellow oleander.
- Common oleander is native to Asia but now is a common ornamental plant in the southern and western USA and other parts of the world.
- Yellow oleander grows in the very southern and southwestern part of the USA but is much more common in Mexico and Central America.
- Oleander contains several cardiac glycosides and ingestion can cause severe cardiac abnormalities and sudden death.
- Intoxication should be considered for any patient presenting for colic in geographic areas where oleander is found.
- The plant remains toxic when dry.

ETIOLOGY/PATHOPHYSIOLOGY

Mechanism of Action

- Toxins cause changes in the resting membrane potential threshold, specifically the Na^+/K^+-ATPase pump, in cardiac muscle cells leading to bradycardia and arrhythmias.

Toxicokinetics

- Oleandrin and thevetin are absorbed through the GI tract after consumption of the oleander plant.
- Fairly rapid onset – 30 minutes to a few hours after ingestion.
- It is widely distributed within the body and is excreted in the feces and urine.

Blackwell's Five-Minute Veterinary Consult Clinical Companion: Equine Toxicology,
First Edition. Edited by Lynn R. Hovda, Dionne Benson, and Robert H. Poppenga.
© 2022 John Wiley & Sons, Inc. Published 2022 by John Wiley & Sons, Inc.
Companion website: www.wiley.com/go/hovda/equine

CHAPTER 64 OLEANDER (*NERIUM OLEANDER* AND *CASCABELA THEVETIA*) **331**

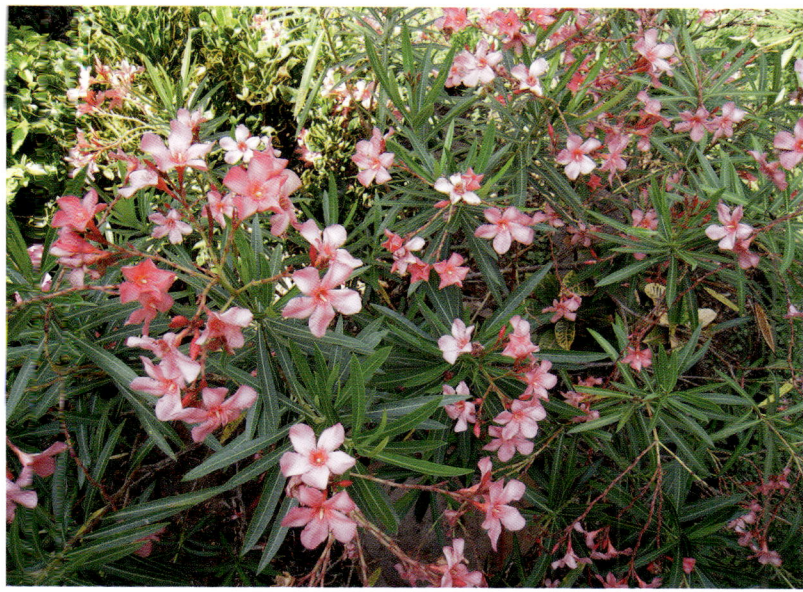

■ **Fig. 64.1.** *Nerium oleander*. Note the distinctive leaves with a prominent midrib. *Source*: Photo courtesy of Tyne K. Hovda.

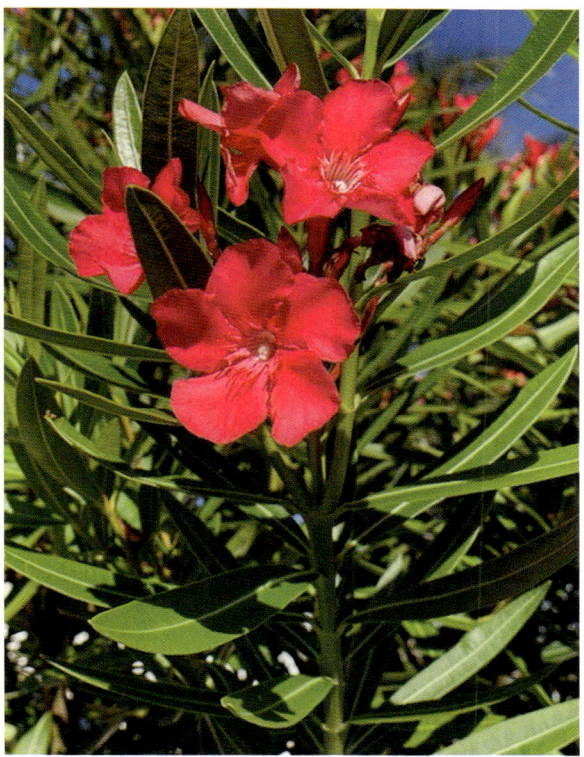

■ **Fig. 64.2** Close-up of *Nerium oleander* flower and leaves. *Source*: Photo courtesy of Tyne K. Hovda.

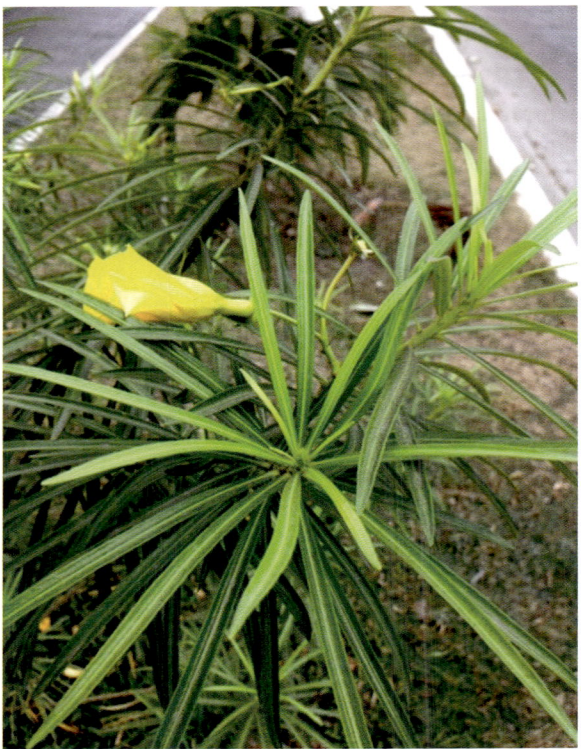

■ **Fig. 64.3.** *Cascabela thevetia* (yellow oleander). The yellow flower is long and bell shaped in contrast to the flatter *Nerium oleander* flower. *Source*: Photo courtesy of Tyne K. Hovda.

Toxicity

- Very low doses are needed to produce clinical signs.
- Ingestion of as little as 0.005% of plant by body weight may be lethal.
- Common oleander (*N. oleander*) – oleandrin and oleandrigenin are the primary toxins.
- Yellow oleander (*C. thevetia*, formerly known as *T. peruviana*) – thevetin A and thevetin B are the primary toxins.
- Yellow oleander is considered by many to be more toxic than common oleander.

Systems Affected

- Cardiovascular.
- Gastrointestinal.
- Nervous.
- Renal/urinary.

 # SIGNALMENT/HISTORY

There is no age, sex, or breed predilection.

Risk Factors

- Exposure to *N. oleander* or *C. thevetia*.
- The plant is stated to be unpalatable, so exposure occurs when there is little else on the pasture for horses to eat or it is consumed dry in hay.

Historical Findings

- History of oleander exposure and evidence of oleander in the ingesta are the most important findings in differentiating oleander toxicosis from other conditions.

Location and Circumstances of Poisoning

- Typically poisonings occur in the southwest United States (California, Arizona, New Mexico, Texas) where these plants are commonly found.
- There are come cultivars that grow farther north, but these are primarily seasonal landscape plants with limited access by horses.

CLINICAL FEATURES

- Anorexia, abdominal pain, colic, diarrhea ± blood.
- Bradycardia or tachycardia (rarely).
- Hypotension, AV block, cardiac arrhythmias.
- Weakness and depression.
- Tremors.
- Pulmonary edema.
- Seizure-like activities.
- Coma.
- Death from asystole.

DIFFERENTIAL DIAGNOSIS

- Other causes of colic, cardiac arrhythmias, and/or renal dysfunction.
- Other cardiotoxic plants (yew, rhododendrons, others).
- Other causes of GI disease, including parasite, viral and bacterial.

DIAGNOSTICS

CBC/Serum Chemistry/Urinalysis

- CBC – generally unremarkable.
- Serum chemistry:
  - Early hyperkalemia, later hypokalemia.
  - Elevated BUN/creatinine.

Other Diagnostic Tests

- Identification of oleander leaves in ingesta.
- Chemical analysis of ingesta or serum for oleandrin or thevetin.
- Serum digoxin concentration.

Pathological Findings

- Gross:
    - Identification of oleander leaves in ingesta.
    - May be no other signs in peracute cases.
- Histopathology:
    - Often no lesions in peracute cases.
    - Endocardial hemorrhages.
    - Increased pericardial fluid.
    - Necrosis of subendocardium, most often involving the left ventricle.
    - Pulmonary edema or hepatic congestion may be present.

THERAPEUTICS

Detoxification

- With suspected ingestion, decontamination including gastric lavage and administration of activated charcoal at 1–4 g/kg body weight is recommended. Consider multidose activated charcoal (two subsequent doses 6–8 hours apart).

Appropriate Health Care

- Supportive care.
- IV fluid therapy as needed, electrolyte and dextrose supplementation as indicated based on laboratory tests.
- Keep the animal quiet with very strict exercise restriction to reduce cardiac metabolic demand.
- Continuous ECG monitoring should be performed and monitoring of renal and electrolyte values while patients are in the hospital.

Antidotes

- No specific antidote for horses is available.
- Digoxin specific Fab antibodies have been used successfully in humans, dogs, and anecdotally in a few oleander equine intoxications.

Drugs of Choice

- Lidocaine 0.25–0.5 mg/kg IV, slowly, q5min; maximum total dose of 2–4 mg/kg for ventricular dysrhythmias.

Precautions/Interactions

- Do not administer potassium in fluids if hyperkalemia is present.
- Avoid calcium-containing solutions and quinidine.

- Avoid the use of beta-blockers and calcium channel blockers as they may have additive effects on AV conduction.
- Renal function should be monitored and the use of nephrotoxic drugs avoided.

Alternative Drugs

- Phenytoin could be considered for treatment of refractory ventricular arrhythmias.

 COMMENTS

Client Education

- Stall confinement should be recommended if any cardiac arrhythmias persist at discharge.

Prevention/Avoidance

- Remove all access to oleander plants.

Possible Complications

- Cardiac arrhythmias may persist following clinical recovery.
- Patients may have decreased renal function long-term following acute kidney injury.

Expected Course and Prognosis

- Mortality rates of 44–50% have been reported when the animal presents to the hospital for treatment. Without emergent medical treatment, prognosis is grave.
- Younger animals with no comorbidities may be more likely to survive but this is anecdotal.

Abbreviations

See Appendix 1 for a complete list.

Internet Resources

Oleander Poisoning of Horses. Available at: https://aces.nmsu.edu/pubs/_b/B712/welcome.html.

Suggested Reading

Bandara V, Weinstein SA, White J, Eddleston M. A review of the natural history, toxinology, diagnosis and clinical management of *Nerium oleander* (common oleander) and *Thevetia peruviana* (yellow oleander) poisoning. Toxicon 2010; 56(3): 273–281.

Butler J, Khan S, Scarzella G. Fatal oleander toxicosis in two miniature horses. J Am Hosp Assoc 2016; 52(6):398–402.

Pao-Franco A, Hammond TN, Weatherton LK, et AL. Successful use of digoxin-specific immune Fab in the treatment of severe *Nerium oleander* toxicosis in a dog. J Vet Emerg Crit Care 2017; 27(5):596–604.

Renier AC, Kass PH, Magdesian KG, et al. Oleander toxicosis in equids: 30 cases (1995-2010). J Am Vet Med Assoc 2013; 242(4):540–549.

Smith PA, Aldridge BM, Kittleson MD. Oleander toxicosis in a donkey. J Vet Intern Med 2003; 17(1):111–114.

Acknowledgement: The author and editors acknowledge the prior contribution of Larry J Thompson.

Author: Emma V. Hummer, DVM
Consulting Editor: Lynn R. Hovda, RPh, DVM, MS, DACVIM

Chapter 65

Pyrrolizidine Alkaloids

DEFINITION/OVERVIEW

- Over 3% of the world's flowering plants contain pyrrolizidine alkaloids (PAs). The most problematic plants are invasive and expansive and as a result they commonly contaminate feeds and food.
- Of the hundreds of PAs, only bioactivated dehydro-pyrrolizidine alkaloids (DHPAs) are toxic.
- Three plant families (Compositae, Leguminosae, and Boraginaceae) account for most PA-containing plants. Clinical disease in the USA is caused by species of the *Senecio*, *Amsinckia*, *Cynoglossum*, and *Crotalaria* genera; however, *Symphytum*, *Echium*, and *Heliotropium* species also have toxic potential (see Table 65.1; Fig 65.1).
- Poisoned animals develop icterus, hyperbilirubinemia, and increased biochemical enzymatic activities with related changes of hepatic damage, hepatic encephalopathy, and photosensitization.
- Intoxications usually occur when horses are fed contaminated hay or forages. Less frequently, horses may be poisoned by grazing contaminated paddocks or pastures. Exposure durations are generally long, over several weeks to months.
- Acute intoxications in horses are rare, primarily because palatability is low, and horses are unlikely to ingest enough plant material to obtain required doses in one or two feedings.
  - High doses can be fatal within days of exposure.
  - Lower doses generally have more prolonged exposures, and it might take several weeks before animals develop liver failure and die.
  - Even lower doses produce transient clinical disease followed by recovery.

ETIOLOGY/PATHOPHYSIOLOGY

Mechanism of Action

- Poisoning requires that DHPAs are bioactivated in the liver where hepatocyte cytochrome P450s produce toxic didehydropyrrolizidine derivatives that can become reactive carbanion intermediates that are potent electrophiles. When these bind to cellular nucleic

---

Blackwell's Five-Minute Veterinary Consult Clinical Companion: Equine Toxicology,
First Edition. Edited by Lynn R. Hovda, Dionne Benson, and Robert H. Poppenga.
© 2022 John Wiley & Sons, Inc. Published 2022 by John Wiley & Sons, Inc.
Companion website: www.wiley.com/go/hovda/equine

TABLE 65.1. Pyrrolizidine alkaloid containing Boraginaceae, Compositae, and Leguminosae plants that have been associated with poisoning. Courtesy Bryan Stegelmeier, USDA/ARS Poisonous Plant Research Laboratory.

Family Compositae	Family Leguminosae
Senecio abyssinicus	Crotalaria anagyroides
S. alpinus,	C. assamica
S. bipinnatisectus	C. equorum
S. brasiliensis	C. goreensis
S. burchelli	C. incana
S. cisplatinus	C. juncea
S. desfontainei	C. laburnoides
S. douglasii var. longilobus	C. mucronata
S. errraticus	C. nana
S. glabellus	C. retusa
S. heterotrichius	C. sagittalis
S. integerrimus	C. saltiana
S. jacobaea	C. spectabilis
S. latifolius	C. verrucosa
S. lobatus	
S. lautus	
S. leptolobus	Family Boraginaceae
S. madagascariensis	Amsinckia intermedia
S. montevidensis	Cynoglossum officinale
S. oxyphyllus	Echium plantagineum
S. pampearus	Heliotropium amplexicale
S. plattensis	H. dasycarpum
S. quadridentatus	H. europaeum
S. raphanifolius	H. lasocarpium
S. retrorsus	H. ovalifolium
S. riddellii	H. scottae
S. sanguisorbae	H. supinum
S. selloi	Symphytum officinale
S. spartioides	S. peregrinum
S. spathulatus	Trichod
S. subalpinus	
S. tweediei	
S. vernalis	
S. vulgaris	

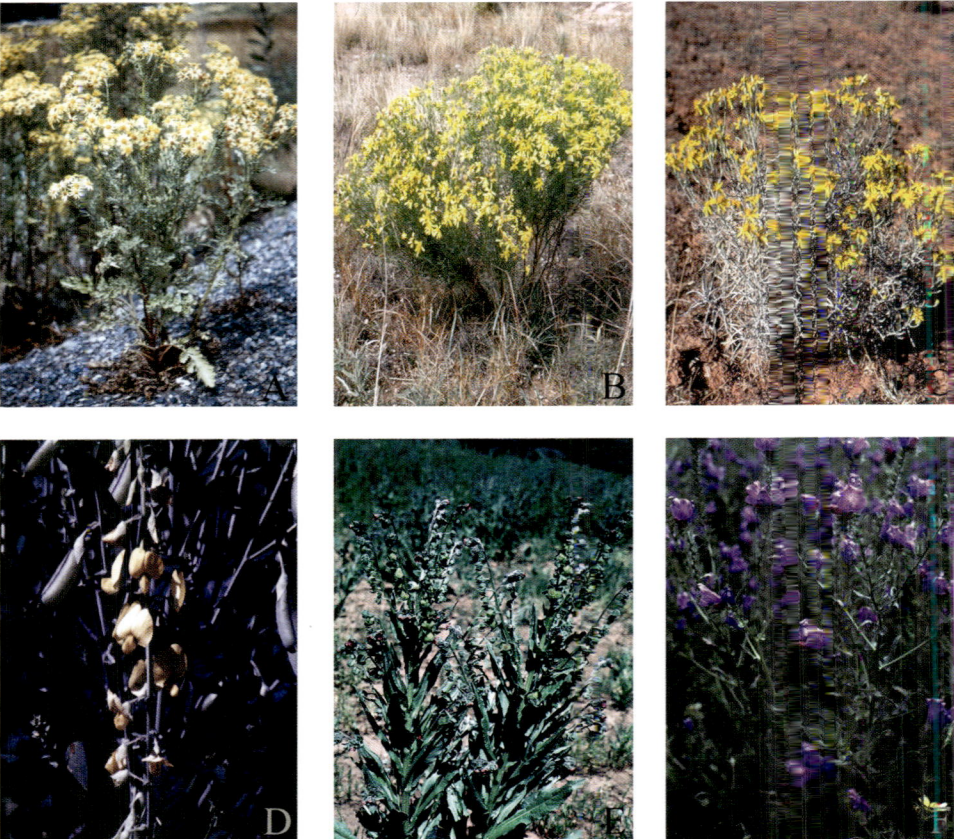

■ **Fig. 65.1.** Selected plants that contain dehyrdropyrrolizidine alkaloids. Photos courtesy of USDA/ARS Poisonous Plant Research Laboratory. A. *Senecio jacobea* (tansy ragwort) grows up to 1.5 M tall with a flowering stalk with terminal clusters of yellow composite flowers. The leaves are up to 20 cm long with 2 to 3 deep pinnate divisions. B *S. riddellii* (Ridcell's groundsel) is a bright green perennial shrub that grows about 0.5 m tall. It has threadlike leaves and glaborous stems. The composite heads have flowers composed of 6 to 8, 1 cm yellow rays. C *S. longilobus* (woolly groundsel) is a low growing, woody perennial found in the North American desert southwest. The leaves and stems are covered with white woolly pubescence. The leaves are about 10 cm long with pinnate locations. It also has flat-topped composite clusters of yellow flowers. D. *Crotalaria spectablilis* (rattlepod) is a pea like legume that was introduce in many areas as a cover crop. It usually grows between 0.5 to 1 m tall. It has simple, 3 to 5 cm long leaves that are covered with short pubescence on both sides. The petioles are winged and generally yellow with a calyx longer than the corolla. The pods are 2-3 cm long that turn black when they mature. It has 2-3 mm long bean shaped seeds that rattle in the dry pods. E *Cyanoglossum officinale* (hound's tongue is a European noxious weed that has been introduced into North America. The first year it usually produces a roset with a deep tap root. In the second year the flowering plant grows from 40 to 90 cm tall. Both years it has long leaves (8-20 cm) that have small hairs on both sides and are oval or tongue shaped. The flowering stalk has terminal cymes that are composed of about 35, blue to purple flowers. When mature, the flowers produce four 6 to 8 mm nutlets that are covered with glochidia (hooks) that allows them to adhere to hair or clothing. F. *Echium plantagineum* salvation Jane or Patterson's curse) is a hardy annual or biennial plant that was originally from Europe, but has become naturalized in Australia and other countries. It has erect, hairy stems that are between 30 and 60 cm tall. The leaves are oval with a prominent mid vein. The flowers are funnel shaped with terminal cymes may be pink as buds, but turn blue or white when they mature.

acids, proteins and other molecules, they are commonly called pyrroles. These pyrroles denature structures damaging cell function and homeostasis.
- With most DHPAs, the bound metabolites or pyrroles are concentrated primarily in the liver, where hepatocytes and hepatic endothelial cells are damaged.
- Some DHPAs also produce extrahepatic damage in the lungs, kidneys, and GI tract.

Toxicokinetics

- Ingested DHPAs are absorbed from the GI tract, metabolized in the liver and secreted in the bile, urine and feces.

Toxicity

- Toxicity is dependent on (1) alkaloid-specific chemistry, (2) plant DHPA concentrations, (3) amount ingested, (4) the duration of exposure, and (5) the species, breed, and condition of the animal poisoned.
- Most DHPA-containing plants are relatively unpalatable and grazing horses avoid eating them; however, toxicity can readily occur if they are present in baled hay.

Systems Affected

- Hepatobiliary – primarily; hepatocytomegaly and necrosis with bile duct proliferation and liver failure.
- Integumentary – primarily; photosensitization.
- Cardiovascular – experimentally; right ventricular hypertrophy and cor pulmonale.
- Respiratory – uncommon in horses; alveolar hemorrhage and edema, pulmonary arteritis and hypertension.
- Renal – not described in horses.

SIGNALMENT/HISTORY

- There are marked differences in species, sex, age and nutritional status on susceptibility to DHPA poisoning. Horses, chickens, pigs, and cattle are much more susceptible to poisoning than goats, sheep and rodents. Males, especially in rodents, are more susceptible than females.
- Foals or young ponies are more susceptible to poisoning. This has been hypothesized to differences in DHPA bioactivation and individual oxidative protection. Other animal factors include smaller body mass, less discriminating eating habits, higher metabolic activity with associated oxidative stress, and higher cellular proliferation.

Risk Factors

- Competition for food especially when fed hay or forages are limited or when animals are kept on poor pastures that lack alternative forages.
- Animals that are nutritionally challenged, especially with reduced protection from oxidative damage, are more likely to develop DHPA poisoning.

Location and Circumstances of Poisoning

- Competition with herd mates and the lack of alternative forages often force animals to eat DHPA-containing forages they might otherwise avoid.

CLINICAL FEATURES

- Clinical poisoning is dose-dependent:
  - High doses produce acute poisoning when animals may have anorexia, depression, icterus, visceral edema, and ascites. These animals have severe hepatic necrosis with hemorrhage and collapse of sinusoids.
  - Lower DHPA doses generally require longer exposure durations as they produce chronic liver disease that may be delayed months or years after initial exposure. Such animals are often clinically normal until they decompensate because of stress or some secondary hepatic injury. There is some evidence that hepatic damage is progressive, and tissue-bound pyrroles may be recycled and continue damaging cellular molecules.

Physical Examination Findings

- Anorexia, weight loss.
- Depression, weakness, lethargy.
- Photodermatitis.
- Icterus.
- Ascites, edema.
- Behavioral abnormalities – mania, derangement, yawning, aimless walking, head pressing, drowsiness, blindness, and ataxia.
- Inspiratory dyspnea – related to paralysis of the pharynx and larynx.
- Gastric impaction.
- Diarrhea with tenesmus.

DIFFERENTIAL DIAGNOSIS

- Poisonous plants – cocklebur, lance-leaf sage, alsike clover and aflatoxins from moldy feeds.
- Hepatic chemicals – chlorinated hydrocarbons, coal tar pitch, phenols, pentachlorophenol.
- Viral encephalitis.
- Other causes of hepatic failure.

DIAGNOSTICS

CBC/Serum Chemistry/Urinalysis

- CBC – inflammatory leukogram.
- Serum chemistry:
  - Hypoproteinemia, hypoalbuminemia,
  - Hyperbilirubinemia.
  - Hyperammonemia.
  - Increased activities of alkaline phosphatase, gamma glutamyl transferase, aspartate aminotransferase, alanine aminotransferase.

Other Diagnostic Tests

- Increased bile acids.
- Abnormalities in clotting factors.
- Abnormal liver biopsy.
- LC-MS detection and quantification of pyrroles in liver or blood. DHPAs may also be identified in feed or stomach contents to document exposure.

Imaging

Ultrasonography may detect extensive hepatic fibrosis.

Pathological Findings

- Gross:
  - Poor body condition with loss of fat, jaundice, ascites and generalized edema, small pale, firm liver with a mottled cut surface, pulmonary edema, interstitial pneumonia.
  - Less common – myocardial necrosis, cecal and colonic edema and hemorrhage, adrenal cortical hypertrophy.
- Histopathological – hepatocyte degeneration, necrosis, fibrosis, biliary epithelial proliferation, megalocytosis, vascular fibrosis or veno-occlusive disease and cirrhosis.

THERAPEUTICS

Detoxification

- The disease is delayed long after exposure, so the use of activated charcoal or cathartics is unlikely to be effective.

Appropriate Health Care

- Primary goal – to provide supportive therapy until enough liver tissue can regenerate and function adequately for the intended use of the horse.
- Many PA-poisoned patients respond poorly to treatment, because hepatic damage is often progressive, overwhelming regenerative compensation.
- IV fluids to correct dehydration.
- Photodermatitis can be treated with appropriate combination of cleansing, hydrotherapy, and debridement, along with restricting exposure to sunlight.
- Consider weekly vitamin B_1, folic acid, and vitamin K_1 supplementation.
- Replace contaminated feed with a high-nutrient diet (easily digestible, high caloric, low protein) divided into four to six daily feedings.

Drugs of Choice

- Neurologic signs:
  - Diazepam – foals 0.1–0.4 mg/kg IV prn; adults 25–50 mg IV prn.
  - Xylazine mg/kg IV or 2.2 mg/kg IM prn.
  - Phenobarbital 16–20 mg/kg IV prn.

- With low blood glucose, a continual 5% dextrose drip may be administered IV at a rate of 2 mL/kg/hour. Dilute the 5% dextrose in normal saline or lactated Ringer's solution if the infusion will last longer than 24–48 hours.
- In animals that develop hepatic encephalopathy, oral neomycin, lactulose, or mineral oil has been used to decrease blood ammonia concentrations, but with varying results.

Precautions/Interactions

- Diarrhea is a common sequela after neomycin or lactulose therapy.
- Exercise care when administering any medication that undergoes extensive hepatic metabolism.

Alternative Drugs

NAC or SAM-e as hepatoprotectants.

COMMENTS

Client Education

- The current recommendation for poisoning is that the source be removed. Affected animals can be monitored biochemically and via biopsies to monitor recovery and to better formulate a prognosis.

Prevention/Avoidance

- Recognize PA-containing plants, both in the field and in feeds. Treatments are generally ineffective in reversing the effects of poisoning, so avoiding exposure is essential.
- Use good management practices and appropriate herbicide control to avoid overexposure of horses to these plants.

Possible Complications

- Pneumonia, cirrhosis and chronic wasting are the most common sequelae.
- PAs have been detected in milk and are hepatotoxic and carcinogenic.
- PAs cross the placenta, causing various fetotoxic effects.

Expected Course and Prognosis

- Most affected horses are given a poor prognosis and are euthanized because of severe debilitation or non-responsive neurologic signs.
- A few animals can recover after several months of care but generally cannot regain their former fitness or activity level.

Abbreviations

See Appendix 1 for a complete list.

Suggested Reading

Burrows GM, Tyrl RJ. Toxic Plants of North America, 2nd edn. Ames, IA: Wiley Blackwell, 2013.
Clayton MJ, Davis TZ, Knoppel EL, et al. Hepatotoxic plants that poison livestock. Vet Clin North Am Food Anim Pract 2020; 36: 715–23.

Pearson EG. Liver failure attributable to pyrrolizidine alkaloid toxicosis and associated with inspiratory dyspnea in ponies: three cases (1982–1988). J Am Vet Med Assoc 1991; 198:1651.

Stegelmeier BL, Davis TZ, Clayton MJ, et al. Identifying plant poisoning in livestock in North America. Vet Clin North Am Food Anim Pract 2020; 36: 661–71.

Stegelmeier BL, Edgar JA, Colegate SM, et al. Pyrrolizidine alkaloid plants, metabolism and toxicity. J Natural Toxins 1999; 8: 95–116.

Acknowledgment: The author and editors acknowledge the prior contribution of Tina Wismer.

Author: Bryan L. Stegelmeier, DVM, PhD, DACVP
Consulting Editor: Lynn R. Hovda, RPh, DVM, MS, DACVIM

Chapter 66

Rayless Goldenrod (*Isocoma pluriflora*)

DEFINITION/OVERVIEW

- Rayless goldenrod is a bushy perennial shrub that grows on range lands throughout Colorado, Arizona, New Mexico, Texas, and northern Mexico.
- Previous scientific names include *Haplopappus heterophyllus*, *H. pluriflorus*, and *Isocoma wrightii*. Common names include jimmyweed and southern goldenbush.
- The plant is 0.6–1.2 m (2–4 ft) tall with erect stems, narrow leaves, and clusters of small yellow flowers atop the stems.
- It contains a group of related compounds collectively known as tremetol, of which tremetone is the major toxin. All parts of the plant are toxic.
- Affected horses develop necrosis of cardiac and skeletal muscle, and possibly secondary acute kidney injury related to myoglobinuria. Clinical signs include depression, weakness, muscle tremors, reluctance to move, stiff gait, profuse sweating, brown urine, tachycardia, cardiac arrhythmia, and sudden death.
- White snakeroot contains the same toxin and produces similar clinical signs.

ETIOLOGY/PATHOPHYSIOLOGY

Mechanism of Action

- The toxin's mechanism of action is unclear. Disruption of oxidative metabolism through Krebs cycle inhibition is suspected.
- Intoxication of horses is uncommon due to the plant's unpalatability. Livestock avoid it unless alternative feed is unavailable.

Toxicokinetics

- Little is known regarding the disposition of tremetol following intestinal absorption.
- Toxicity of tremetone requires microsomal activation by hepatic cytochrome P450.
- Some tremetol is secreted in milk, putting nursing foals at risk of toxicity.

Toxicity

- Data are insufficient to predict a toxic dose and estimates are confounded by variation in plant tremetol content.

Blackwell's Five-Minute Veterinary Consult Clinical Companion: Equine Toxicology, First Edition. Edited by Lynn R. Hovda, Dionne Benson, and Robert H. Poppenga.
© 2022 John Wiley & Sons, Inc. Published 2022 by John Wiley & Sons, Inc.
Companion website: www.wiley.com/go/hovda/equine

- Field observations indicate that consumption of tremetol-containing plants at 0.5–2% of body weight over 1–3 weeks is sufficient to induce lethal toxicity.
- In the single available report of experimental toxicosis, feeding rayless goldenrod at 3% of body weight for 7–10 days resulted in clinical, laboratory, and necropsy abnormalities typical of tremetol toxicity. Feeding at 1.5% of body weight for 14 days resulted in intermittent arrhythmias and multifocal degeneration and necrosis of myofibers on histology.

Systems Affected

- Cardiovascular – tachycardia, arrhythmia, possible progression to cardiomyopathy and congestive heart failure.
- Musculoskeletal – weakness, muscle tremors, reluctance to move, stiff gait, possible muscle pain, recumbency.
- Nervous – depression.
- Skin/exocrine – sweating.
- Renal/urologic – myoglobinuria, secondary tubular necrosis.
- Gastrointestinal – inappetance, dysphagia, and esophageal obstruction occasionally reported.

SIGNALMENT/HISTORY

- Horses of any age, breed or sex may be affected.
- Because tremetol is excreted in milk, nursing foals may develop clinical signs of toxicity before signs are observed in the dam.
- Cattle, sheep, and goats are also susceptible. Humans may be poisoned by the milk of affected livestock.

Historical Findings

- Consumption of rayless goldenrod may not have been witnessed.

Location and Circumstances of Poisoning

- Owners may be unaware of the presence of toxic plants on their property or rangeland, necessitating inspection by a qualified veterinarian or extension agent.

CLINICAL FEATURES

- There are no reports of naturally occurring disease in the horse. However, the toxin is the same as that in white snakeroot, and field observations, together with one report of experimental toxicosis, support clinical signs consistent with severe non-exertional rhabdomyolysis – depression, weakness, muscle tremors, reluctance to move, stiff gait, profuse sweating, and myoglobinuria.
- Cardiac involvement results in arrhythmia and/or signs of heart failure – tachycardia, jugular distension and pulsation, and ventral edema.
- Affected horses may be found recumbent or dead.

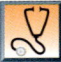

DIFFERENTIAL DIAGNOSIS

- Exertional rhabdomyolysis.
- Other causes of non-exertional rhabdomyolysis:
  - Nutritional deficiency of selenium and/or vitamin E.
  - *Anaplasma phagocytophilum* infection.
  - Myosin heavy chain myopathy (MYH1 mutation).
  - Pasture myopathy – ingestion of hypoglycin A in seeds of the box elder tree (*Acer negundo*; North America) or sycamore maple tree (*Acer pseudoplatanus*; Europe).
  - Toxic plants – *Ageratina altissima* (white snakeroot), *Senna obtusifolia* (sicklepod) seeds, *Malva parviflora* (marshmallow).
- Other causes of acute arrythmia and cardiac dysfunction:
  - Sepsis, endotoxemia, electrolyte derangement.
  - Progression of unrecognized cardiac disease – pericarditis, congenital abnormalities, myocarditis, valvular disease, great vessel rupture.
  - Other cardiotoxins:
    - Ionophores.
    - Oleander.
    - Yew.
    - Rattlesnake envenomation.
- Other causes of muscle tremors, generalized weakness, and recumbency:
  - Botulism.
  - Hyperkalemic periodic paralysis.
  - Vitamin E-deficient myopathy.
  - Equine motor neuron disease.
  - Tick paralysis.
  - Primary brain or spinal cord disease – trauma, rabies, viral encephalitides.
- Other causes of pigmenturia:
  - Myoglobinuria – infarctive purpura hemorrhagica, clostridial myonecrosis.
  - Hemoglobinuria – red maple toxicosis, leptospirosis, piroplasmosis, hypotonic IV fluids, IV DMSO.

DIAGNOSTICS

- Diagnosis is presumptive based on clinical signs, laboratory findings (marked elevation of CK and AST, myoglobinuria), necropsy findings, and consumption of, or access to, rayless goldenrod.
- Tremetone may be detected in the urine and possibly the blood, kidney, liver, and intestinal contents of affected animals, but testing is not readily available
- ECG abnormalities include AV block, ventricular premature beats, and marked ST-segment depression.
- Cardiac troponin I is a sensitive marker of myocardial injury, but elevations are not specific for tremetol toxicity.

Pathological Findings

- Based on findings in white snakeroot toxicosis and a single report of experimentally induced rayless goldenrod toxicosis, gross findings include pallor and necrosis of skeletal and cardiac muscle, pulmonary congestion, and hepatopathy.
- Macroscopic lesions of the heart include pale areas and linear streaks throughout the myocardium. Histological lesions include myocardial degeneration, necrosis, and fibrosis.
- Histopathologic findings may also include centrilobular hepatic necrosis and mild renal tubular necrosis.

THERAPEUTICS

- Treatment is symptomatic and supportive.
- Goals of therapy are to prevent further toxin consumption; decontaminate the gut; optimize tissue perfusion and correct metabolic derangements; manage pain as needed; and prevent/treat complications.

Detoxification

- If acute/subacute exposure is suspected, a single dose of AC and a cathartic agent (magnesium sulfate; Epsom salts) may be beneficial:
  - Administer AC (1–3 g/kg) by NG tube as a slurry in water or magnesium sulfate solution.
  - If AC is unavailable, administer DTO smectite (BioSponge®; 3 g/kg) by NG tube as a slurry in water or magnesium sulfate solution.
  - Administer a single dose of Epsom salts (500 mg to 1 g/kg dissolved in 4 L of warm water by NG tube).
- Gastric lavage is unlikely to be helpful and not recommended.

Appropriate Health Care

- Hospitalize affected horses for provision of supportive care.
- IV fluids are indicated to address dehydration, metabolic acidosis, and electrolyte derangement; maintain tissue perfusion; and reduce the risk of pigment nephropathy.
- Administer analgesics if myonecrosis is associated with pain.
- ECG monitoring if the patient's heart rate is unexpectedly high, low, or irregular. Treat significant arrhythmias.

Antidotes

- No known antidote.

Drugs of Choice

- IV fluid therapy – balanced polyionic solution (LRS).
- NSAIDs to control pain, if needed. Clinical signs associated with this condition make it difficult to determine whether or not a horse is experiencing significant pain. If in doubt, assess the horse's response to analgesic agents:
  - Flunixin (1.1 mg/kg IV or PO q12–24h).
  - Phenylbutazone (2.2–4.4 mg/kg IV or PO q12–24h).
  - Ketoprofen (2.2 mg/kg IV q24h).

- Note that NSAIDs increase the risk of renal injury in patients with dehydration and/or existing renal compromise. If it is unclear whether significant pain is present, or if NSAIDs alone are insufficient to control pain, consider alternative analgesic agents such lidocaine and/or opioids (butorphanol, morphine):
  - Lidocaine CRI – 1.3 mg/kg slow IV injection loading dose followed by continuous rate infusion at 0.05 mg/kg/min.
  - Butorphanol (0.01–0.04 mg/kg IV or IM q2–4h).
  - Butorphanol CRI – standard IV loading dose followed by continuous rate infusion at 13–22 µg/kg/h IV.
  - Morphine (0.05–0.1 mg/kg IV or IM q4–6h).

COMMENTS

Client Education

- For down horses, advise owners of the extensive nursing care required for humane management in the farm setting.
- Rayless goldenrod is also toxic to cattle, sheep, and goats.

Patient Monitoring

- Horses with myoglobinuria and dehydration are at risk for acute kidney injury – urine output should be monitored.
- Daily serum chemistry in severe cases to monitor for improvements in muscle enzymes, metabolic acidosis, and renal function; consider urinalysis.

Prevention/Avoidance

- Avoid grazing horses on infested ranges.
- If this is not possible or practical, avoid overgrazing, which encourages consumption of toxic plants, and provide supplemental forage.
- Herbicides may be used for chemical control.

Expected Course and Prognosis

- Prognosis for severe cases is poor, with death occurring 1–3 days after onset of signs.
- Horses that survive may take weeks to recover. Some go on to develop cardiomyopathy and congestive heart failure.
- Mildly affected horses with no cardiac involvement may recover fully in 2 weeks with rest and appropriate supportive care.

See Also

White Snakeroot (*Ageratina altissima*)

Abbreviations

See Appendix 1 for a complete list.

Suggested Reading

Davis TZ, Stegelmeier BL, Lee ST, Green BT, Hall JO. Experimental rayless goldenrod (*Isocoma pluriflora*) toxicosis in horses. Toxicon 2013; 73:88–95.

Meerdink GL, Frederickson RL, Bordson GO. Tremetone. In: Plumlee KH, ed. Clinical Veterinary Toxicology. St Louis, MO: Mosby, 2004; pp. 348–350.

Panter KE, Welch KD, Gardner DR, Lee ST, Green BT, Pfister JA, Cook D, Davis TZ, Stegelmeier BL. Poisonous plants of the United States. In: Gupta RC, ed. Veterinary Toxicology: Basic and Clinical Principles, 3rd edn. San Diego, CA: Academic Press, 2018; pp. 867–868.

Talcott P. Toxicologic problems. In: Reed SM, Bayly WM, Sellon DC, eds. Equine Internal Medicine, 4th edn. St Louis, MO: Elsevier, 2018; pp. 1484–1485.

Author: Christie Ward, DVM, MVSc, PhD, DACVIM
Consulting Editor: Lynn R. Hovda, RPh, DVM, MS, DACVIM

Chapter 67

Rhododendron spp.

DEFINITION/OVERVIEW

- *Rhododendron* spp. has 700–1,000 species, and multiple cultivars. Distribution is primarily in cool-to-temperate regions of the northern hemisphere, and into the southern hemisphere of Southeast Asia.
- The species is divided into eight subgenera with a large number of common names: rhododendron, azalea, rosebay, laurel, and others. They are all members of the Ericaceae (Heath) family:
  - Deciduous species are referred to as azalea, while the evergreens as rhododendron but there are exceptions.
  - The plants are shrubs or occasionally small trees; evergreen or deciduous.
- Leaves are alternate or in false whorls at the branch ends. The blades have a variety of shapes and the leaf surface is glabrous or variously indumented; margins are entire or minutely crenulate (see Fig. 67.1).
- Flowers are radially or bilaterally symmetrical. Petals are fused, usually five, and of various colors, except blue (see Fig. 67.2).
- The stems are erect or ascending, occasionally prostrate. Bark is either rough or smooth.
- Toxic agent is generally regarded to be water-soluble diterpenoid. Toxins are found throughout the plants, in all parts of the plant – blooms, nectar, stems – and especially in the leaves.

ETIOLOGY/PATHOPHYSIOLOGY

Mechanism of Action

- Grayanotoxins most profoundly affect the sodium channels in excitable cell membranes of the nerve cells, skeletal, and cardiac muscles.
- They bind to group II receptor sites in the voltage-gated sodium channels, increasing the permeability of sodium ions ceasing prolonged cell membrane depolarization.

Toxicokinetics

- Rapid onset of action (2+ hours).
- Rapidly absorbed from the GI tract when ingested.
- Acute signs may last for 24 hours, but weakness and neurological effects may last for 2–3 days.

Blackwell's Five-Minute Veterinary Consult Clinical Companion: Equine Toxicology,
First Edition. Edited by Lynn R. Hovda, Dionne Benson, and Robert H. Poppenga.
© 2022 John Wiley & Sons, Inc. Published 2022 by John Wiley & Sons, Inc.
Companion website: www.wiley.com/go/hovda/equine

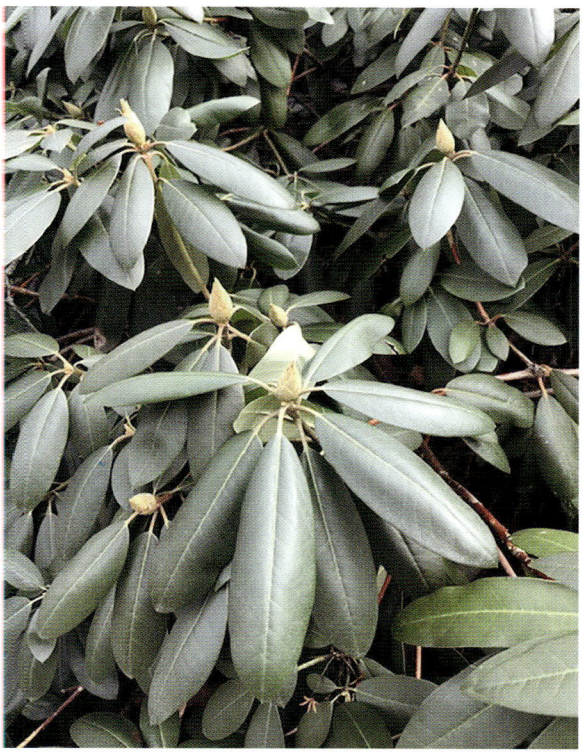

■ **Fig. 67.1.** Rhododendron leaves arranged around a single center bud. *Source:* Photo courtesy of Tyne K. Hovda.

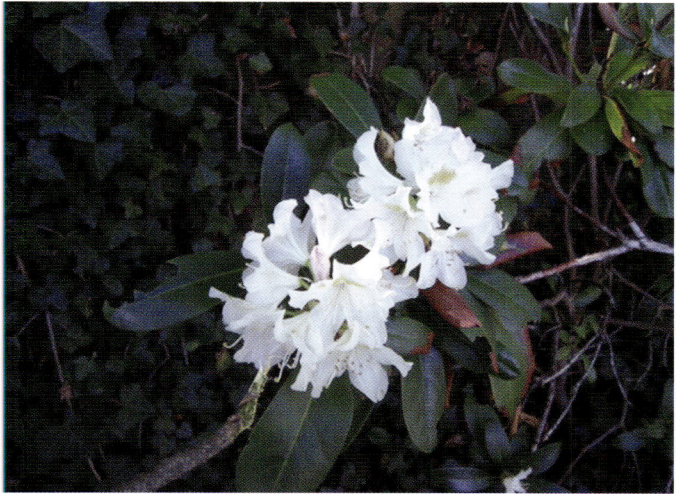

■ **Fig. 67.2.** Rhododendron flower. Note woody stems on shrub. *Source:* Photo courtesy of Tyne K. Hovda.

Toxicity

- The toxins are known collectively as grayanotoxins, consisting of a variety of grayanotoxins (I–XXV). The concentration varies depending upon the cultivar. Synonyms include andromedotoxin, acetylandromedol, rhodotoxin, asebotoxin, and polyhydroxylated diterpenes.
- Those species considered to be rhododendron (not azaleas) are generally regarded as more toxic, but this is variable.

Systems Affected

- Gastrointestinal.
- Cardiovascular.
- Nervous.

SIGNALMENT/HISTORY

- No known breed, sex, or age predispositions.

Risk Factors

- Consumption of *Rhododendron* spp. of plants or other plants containing grayanotoxins.
- Lack of adequate feed and boredom.

Historical Findings

- The plants are not especially palatable to horses. Evergreen plants are more attractive to horses in the winter time, as they may be the only green substance available to them. Also, horses will sample forages out of boredom.

CLINICAL FEATURES

- Profuse salivation, copious nasal secretions, repeated swallowing, bloat, colic and/or severe abdominal pain, and irregular respiration. Weakness and profuse salivation may result in aspiration pneumonia.
- Hypotension and changes in heart rate and rhythm (bradycardia, tachycardia [rarely], AV block, arrhythmias).
- Respiratory depression.
- Marked loss of body condition.
- Weakness, reluctance to rise, or inability to stand.

DIFFERENTIAL DIAGNOSIS

- Any other plant in the Ericaceae family, which contains about 1,350 species widely distributed in all continents. Plants in the Ericaceae family besides *Rhododendron* species are: *Kalmia* species (mountain laurel, sheep laurel, lambkill, sheepkill, dwarf laurel, calico bush), *Pieris* species (Japanese pieris, mountain pieris), *Leucothoe* species (dog hobble, dog laurel, fetter bush, black laurel), and *Lyonia* species (fetter bush, maleberry, staggerbush).
- Underlying GI or cardiovascular disease.

DIAGNOSTICS

CBC/Serum Chemistry/Urinalysis

- Elevation in AST and ALT.
- Acidosis may be noted if the animal has had seizures.

Other Diagnostic Tests

- The presence of grayanotoxins in serum, urine, and GI contents, plant material and honey can be determined with chromatographic methods.
- Stomach contents should be collected as soon after death as possible and frozen immediately. The contents should be shipped to a diagnostic laboratory in such a fashion as to remain frozen. A TLC method yields results in approximately 4 hours.
- Microscopic examination of the stomach contents may yield evidence of the plant, especially leaves and leaf fragments.
- Grayanotoxins can be detected in urine of exposed animals up to 3–5 days after exposure using LC-MS technology. This method allows the detection at the ng/g level of grayanotoxins I, II, and III in serum or urine.

Pathological Findings

- Gross – plant parts, especially leaves, may be found in the stomach contents.
- Histopathology changes are not distinct and are mild, if present. These include edema of lungs and renal tubular and hepatocellular necrosis.

THERAPEUTICS

Detoxification

- Administration of AC (2–4 g/kg in a water slurry) may be of some benefit in limiting further absorption of the toxins.

Appropriate Health Care

- Treatment is directed at treatment and relief of clinical signs.
- Passage of nasogastric tube if bloat is present.
- IV fluids as needed for dehydration and maintenance of blood pressure.
- Monitor closely for evidence of aspiration pneumonia and treat accordingly.
- Monitor vital signs.
- Bradycardia and hypersalivation may be responsive to atropine but use with caution as it may decrease GI l movement in the horse.

Antidotes

- There is no specific antidote.

Drugs of Choice

- Bradycardia – atropine 0.01–0.02 mg/kg IV.
- GI protectants:

- Omeprazole 4 mg/kg PO q24h.
- Sucralfate 10–20 mg/kg PO q6–8h.
■ Antibiotics for aspiration pneumonia:
- Based on culture and sensitivity.

Precautions/Interactions

■ Judicious use of atropine to avoid adverse GI effects.

COMMENTS

Client Education

■ Do not throw azalea or rhododendron clippings into the pasture, paddock, or turnout area.
■ Do not plant these as ornamental shrubs in the pasture or adjacent to the fence line.

Prevention/Avoidance

■ Ensure appropriate feed, and other activities to avoid boredom.

Possible Complications

■ Aspiration pneumonia.
■ Rarely horses are found dead.

Expected Course and Prognosis

■ Recovery without complications should occur with supportive treatment in approximately a week.

Abbreviations

See Appendix 1 for a complete list.

Internet Resources

Rhododendron. Available at: https://csuvth.colostate.edu/poisonous_plants/Plants.Details/111.

Suggested Reading

Burrow GE, Tyrl RJ. Toxic Plants of North America. Ames, IA: Iowa State University Press, 2006; pp. 444–449.
Jansen SA, Kleerekooper I, Hofman ZL, et al. Grayanotoxin poisoning: 'mad honey disease' and beyond. Cardiovascular Toxicol. 2012; 12(3):208–215.
Plumlee, KH. Clinical Veterinary Toxicology. Mosby, 2004; pp 337–338.

Author: Tam Garland, DVM, PhD, DABVT
Consulting Editor: Lynn R. Hovda, RPh, DVM, MS, DACVIM

Chapter 68

Sudangrass (*Sorghum* spp.)

DEFINITION/OVERVIEW

- Chronic ingestion of *Sorghum vulgare* var. *sudanense* (sudangrass or hybrid sudangrass) causes urinary incontinence with cystitis, rear limb ataxia, and teratogenesis in horses.
- Grazing on sudan pastures and ingestion of freshly cut hay are associated with the syndrome, but feeding cured hay is not.
- Geographically, sudangrass is most commonly used as a forage in the southwestern and central USA.
- Generally, intoxication occurs during periods of high rainfall and rapid plant growth. Plant and pasture fertilization have no effect on toxicity.
- Ingestion of *Sorghum* spp. is also associated with cyanide and nitrate toxicoses; see chapters on cyanide toxicosis (Ch. 49) and nitrate/nitrite toxicosis (Ch. 29) for more in-depth discussion of these intoxications.

ETIOLOGY/PATHOPHYSIOLOGY

Mechanism of Action

- Toxin causes axonal degeneration and myelomalacia in the spinal cord.

Toxicokinetics

- Onset of clinical signs occurs after weeks to months (average of 8 weeks) of grazing a sudangrass pasture.

Toxicity

- The toxin is believed to be a lathyrogenic agent, γ-glutamyl-β-cyanoalanine.

Systems Affected

- Nervous.
- Urinary.
- Reproductive.

Blackwell's Five-Minute Veterinary Consult Clinical Companion: Equine Toxicology,
First Edition. Edited by Lynn R. Hovda, Dionne Benson, and Robert H. Poppenga.
© 2022 John Wiley & Sons, Inc. Published 2022 by John Wiley & Sons, Inc.
Companion website: www.wiley.com/go/hovda/equine

SIGNALMENT/HISTORY

- Both sexes, all ages, and all breeds may be affected.

Risk Factors

- Grazing sudangrass or freshly cut hay.
- Johnson grass has also been implicated.

Historical Findings

- Grazing for weeks to months on sudangrass pasture or freshly cut hay.

Location and Circumstances of Poisoning

- Southwestern and central USA.

CLINICAL FEATURES

- Posterior ataxia and incoordination; forced movement enhances ataxia.
- Falling when backed up.
- Recumbency.
- Full bladder with constant urine dribbling.
- Urine scalding and evidence of cystitis.
- Frequent opening and closing of vulva (winking).
- Mares may appear to be in constant estrus.
- Fetal malformations (extreme flexion of joint or ankylosis) when mares graze sudangrass between days 20 and 50 of gestation.
- Secondary complications of urinary tract and kidney infection.

DIFFERENTIAL DIAGNOSIS

- Polyneuritis equi (cauda equina neuritis).
- Cystitis from other causes.
- Trauma.
- Infectious – abscess, equine viral or bacterial encephalitis, equine herpesvirus-1 myeloencephalitis (EHM), EPM.
- Neoplasia.
- Rabies.

DIAGNOSTICS

CBC/Serum Chemistry/Urinalysis

- Urinalysis – leukocytes, epithelial cells hyaline casts, crystals, bacteria, red blood cells.

Imaging

- Cystoscopy.

Pathological Findings

- Gross – cystitis with marked thickening of the bladder wall:
  - Full bladder.
  - Ulcerations of the bladder mucosa.
  - Hyperemic urethra and ureters.
  - Vaginal hyperemia.
  - External abrasions from falling.
  - Areas of urine-scalded skin.
  - Pyelonephritis.
- Histopathology – necrotizing cystitis:
  - Pyelonephritis.
  - Inflammation of the ureters, urethra, bladder, and vagina.
  - Axonal degeneration of the spinal cord and cerebellum.
  - Myelomalacia of the spinal cord and cerebellum.

THERAPEUTICS

Detoxification

- The use of activated charcoal or cathartics is not recommended as this is a chronic disease that develops over weeks to months.

Appropriate Health Care

- Outpatient primarily; rarely is hospitalization needed.
- Prevent further exposure by removing horses from and preventing access to sudangrass.
- Cystitis/pyelonephritis can be treated, but recurrence of signs generally occurs 2–3 weeks after therapy is stopped.
- Treatment is unsuccessful in horses that exhibit incoordination and/or urine dribbling.
- Protective ointment for urine scalded areas.
- Monitor urine for evidence of bacteria/cystitis twice weekly during and after antibiotic therapy.

Antidotes

- There is no antidote.

Drugs of Choice

- Antimicrobial therapy for cystitis/pyelonephritis should be based upon culture and sensitivity tests.

COMMENTS

Client Education

- Monitor pastures and hay for sudangrass.

Prevention/Avoidance

- Avoid exposure to sudangrass pastures.
- Don't feed freshly cut hay.

Possible Complications

- Fetal malformations (extreme flexion of joints or ankylosis) occur when mares graze sudangrass between days 20 and 50 of gestation.
- With severe ulceration and necrosis, scarring and strictures are possible.

Expected Course and Prognosis

- Recovery of clinically effected horses is extremely rare.
- Horses may still be used for breeding, but cystitis, vaginitis, or urethritis can complicate breeding efforts.
- Horses that survive and have recurrent cystitis should not be used for work or riding owing to residual nervous system damage.

Abbreviations

See Appendix 1 for a complete list.

Suggested Reading

Burrows GE, Tyrl RJ. Toxic Plants of North America. Ames, IA: Iowa State University Press, 2001; p. 929.
Knight AP, Walter RG. A Guide to Plant Poisoning in North America. Jackson, WY: Teton NewMedia, 2001; pp. 242–243.
Morgan SE, Johnson B, Brewer B, Walker J. Sorghum cystitis ataxia syndrome in horses. Vet Hum Toxicol 1990; 32(6):582.
Van Kampen KR. Sudan grass and sorghum poisoning of horses: a possible lathyrogenic disease. J Am Vet Med Assoc 1970; 156:629–630.

Acknowledgment: The author and editors acknowledge the prior contribution of Jeffery O Hall.

Author: Lynn R. Hovda, RPh, DVM, MS, DACVIM
Consulting Editor: Lynn R. Hovda, RPh, DVM, MS, DACVIM

Chapter 69

Tansy Ragwort (*Senecio jacobaea*)

DEFINITION/OVERVIEW

- Tansy ragwort (*Senecio jacobaea*, syn. *Jacobaea vulgaris*) is one of a number of plants causing pyrrolizidine alkaloid (PA) toxicity and hepatic failure.
- Intoxication with tansy ragwort most commonly occurs when horses graze contaminated pastures or consume hay contaminated with *Senecio*. Acute intoxications are rare due to the amount of *Senecio* that would need to be ingested at a single feeding.
- Ragwort is a biennial plant and herbicide-killed ragwort maintains its toxicity; the only means of eliminating the plant is to uproot it. All parts of the ragwort plant are toxic, and the toxic principle is maintained in the dried plant.
- Tansy ragwort is found primarily in the northwestern and northeastern United States.

ETIOLOGY/PATHOPHYSIOLOGY

Mechanism of Action

- Rapidly absorbed from the GI tract. They is subject to extensive hepatic metabolism by mixed-function oxidases.
- The primary toxin in ragwort is jacobine.
- Jacobine and other PAs are converted to toxic pyrrole derivatives in the liver, primarily through dehydrogenation.
- Pyrroles alkylate DNA, leading to inhibition of mitosis. Though mitosis is prevented, expansion of hepatocyte cytoplasm and nuclei occurs, which leads to megalocyte formation. Necrotic megalocytes are eventually replaced by fibrous tissue, leading to cirrhosis.
- Hepatic changes may worsen over time even if the toxic plant is removed from the diet.
- The toxic dose for horses is thought to be 0.05–0.2 kg/kg.

Systems Affected

- Hepatic – the hepatobiliary system is the most commonly affected, with hepatocyte megalocytosis, necrosis and fibrosis and bile duct proliferation and fibrosis. Centrilobular and hepatic vein endothelial proliferation may also occur.
- Neurologic – various neurologic signs and behavioral changes are often seen secondary to hepatic encephalopathy, but gross CNS lesions are absent.

Blackwell's Five-Minute Veterinary Consult Clinical Companion: Equine Toxicology,
First Edition. Edited by Lynn R. Hovda, Dionne Benson, and Robert H. Poppenga.
© 2022 John Wiley & Sons, Inc. Published 2022 by John Wiley & Sons, Inc.
Companion website: www.wiley.com/go/hovda/equine

- Pulmonary – in rare cases, the lungs may be affected; alveolar edema and hemorrhage, proliferation of alveolar walls, pulmonary arteritis and hypertension may be evident.
- Reproductive – abortion may occur in pregnant mares, but long-term fertility appears unimpaired.

SIGNALMENT/HISTORY

- There is no breed or sex predilection; grazing equids of any age may be affected. Foals suckling exposed mares do not appear to be affected.
- Most cases in pastured animals are seen in spring, summer and fall, but cases linked to hay may appear at any time.

Risk Factors
- Risk factors include overgrazing of pastures, as the plant is poorly palatable and generally avoided if adequate forage is present. The incidence of ragwort toxicity is unknown.

Historical Findings
- Most affected equids present with chronic weight loss, inappetence, and behavioral changes.
- Behavioral changes may include somnolence, yawning, aimless walking, ataxia, head pressing, or mania.
- Some may present with signs of colic.
- Exercise intolerance may be reported.

Location and Circumstances of Poisoning
- Investigation of pastures or hay may reveal *Senecio* spp.
- Ingestion of the toxic plant often occurs weeks or months prior to the onset of clinical signs.
- Onset of clinical signs is often acute.

CLINICAL FEATURES

- Weight loss.
- Inappetence.
- Exercise intolerance.
- Behavioral changes.
- Icterus.
- Gastric impaction.
- Ascites.
- Diarrhea.
- Laryngeal hemiplegia.
- Photosensitization.

DIFFERENTIAL DIAGNOSIS

- Acute hepatitis/Theiler's disease.
- Chronic active hepatitis.
- Cholangiohepatitis.
- Liver abscess.
- Viral encephalitis.
- Nigropallidal encephalomalacia.
- Leukoencephalomalacia.
- EPM.
- Alsike clover/red clover intoxication.
- Other hepatotoxins (acute): carbon tetrachloride, chlorinated hydrocarbons, coal tar, phenol, etc.

DIAGNOSTICS

CBC/Serum Chemistry/Urinalysis

- Serum chemistry – increases in GGT, ALP, AST and bilirubin, possible hypoalbuminemia.
- Increased bile acids and hyperammonemia may occur.
- Serum bile acids > 50 µmol/L indicates a poor prognosis.

Other Diagnostic Tests

- Ultrasonography may demonstrate a small hyperechoic liver.
- Liver biopsy will show bridging fibrosis, megalocytosis, and bile duct proliferation.

Pathological Findings

- Gross necropsy findings may include poor body condition, icterus, ascites/edema, gastric impaction, and/or pale and small liver mottled on cut surface.
- Histologic findings include megalocytosis with necrosis, centrilobular and periportal bridging fibrosis, biliary hyperplasia, pulmonary edema, and interstitial pneumonia.

THERAPEUTICS

Detoxification

- Tansy ragwort remains toxic even after drying or herbicide killing; no viable means of detoxification exists for equine consumption.

Appropriate Health Care

- Treatment involves removal of the alkaloid-containing plant from the diet and supportive care; no specific antidote is available.

- Supportive therapy is needed until the liver can regenerate sufficiently. However the prognosis is poor as in most cases irreversible liver damage has occurred by the time the disease is diagnosed and regeneration is no longer possible.
- Therapy includes providing a highly digestible, low-protein diet in several small feedings per day. A combination of 1–2 parts beet pulp, sorghum or milo to 0.5–1 part cracked corn mixed with molasses and fed at 2.5 kg per 45 kg (100 lb) BW has been suggested. Oat or grass hay is recommended as a roughage source; alfalfa should be avoided. Supplementation of vitamins B_1, folic acid and K_1 may be beneficial.

Antidotes

- No antidote is available.

Drugs of Choice

- For cases demonstrating clinical signs, IV fluid therapy may be needed. Dextrose (2 mL/kg/hour of 5% dextrose) may be administered if low blood glucose is present.
- For neurologic signs, diazepam (adults 25–50mg IV; foals 0.05–0.4 mg/kg IV) or xylazine (1.1 mg/kg IV or 2.2 mg/kg IM) may be given.
- If hepatic encephalopathy is suspected, lactulose (0.3 ml/kg PO QID) or neomycin (50–100 mg/kg PO QID) may be given; diarrhea is a common side effect of these medications.
- If photodermatitis is present, prevention of exposure to sunlight is important. Lesions may be treated with appropriate cleaning, hydrotherapy and debridement with topical or oral antibiotics used as necessary.

Precautions/Interactions

- Avoid drugs with extensive hepatic metabolism.
- Excessive dietary copper should be avoided.

COMMENTS

Client Education

- Clients should be educated on the appearance of tansy ragwort and advised to inspect their pastures for the plant and remove it if present.
- Forage extension agents may be helpful.

Patient Monitoring

- Affected equids should have weight, appetite, serum liver enzymes, and bile acids monitored every 2–4 weeks.
- Magnitude of enzyme increase does not necessarily correlate with degree of hepatic impairment.
- Trends may be helpful in determining prognosis, particularly AST and bile acids.
- Serum urea nitrogen often decreases in the terminal stage.
- Other equids exposed to the same pasture as an affected equid should be examined for the presence of signs of toxicity, and clinicopathologic tests may be considered

Prevention/Avoidance

- Adequate forage should be provided to limit overgrazing of pastures and prevent ingestion of tansy ragwort.
- Hay should be inspected for the presence of ragwort; affected lots should be disposed of or fed to sheep, which are relatively resistant to tansy ragwort.
- Sheep may be used to graze heavily infested pastures.

Possible Complications

- Affected animals tend to be poor doers and chronic wasting is common.
- Pneumonia may also be seen.

Expected Course and Prognosis

- Overall prognosis is poor due to the degree of hepatic destruction present when cases are typically diagnosed.
- Most horses are euthanized within a short time period (weeks to months) for chronic debilitation or persistent neurologic signs.
- A small percentage of horses may recover after several months but usually fail to return to full performance.

Abbreviations

See Appendix 1 for a complete list.

Suggested Reading

Divers TJ and Barton MH. Diseases of the Liver. In: Reed SM, Bayly WM, eds. Equine Internal Medicine, 4th edn. Philadelphia: WB Saunders, 2018; pp. 843–887.
Giles CJ. Outbreak of ragwort (*Senecio jacobaea*) poisoning in horses. Equine Vet J 1983; 15(3):248–250.
Love A and Love D. Senecio L. and Packera. In Burrows GE and Tyrl RJ (eds.). Toxic Plants of North America, 2nd edn. Ames, IA: John Wiley & Sons, 2013; pp. 202–214.
Mendel VE, Will MR, Gitchell BS et al. Pyrrolizidine alkaloid-induced liver disease in horses: an early diagnosis. Am J Vet Res 1988; 49(4):572–578.
Milne EM, Fogson DM, Doxey DL. Secondary gastric impaction associated with ragwort poisoning in three ponies. Vet Record 1990; 126(20):502–504.

Author: Tamara Gull, DVM, PhD, DACVIM (LAIM), DACVPM, DACVM
Consulting Editor: Lynn R. Hovda, RPh, DVM, MS, DACVIM

Chapter 70

White Snakeroot (*Ageratina altissima*)

DEFINITION/OVERVIEW

- White snakeroot is a perennial common throughout eastern and central North America. It was previously known as *Eupatorium rugosum*; common names include richweed and white sanicle.
- The plant is 0.6–1.2 m (2–4 ft) tall and has large heart-shaped leaves with serrated edges. Clusters of small white flowers bloom from midsummer through fall.
- It prefers moist shady areas and is often found in woods and brush adjacent to pastures.
- It contains a group of related compounds collectively known as tremetol, of which tremetone is the major toxin. All parts of the plant are toxic.
- Affected horses develop necrosis of cardiac and skeletal muscle, and possibly secondary acute kidney injury related to myoglobinuria. Common clinical signs include depression, weakness, muscle tremors, reluctance to move, stiff gait, profuse sweating, brown urine, tachycardia, cardiac arrhythmia, and sudden death.
- *Isocoma pluriflora* (rayless goldenrod) contains the same toxin and produces similar clinical signs.

ETIOLOGY/PATHOPHYSIOLOGY

Mechanism of Action

- The toxin's mechanism of action is unclear. Disruption of oxidative metabolism through Krebs cycle inhibition is suspected.
- Despite widespread distribution and the palatability of white snakeroot, incidence of toxicity is sporadic due to variability in plant toxin content.

Toxicokinetics

- Little is known regarding the disposition of tremetol following intestinal absorption.
- Toxicity of tremetone requires microsomal activation by cytochrome P450 in the liver.
- Some tremetol is secreted in milk, putting nursing foals at risk of toxicity.

Blackwell's Five-Minute Veterinary Consult Clinical Companion: Equine Toxicology, First Edition. Edited by Lynn R. Hovda, Dionne Benson, and Robert H. Poppenga. © 2022 John Wiley & Sons, Inc. Published 2022 by John Wiley & Sons, Inc. Companion website: www.wiley.com/go/hovda/equine

Toxicity

- Data are insufficient to predict a toxic dose with accuracy, and estimates are confounded by variation in plant tremetol content.
- Field observations indicate that consumption of tremetol-containing plants at 0.5–2% of body weight over 1–3 weeks is sufficient to induce lethal toxicity.
- The entire plant is toxic whether fresh (green) or dried (in hay or dead in the field).

Systems Affected

- Cardiovascular – tachycardia, arrhythmia, possible progression to cardiomyopathy and congestive heart failure.
- Musculoskeletal – weakness, muscle tremors, reluctance to move, stiff gait, possible muscle pain, recumbency.
- Nervous – depression.
- Skin/exocrine – sweating.
- Renal/urologic – myoglobinuria, secondary tubular necrosis.
- Gastrointestinal – inappetance, dysphagia, and esophageal obstruction occasionally reported.

SIGNALMENT/HISTORY

- Horses of any age, breed or sex may be affected.
- Because tremetol is excreted in milk, nursing foals may develop clinical signs of toxicity before signs are observed in the dam.
- Cattle, sheep, and goats are also susceptible. Humans may be poisoned by the milk of affected livestock.

Risk Factors

- Stress may precipitate onset of clinical signs in exposed horses.

Historical Findings

- Consumption of white snakeroot may not have been witnessed.

Location and Circumstances of Poisoning

- Owners may be unaware of the presence of toxic plants on their property, necessitating inspection by a qualified veterinarian or extension agent.

CLINICAL FEATURES

- In both natural and experimental disease, clinical signs are consistent with severe non-exertional rhabdomyolysis – depression, weakness, muscle tremors, reluctance to move, stiff gait, profuse sweating, and myoglobinuria.
- Significant cardiac involvement results in arrhythmia and/or signs of congestive heart failure – tachycardia, jugular distension and pulsation, and ventral edema.
- Affected horses may be found recumbent or dead.

DIFFERENTIAL DIAGNOSIS

- Other causes of non-exertional rhabdomyolysis:
  - Nutritional deficiency of selenium and/or vitamin E.
  - *Anaplasma phagocytophilum* infection.
  - Myosin heavy chain myopathy (MYH1 mutation).
  - Pasture myopathy – ingestion of hypoglycin A in seeds of the box elder tree (*Acer negundo*; North America) or sycamore maple tree (*Acer pseudoplatanus*; Europe).
  - Toxic plants – *Isocoma pluriflora* (rayless goldenrod), *Senna obtusifolia* (sicklepod) seeds, *Malva parviflora* (marshmallow).
- Other causes of acute arrythmia and cardiac dysfunction:
  - Sepsis, endotoxemia, electrolyte derangement.
  - Progression of previously unrecognized cardiac disease – pericarditis, congenital abnormalities, myocarditis, valvular disease, great vessel rupture, congestive heart failure.
  - Other cardiotoxins:
    - Ionophores.
    - Oleander.
    - Yew.
    - Rattlesnake envenomation.
- Other causes of muscle tremors generalized weakness, and recumbency:
  - Botulism.
  - Hyperkalemic periodic paralysis.
  - Vitamin E-deficient myopathy.
  - Equine motor neuron disease.
  - Tick paralysis.
  - Primary brain or spinal cord disease – trauma, rabies, viral encephalitides.
- Other causes of pigmenturia:
  - Myoglobinuria – infarctive purpura hemorrhagica, clostridial myonecrosis.
  - Hemoglobinuria – red maple toxicosis, leptospirosis, piroplasmosis, hypotonic IV fluids, IV DMSO.

DIAGNOSTICS

CBC/Serum Chemistry/Urinalysis

- Diagnosis is presumptive based on clinical signs, laboratory findings (marked elevation of CK and AST consistent with myonecrosis; myoglobinuria), necropsy findings, and consumption of, or access to, white snakeroot.

Other Diagnostic Tests

- Tremetone may be detected in the urine and possibly the blood, kidney, liver, and intestinal contents of affected animals, but testing is not readily available.
- ECG abnormalities include AV block, ventricular premature beats, and marked ST-segment depression.
- Cardiac troponin I is a sensitive marker of myocardial injury, but elevations are not specific for tremetol toxicity.

Pathological Findings

- Gross findings include pallor and necrosis of skeletal and cardiac muscle, pulmonary congestion and hepatopathy.
- Macroscopic lesions of the heart include pale areas and linear streaks throughout the myocardium. Histological lesions include myocardial degeneration, necrosis, fibrosis, and calcification.
- Histopathologic findings may also include centrilobular hepatic necrosis and mild renal tubular necrosis.

THERAPEUTICS

- Treatment is symptomatic and supportive.
- Goals of therapy are to prevent further toxin consumption; decontaminate the gut; optimize tissue perfusion and correct metabolic derangements; manage pain as needed; and prevent/treat complications.

Detoxification

- Give AC and a single dose of cathartic agent (magnesium sulfate; Epsom salts):
  - Administer AC (1–3 g/kg) by NG tube as a slurry in water or Epsom salts (500 mg to 1 g/kg magnesium sulfate dissolved in 4 L of warm water).
  - If AC is unavailable, administer DTO smectite (BioSponge®; 3 g/kg) by NG tube as a slurry in water or Epsom salts.
- Gastric lavage is unlikely to be helpful and is not recommended.

Appropriate Health Care

- Hospitalize affected horses for provision of supportive care.
- IV fluids are indicated to address dehydration, metabolic acidosis, and electrolyte derangement; maintain tissue perfusion; and reduce the risk of pigment nephropathy.
- Administer analgesics if myonecrosis is associated with pain.
- ECG monitoring if the patient's heart rate is unexpectedly high, low, or irregular. Treat significant arrhythmias.
- Horses with myoglobinuria and dehydration are at risk of acute kidney injury – urine output should be monitored.
- Daily serum chemistry to monitor for improvements in muscle enzymes, metabolic acidosis, and renal function; consider urinalysis.

Antidotes

- No known antidote.

Drugs of Choice

- IV fluid therapy – balanced polyionic solution (LRS).
- NSAIDs to control pain, if needed. Clinical signs associated with this condition make it difficult to determine whether or not a horse is experiencing significant pain. If in doubt, assess the horse's response to analgesic agents:
  - Flunixin (1.1 mg/kg IV or PO q12–24h).

- Phenylbutazone (2.2–4.4 mg/kg IV or PO q12–24h).
- Ketoprofen (2.2 mg/kg IV q24h).

■ Note that NSAIDs increase the risk of renal injury in patients with dehydration and/or existing renal compromise. If it is unclear whether significant pain is present, or if NSAIDs alone are insufficient to control pain, consider alternative analgesic agents such lidocaine and/or opioids (butorphanol, morphine):
- Lidocaine (1.3 mg/kg slow IV injection loading dose followed by 0.05 mg/kg/min CRI).
- Butorphanol (0.01–0.04 mg/kg IV or IM q2–4h)
- Butorphanol CRI – 0.02 mg/kg IV loading dose followed by continuous rate infusion at 13–22 µg/kg/h IV.
- Morphine (0.05–0.1 mg/kg IV or IM q4–6h).

COMMENTS

Client Education

■ For down horses, advise owners of the extensive nursing care required for humane management in the farm setting.
■ White snakeroot is also toxic to cattle, sheep, and goats.

Prevention/Avoidance

■ Avoid grazing horses on infested pastures.
■ Plants should be pulled out by the roots and burned; identification of the white blossoms is easiest in late summer and early fall.
■ Herbicides may be used for chemical control.

Expected Course and Prognosis

■ Prognosis for severe cases is poor, with death occurring in 1–3 days.
■ Horses that survive may take weeks to recover, and some go on to develop cardiomyopathy and congestive heart failure.
■ Mildly affected horses with no cardiac involvement may recover fully in 2 weeks with rest and appropriate supportive care.

Abbreviations

See Appendix 1 for a complete list.

Suggested Reading

Meerdink GL, Frederickson RL, Bordson GO. Tremetone. In: Plumlee KH, ed. Clinical Veterinary Toxicology. St Louis, MO: Mosby, 2004; pp. 348–350.
Sanders M. White snakeroot poisoning in a foal: a case report. J Equine Vet Sci 1983; 3:128–131.
Smetzer DL, Coppock RW, Ely RW, Duckett WM, Buck WB. Cardiac effects of white snakeroot intoxication in horses. Equine Pract 1983; 5: 26–32.
Talcott P. Toxicologic problems. In: Reed SM, Bayly WM, Sellon DC, eds. Equine Internal Medicine, 4th edn. St Louis, MO: Elsevier, 2018; pp. 1484–1485.

Author: Christie Ward, DVM, MVSc, PhD, DACVIM
Consulting Editor: Lynn R. Hovda, RPh, DVM, MS, DACVIM

Yellow Star Thistle (*Centaurea solstitialis*) and Russian Knapweed (*Acroptilon repens*)

Chapter 71

DEFINITION/OVERVIEW

- *Centaurea solstitialis* (yellow star thistle) and *Acroptilon repens* (Russian knapweed) are both weed plants found in the western USA (see Figs 71.1 and 71.2).
- Russian knapweed is also known as *Rhaponticum repens*.
- Chronic ingestion of either plant can result in equine nigropallidal encephalomalacia, a neurologic disease with characteristic clinical signs of dystonia/hypertonicity of the lips and tongue, generalized depression, inability to prehend food or drink water, and locomotor deficits.
- Disease eventually leads to death by starvation and/or dehydration.
- There is currently no cure or specific treatment for this disease, and in mild cases supportive care may be successful. In more advanced cases prognosis is grave.

ETIOLOGY/PATHOPHYSIOLOGY

Mechanism of Action

- The specific mechanism of action has not been identified, but it is suspected that repin, a sesquiterpene lactone present in both plants, is the toxin.
- The neurotoxin causes necrosis of the globus pallidus and substantia nigra.
- It affects the dopaminergic pathways of cranial nerves V, VII ad IX

Toxicokinetics

- Chronic toxicity usually taking a minimum of 60–90 days of grazing.

Toxicity

- Yellow star thistle – lethal dose of fresh plant material is 2.3–2.6 kg/100 kg BW.
- Russian knapweed – lethal dose of fresh plant material is 1.8–2.5kg/100 kg BW.
- Dried plants may also be toxic.
- Toxicity only occurs after chronic ingestion.

Blackwell's Five-Minute Veterinary Consult Clinical Companion: Equine Toxicology,
First Edition. Edited by Lynn R. Hovda, Dionne Benson, and Robert H. Poppenga.
© 2022 John Wiley & Sons, Inc. Published 2022 by John Wiley & Sons, Inc.
Companion website: www.wiley.com/go/hovda/equine

370 PLANTS AND BIOTOXINS

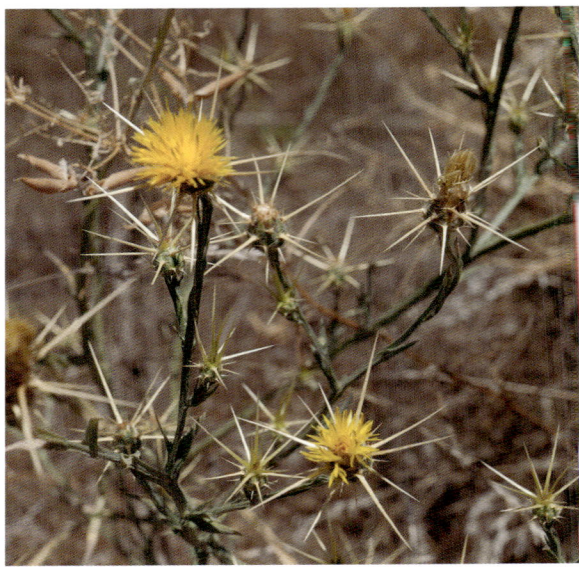

■ **Fig. 71.1.** Yellow star thistle (*Centaurea solstitialis*). *Source:* Franco Folini (https://commons.wikimedia.org/w/index.php?curid=33653694).

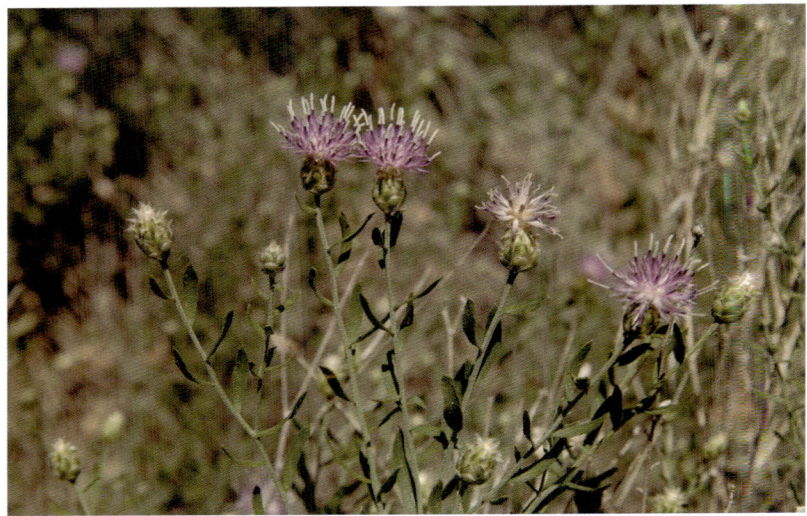

■ **Fig. 71.2.** Russian knapweed (*Acroptilon repens* or *Rhaponticum repens*). *Source:* Bob Nichols (https://commons.wikimedia.org/wiki/File:R.repens-USDA-1.jpg).

Systems Affected
- Nervous (specifically the brain).

 SIGNALMENT/HISTORY

- Any breed, sex, or age horse may become affected.

Risk Factors

- Primary risk is chronic exposure to the plant.
- Lack of access to other available feed sources could be considered a contributing factor, as most horses will avoid ingestion of these plants unless there is little else available.

Historical Findings

- Owners generally report nonspecific signs such loss of body condition and lethargy.
- More apparent neurologic signs and noticeable difficulties with prehension and mastication of food usually appear abruptly following chronic ingestion of either plant.

Location and Circumstances of Poisoning

- *Centaurea solstitialis* is a winter annual that generally grows in dry, light-intensive areas below 7,000 ft of elevation.
- *Acroptilon repens* is a perennial weed that is more tolerant of wet climates than *C. solstitialis* but tends not to grow past elevations of 6,200 ft or greater.
- *Acroptilon repens* can also be found in some areas of the eastern United States but is not nearly as common as on the west coast. A very small number of cases have been reported in Australia.

CLINICAL FEATURES

- Loss of body condition.
- Altered mentation, head pressing, aimless walking, ataxia.
- Tongue lolling and hypertonicity of facial and lip muscles.
- Altered mentation/depression/drowsiness/lethargy.
- Difficulty eating and drinking; horse may submerge entire head in water bucket to drink.
- Dehydration and associated signs – dry mucous membranes, increased CRT, decreased skin turgor, sinus tachycardia, and decreased pulse quality.

DIFFERENTIAL DIAGNOSIS

- Chronic disease process leading to loss of body condition.
- Dental or oral disease such as tooth root abscess or oral ulceration, causing difficulties in prehending food.
- Hepatic encephalopathy.
- Bacterial and viral encephalitis, WNV encephalitis, EPM.
- Rabies virus.
- Botulism toxicosis.

DIAGNOSTICS

CBC/Serum Chemistry/Urinalysis

- CBC – elevated PCV consistent with dehydration.
- Serum chemistry – elevated BUN and creatinine consistent with dehydration.

Imaging

- MRI has been used successfully to diagnose equine nigropallidal encephalomalacia. Lesions can be seen on T1-weighted, T2-weighted, and proton density images.
- The usefulness of MRI is limited to confirming the diagnosis and preventing unnecessary suffering of the patient, while further diagnostics are pursued to rule out other causes of the clinical signs.
- No other diagnostics have proven valuable to support the diagnosis.

Pathological Findings

- Gross – degeneration and necrosis of the globus pallidus and substantia nigra.
- Histopathology – confirms presence of degeneration and necrosis of the globus pallidus and substantia nigra.

THERAPEUTICS

Detoxification

- There are no decontamination recommendations as signs result from chronic ingestion.

Appropriate Health Care

- For very mild cases, treatment consists primarily of supportive care, including IV fluid therapy and nutritional supplementation, which may be successful. However, residual neurologic signs will persist.
- As toxicity causes irreversible changes to the brain, euthanasia is recommended in most affected cases.

Antidote

- There is no antidote available.

COMMENTS

Client Education

- Clients with affected animals should be made aware of the description of *A. repens* and *C. solstitialis* so they can remove plants from grazing areas.

Prevention/Avoidance

- Prevent access to *A. repens* and *C. solstitialis* plants and provide alternative nutrition sources.

Expected Course and Prognosis

- Once significant neurologic signs are present, prognosis is grave, and euthanasia should be recommended if other differentials have been ruled out.

Abbreviations

See Appendix 1 for a complete list.

Suggested Reading

Burrows GE, Tyrl RJ. Toxic Plants of North America, 2nd edn. Ames, Iowa: John Wiley & Sons, Inc, 2013.

Chang HT, Rumbeiha WK, Patterson JS, et al. Toxic equine parkinsonism: an immunohistochemical study of 12 horses with nigropallidal encephalomalacia. Vet Pathol 2012; 49(2):398–402.

Elliott CR, McCowan CI. Nigropallidal encephalomalacia in horses grazing *Rhaponticum repens* (creeping knapweed). Aust Vet J. 2012; 90(4):151–154.

Sanders SG, Tucker RL, Bagley RS, Gavin PR. Magnetic resonance imaging features of equine nigropallidal encephalomalacia. Vet Radiol Ultrasound 2001; 42(4):291–296.

Acknowledgement: The author and editors acknowledge the prior contribution of Larry Thompson.

Author: Emma V. Hummer, DVM
Consulting Editor: Lynn R. Hovda, RPh, DVM, MS, DACVIM

Chapter 72

Yew (*Taxus* spp.)

DEFINITION/OVERVIEW

- Yews (*Taxus* spp.) are evergreen trees and shrubs that grow natively throughout the northern hemisphere. Ornamental varieties are widely used in landscaping because they stay green year-round, require little maintenance, and the dense foliage is well suited to borders and hedges.
- Ornamental yews account for most cases of equine intoxication, usually through inadvertent consumption of landscape plants or inappropriate disposal of trimmings in pastures or paddocks.
- Relevant species include the Japanese yew (*T. cuspidata*), American yew (*T. canadensis*; ground hemlock), English yew (*T. baccata*), and Pacific or Western yew (*T. brevifolia*). All varieties should be considered toxic.
- Yew leaves, seeds, and bark contain cardiotoxic taxine alkaloids; only the bright red flesh of the berry-like aril is nontoxic (see Figs 72.1 and 72.2).
- Toxicity persists after plant material has been cut and dried.

ETIOLOGY/PATHOPHYSIOLOGY

- Exposed animals typically die of heart failure within several hours of yew consumption.
- Most affected horses are found dead.

Mechanism of Action

- Yews contain several taxine alkaloids, of which taxine B is the major toxic agent.
- Taxines antagonize myocardial calcium and sodium channels, leading to increased cytoplasmic calcium, cardiac conduction disturbances, and death from cardiac arrest or cardiogenic shock.
- In animal models, bradycardia, AV block, and prolonged QRS complexes have been reported.
- In cases of human poisoning ventricular tachycardia is often the initial arrhythmia, followed by variable ECG abnormalities reflecting AV block, delayed and aberrant ventricular depolarization and repolarization, ventricular fibrillation, and asystole.

Blackwell's Five-Minute Veterinary Consult Clinical Companion: Equine Toxicology,
First Edition. Edited by Lynn R. Hovda, Dionne Benson, and Robert H. Poppenga.
© 2022 John Wiley & Sons, Inc. Published 2022 by John Wiley & Sons, Inc.
Companion website: www.wiley.com/go/hovda/equine

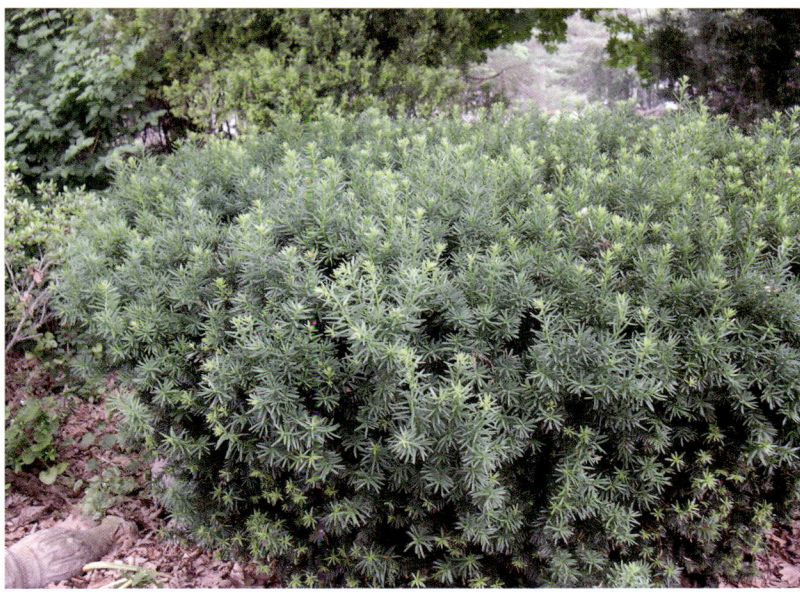

■ **Fig. 72.1.** Japanese yew (*Taxus cuspidata*) shrub. All parts except the fleshy red fruit are poisonous. *Source:* Photo courtesy of Tyne K. Hovda.

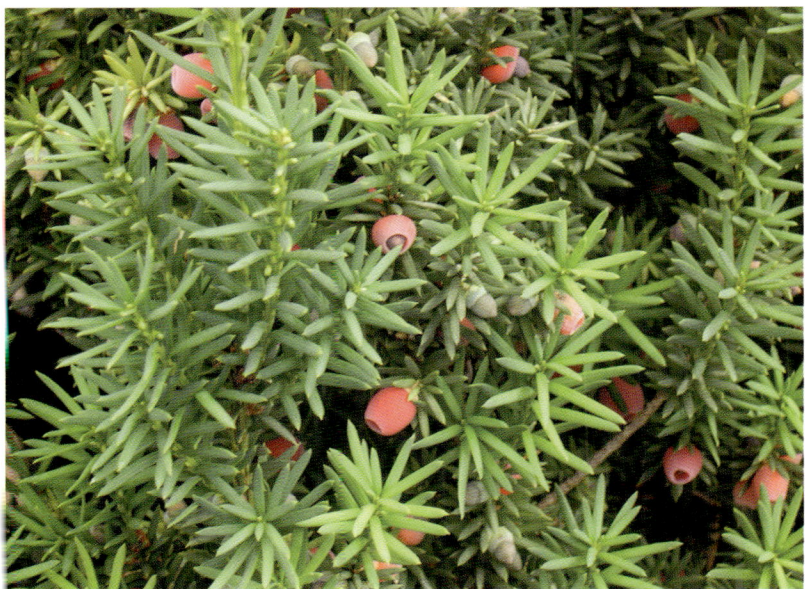

■ **Fig. 72.2.** Japanese yew (*Taxus cuspidata*) berries (arils). The fleshy red part is edible; the seed inside is deadly. *Source:* Photo courtesy of Tyne K. Hovda.

- Ventricular tachycardia has not been specifically reported in equine yew poisoning, but this may reflect the rarity of antemortem diagnosis and treatment.
- Yews also contain irritant volatile compounds that may cause colic and diarrhea in horses that consume a sublethal dose.

Toxicokinetics

- Taxines are rapidly absorbed and widely distributed.
- They are metabolized by hepatic P450 enzymes, and then excreted in bile and, to a lesser extent, urine.

Toxicity

- All livestock species are susceptible, with horses considered most susceptible.
- The minimum lethal dose of taxine is estimated at 1–2 mg/kg.
- Yews contain variable levels of taxine, but the minimum lethal dose of yew is estimated at 0.2–0.4 g yew leaves/kg body weight, or as little as 90 g of leaves for a 450-kg horse.
- Yew is also toxic to companion animals and humans, but incidence of poisoning is much lower in those species.

Systems Affected

- Cardiovascular – bradycardia, arrhythmia, cardiac arrest.
- Gastrointestinal – possible colic and diarrhea in animals that survive subacute exposure.
- Nervous – agitation, incoordination, trembling, terminal convulsions.
- Neuromuscular – weakness, collapse.
- Respiratory – pulmonary edema, dyspnea.

SIGNALMENT/HISTORY

- Horses of any age, breed, or sex.
- Owners typically report sudden death of one or more animals with no premonitory signs.

CLINICAL FEATURES

- Poisoned animals develop arrhythmias, myocardial dysfunction, and die of cardiac arrest or cardiogenic shock within several hours of yew consumption.
- When clinical signs are observed, as with experimental intoxication or sublethal ingestion, animals exhibit muscle tremors, bradycardia, cardiac arrhythmias, jugular distension and pulsation, dyspnea, collapse, and terminal convulsions.
- Horses that survive acute cardiac effects may develop colic or diarrhea from the irritant compounds in yew.

DIFFERENTIAL DIAGNOSIS

- Other cardiotoxins:
  - Plants containing cardiac glycosides: oleander (*Nerium oleander*), summer pheasant's eye (*Adonis aestivalis*), foxglove (*Digitalis purpurea*), lily-of-the-valley (*Convallaria majalis*), dogbane (*Apocynum* spp.).

- Rhododendron (*Rhododendron ponticum*).
- Death camas (*Zigadenus venenosus*).
- Avocado (*Persea* spp.).
- Ionophores (monensin, lasalocid, salinomycin).
■ Other toxic causes of sudden death:
- Cantharidin (blister beetles).
- Acute selenium toxicity.
- Organophosphate and carbamate insecticides.
- Box elder seeds (*Acer negundo*).
- Red maple (*Acer rubrum*).
■ Primary cardiac disease:
- Myocarditis, aortic root rupture, pulmonary artery rupture, endocarditis, acute severe valvular insufficiency (e.g., chordal rupture), acute decompensation of chronic heart failure.

DIAGNOSTICS

■ Presumptive diagnosis is based on consistent clinical signs or sudden death, presence of yew in the animal's environment, and gross or microscopic identification of yew material in the stomach or intestine.
■ Definitive diagnosis is by GC-MS demonstration of taxine alkaloids in stomach or intestinal contents.
■ Confirmatory testing in humans is based on GC-MS detection of 3,5-dimethoxyphenol, a marker of yew consumption, in urine, blood, and gastric contents. There are no reports of this test's application in horses, however.

Pathological Findings

■ Cases of peracute death exhibit no definitive gross lesions.
■ Histopathology may reveal mutifocal myocardial necrosis.
■ Two calves that survived initial yew exposure died later with microscopic evidence of myocardial necrosis (6 days post-exposure) and extensive myocardial fibrosis (18 days post-exposure). While this has not been reported for horses, it should be considered a possible outcome of sublethal exposure.

THERAPEUTICS

■ Opportunities for treatment are rare, given rapid progression to collapse and death.
■ Treatment is symptomatic and supportive.
■ Goals of therapy are to halt toxin ingestion, decontaminate the gut, treat arrythmias, and maintain blood pressure and tissue perfusion.

Detoxification

■ Give AC and a single dose of cathartic agent (magnesium sulfate; Epsom salts):
- Administer AC (1–3 g/kg) by NG tube as a slurry in water or Epsom salts (500 mg to 1 g/kg magnesium sulfate dissolved in 4 L of warm water).

- If AC is unavailable, administer DTO smectite (BioSponge®; 3 g/kg) by NG tube as a slurry in water or Epsom salts.
- Note that stress of treatment may precipitate clinical signs or cardiac arrest

Appropriate Health Care

- Continuous ECG monitoring for 48 hours, with treatment of any clinically significant arrhythmia.
- Minimize stress, excitement, and activity, particularly once clinical signs appear.

Antidotes

- No specific antidote.

Drugs of Choice

- IV fluids to maintain blood pressure and tissue perfusion.
- Antiarrhythmic medications as needed.
  - Recommendations for medical treatment of specific dysrhythmias are provided below. Note that all antiarrhythmic agents carry a risk of proarrhythmic effects, seizures, and sudden death. Treatment must therefore be tailored to the individual patient and guided by continuous ECG monitoring.
- For bradycardia and complete (third-degree) AV block:
  - Atropine (0.005–0.01 mg/kg IV).
  - Glycopyrrolate (0.005–0.01 mg/kg IV).
- For ventricular tachycardia, administer medications in the order presented below (as available) until conversion to sinus rhythm is confirmed:
  - Lidocaine (0.25–0.5 mg/kg slow IV. Repeat in 5–10 minutes to effect up to a maximum total dose of 1.5 mg/kg, followed by 0.05 mg/kg/min CRI).
  - Magnesium sulfate (2–6 mg/kg/min to effect, up to a maximum total dose of 55 mg/kg)
  - Procainamide (1 mg/kg/min IV up to a maximum total dose of 20 mg/kg).
  - Amiodarone (5 mg/kg/hour IV for 1 hour, followed by 0.83 mg/kg/hour for 23 hours, and subsequently 1.9 mg/kg/hour for 30 hours or to effect).
  - Quinidine gluconate (1–2.2 mg/kg IV q10min to effect; not to exceed a maximum total dose of 12 mg/kg).
  - If pulmonary edema develops, give furosemide (1–2 mg/kg IV) and intranasal oxygen.

Alternate Drugs

- Digoxin-specific Fab antibody fragments have been used to manage human patients based on structural similarities between taxine and digoxin, but this is unlikely to be available or practical for use in the veterinary setting.

COMMENTS

Client Education

Yew is also toxic to other livestock species (cattle, goats, sheep, pigs, camelids), companion animals, and humans.

Prevention/Avoidance

- Yews are sufficiently palatable that livestock will consume it even when appropriate feed is available, so access to these plants must be prevented.
- Remove all yews near paddocks or pastures, and ideally from anywhere on a horse property lest horses escape their enclosures and gain access to them.
- Do not plant yews when landscaping horse properties and show facilities.
- Do not allow horses to graze landscape plants at show and sale facilities.
- Dispose of clippings safely where they cannot be accessed by livestock or pets. Consider composting, burning, or landfill disposal.
- The green foliage and red berries make yew a popular choice for holiday wreaths and decorations, but these should never be used for barns or paddocks.

Expected Course and Prognosis

- Poor prognosis; animals poisoned with yew are usually found dead.
- Onset of clinical signs and cardiac dysfunction is so rapid that treatment is usually too late and ineffective.
- Horses that consume a sublethal dose and survive beyond 48 hours may recover, but evidence from calves supports the possibility of residual cardiac pathology.

See Also

Cardiotoxic Plants
Oleander (*Nerium oleander* and *Cascabela thevetia*)
Rhododendron spp.

Abbreviations

See Appendix 1 for a complete list.

Suggested Reading

Burcham GN, Becker KJ, Tahara JM, et al. Myocardial fibrosis associated with previous ingestion of yew (*Taxus* sp.) in a Holstein heifer: evidence for chronic yew toxicity in cattle. J Vet Diagn Invest 2013; 25:147–152.
Casteel SW. Taxine alkaloids. In: Plumlee KH, ed. Clinical Veterinary Toxicology. St. Louis, MO: Mosby, 2004; pp 379–381.
Lowe JE, Hintz HF, Schryver HF, Kingsbury JM. *Taxus cuspidata* (Japanese yew) poisoning in horses. Cornell Vet 1970; 60:36–39.
Tiwary AK, Puschner B, Kinde H, Tor ER. Diagnosis of *Taxus* (yew) poisoning in a horse. J Vet Diagn Invest 2005 17:252–255.
Wilson CR, Hooser SB. Toxicity of yew (*Taxus* spp.) alkaloids. In: Gupta RC, ed. Veterinary Toxicology: Basic and Clinical Principles, 3rd edn. San Diego, CA: Academic Press, 2018; pp. 947–953.

Author: Christie Ward, DVM, MVSc, PhD, DACVIM
Consulting Editor: Lynn R. Hovda, RPh, DVM, MS, DACVIM

Rodenticides

Chapter 73

Anticoagulants

DEFINITION/OVERVIEW

- Ingestion of anticoagulant rodenticides leads to coagulopathy and hemorrhage due to the reduction of vitamin K1 coagulation factors in circulation.
- Anticoagulant rodenticides are typically available as pelleted or block products. The palatability of the bait may increase the incidence of toxicity in non-target species.
- Products available are classified as either first-generation anticoagulants (FGAR) or second-generation anticoagulants (SGAR). SGAR (also known as "super warfarins") were developed in response to the development of resistance to FGAR products in rodents. Recent EPA restrictions have limited the availability of consumer products containing SGAR.
- The EPA ruled in 2008 that by the year 2011 consumer products may not be sold in containers larger than 1 lb and may not contain SGAR, including brodifacoum, difethialone, difenacoum, and bromadiolone. They may contain non-anticoagulants or FGAR, including warfarin, diphacinone, chlorphacinone, and dicoumarol.
- SGAR, however, may be still be used by pest control officers or sold for agricultural use.
- FGAR have a shorter duration of action (days); SGAR have a much longer duration of action (weeks)

ETIOLOGY/PATHOPHYSIOLOGY

Mechanism of Action

- Clotting factors II, VII, IX, and X bind with Ca in active clot formation. Carboxylation of clotting factor precursors using vitamin K1 hydroquinone as a cofactor is required to permit Ca-binding ability.
- Vitamin K1 hydroquinone is converted to its epoxide form, vitamin K1 2,3 epoxide in the vitamin K-dependent carboxylase reaction.
- Vitamin K1 2,3 epoxide is then reduced to vitamin K1 and recycled by enzyme epoxide reductase.
- Anticoagulant rodenticides interfere with the vitamin K1 epoxide reductase enzyme resulting in the depletion of vitamin K1. This impairs the synthesis of carboxylated clotting factors II, VII, IX, and X.
- This does not allow for active clot formation and leads to clinical coagulopathy.

Blackwell's Five-Minute Veterinary Consult Clinical Companion: Equine Toxicology,
First Edition. Edited by Lynn R. Hovda, Dionne Benson, and Robert H. Poppenga.
© 2022 John Wiley & Sons, Inc. Published 2022 by John Wiley & Sons, Inc.
Companion website: www.wiley.com/go/hovda/equine

Toxicokinetics

- Rapidly well absorbed from the GI tract.
- After absorption, rapidly distributed; may be detected in stable form in the liver and kidneys.
- Peak plasma levels:
    - Warfarin (FGAR): reached 3–11 hours after ingestion when given with food.
    - Brodifacoum (SGAR): reached 2–3 hours after ingestion.
- Stored and metabolized in the liver.
- Metabolites are eliminated renally.
- Terminal half-life depends on specific FGAR or SGAR.

Toxicity

- Brodifacoum is the SGAR with the lowest reported oral median lethal dose in horses.
- LD_{50} (brodifacoum 0.005%): 50–100 mg/adult horse or about 1–2 kg of finished product/adult horse.
- Toxic dose: 0.1–0.2 mg/kg PO in one source; 0.125 mg/kg PO in another.

Systems Affected

- Hemic/lymphatic/immune – depletion of activated clotting factors, resulting in hemorrhage in a variety of locations.
- Gastrointestinal – anorexia, weight loss, oral, gastric, or intestinal bleeding, colic, epistaxis.
- Cardiovascular – hemopericardium, resulting in arrhythmia, tachycardia, hypotension.
- Neuromuscular – bleeding into the CNS may cause nystagmus, tremor, gait changes.
- Reproductive – may result in placental bleeding, abortion.
- Respiratory – pulmonary hemorrhage and hemothorax.
- Musculoskeletal – hemarthrosis resulting in lameness; hemoperitoneum resulting in abdominal distention.
- Nervous – depression, restlessness.

SIGNALMENT/HISTORY

- No breed, gender, or age predilection.

Risk Factors

- Risk of exposure to SGAR may be decreased in urban settings following new EPA regulations, but due to their permitted use in agricultural settings, horses may continue to be exposed.
- Rodenticides are most commonly used in spring and fall, with exposure increasing during those times.

Historical Findings

- Products may be seen in the environment or feed, present as blue, green, red, or brown/tan pellets or blocks. The color of the bait is not always correlated with bait color, and caution should be taken with bait identification if product packaging is not available.

- Lethargy restlessness, pawing, anorexia, and exercise intolerance may be the first signs noted.
- Sudden death may result in some cases.

Location and Circumstances of Poisoning

- May occur in and around building where rodents are present and baits are placed.
- Chance of exposure increases when protective baits stations are not used, or bulk bait products are present.
- Bait may be accidentally mixed with feed, leading to exposure.
- Exposure may be a single, acute dose or multiple small, chronic doses.

CLINICAL FEATURES

- Tachycardia, hypotension, pallor, poor pulse quality.
- Hemarthrosis, lameness.
- Bleeding from any body orifice – epistaxis, oral, vaginal or rectal bleeding, melena.
- Tachypnea, dyspnea.
- Petechiae or ecchymosis.
- Hematomas or excessive bleeding at venepuncture sites.
- Abdominal distension.
- Weight loss, lethargy, restlessness, poor appetite.

DIAGNOSTICS

CBC/Serum Chemistry/Urinalysis

- Anemia – decreased hematocrit, hemoglobin, erythrocyte count by 8 days post-ingestion; often acute, non-regenerative anemia.
- Thrombocytopenia secondary to consumptive bleeding/hemorrhage.
- Blood chemistry panel may show hypoproteinemia, hypoalbuminemia secondary to hemorrhage, increased total bilirubin, urea, creatinine, and creatinine kinase.
- Hepatic dysfunction may impede metabolism and excretion, and may exacerbate toxicity.
- Urinalysis may show hematuria, proteinuria.

Other Diagnostic Tests

- Prolonged coagulation factors (SGAR):
    - PTT increased by 24 hours, four-fold increase by day 4.
    - PT increased by 48 hours, two-fold increase by day 6.
- Abdominocentesis may confirm hemoabdomen, hemorrhagic peritoneal fluid.
- Thoracocentesis may confirm hemothorax in dyspneic patients.
- Arthrocentesis to confirm hemarthrosis.

Pathological Findings

- Evidence of hemorrhage, free blood in the thorax, pericardium, abdominal cavity.
- Multifocal hemorrhage in SC tissue, muscle bellies, serosal membranes, meninges.
- Evidence of anticoagulant rodenticides in liver, tissue analysis performed by LC-MS/MS.

THERAPEUTICS

- Therapy is aimed at initial detoxification (if appropriate, given time-frame and patient presentation).
- The antidote, vitamin K1, should be started as soon as possible.

Detoxification

- If recent ingestion, activated charcoal (1–3 g/kg as a watery slurry) or a cathartic (magnesium sulfate 250–500 mg/kg in 2–4 L of warm water) may be administered via nasogastric tube
- If clinical signs have already developed or the patient has become coagulopathic, decontamination may not be effective.

Appropriate Health Care

- Depending on the amount ingested and clinical signs, treatment may be effective at home.
- In-patient care will be needed for a patient in acute crisis.
- Patient stabilization is accomplished using IV fluid therapy, additional blood products, and supportive care as needed.
- Fluid therapy to correct hypotension, hemorrhagic shock.
- Whole-blood or plasma transfusions may be given to clinically coagulopathic patients.
- Stall rest is recommended to decrease potential for trauma or injury in coagulopathic patients.

Antidote

- Vitamin K1 (phytonadione) is the antidote for both FGAR and SGAR toxicity. Oral dosing may be cost-prohibitive.
- Many different equine vitamin K1 dosing regiments have been suggested.
- FGAR:
  - Initial IV dose of 0.3–0.5 mg/kg IV, followed by PO dosing (0.25–2.5 mg/kg × 7 days).
  - 0.5–2.5 mg/kg IM or SC × 7–14 days.
- SGAR:
  - 2.5 mg/kg SC q12h × 36 hours, then PO q12h × 23 days.
  - 2.5 mg/kg SC q24h × 3 days, then 1 mg/kg SC q24h × 21 days.
  - 0.5–2.5 mg/kg IM or SC once daily until normal Pt/PTT.
- PT/PTT monitoring:
  - Recheck PT/PTT after 7–10 days of oral vitamin K1 therapy for FGAR and 14–21 days for SGAR. If still prolonged, continue therapy for 10–14 more days.
- Do not discontinue vitamin K1 therapy, even if patient appears clinically normal, until full duration of therapy has been completed.
- Alfalfa hay may be given as an additional source of vitamin K.

Drugs of Choice

- Depends on clinical signs for each individual horse.

Precautions/Interactions

- Vitamin K3 (menadione) is *not* recommended. It is not efficacious and may lead to renal tubular necrosis.
- Some drugs may increase the toxic effects of anticoagulant rodenticides- NSAIDs, phenylbutazone, oxyphenbutazone, heparin, phenytoin, salicylates, quinidine, potentated sulfas, penicillin, streptomycin, corticosteroids.

- Strenuous exercise may be associated with fatal, acute hemorrhage in exposed patients.
- Minimize venepuncture or invasive sampling procedures to avoid catastrophic bleeding or hematoma formation.

COMMENTS

Prevention/Avoidance

- Do not allow animal access to anticoagulant rodenticide products; use caution to avoid contamination of feed stuffs with products.
- Re-exposure may be a concern; bait should be removed from the animal's environment.

Possible Complications

- Pregnant animals may abort secondary to placental hemorrhage.
- The toxin is lipophilic and may be transmitted in milk to foals who are nursing. The amount is unknown and may be negligible, but nursing foals should be weaned or treated if the mare ingested a toxic dose.

Expected Course and Prognosis

- Depending on specific rodenticide and amount ingested, treatment may be as short as 5–7 days or several weeks.
- Prompt treatment and administration of vitamin K1 decreases potential for clinical coagulopathy to arise and improves prognosis.

Abbreviations

See Appendix 1 for a complete list.

Internet Resources

Rodent control pesticide Safety Review. Available at: https://www.epa.gov/rodenticides/rodent-control-pesticide-safety-review (6 April 2017).

Suggested Reading

Ayala I, Rodriguez J, Martos N, et al. Fatal brodifacoum poisoning in a pony. Can J Vet Res 2007; 48(6):627–629.
Boermans HJ, Johnstone I, Black WD. Clinical signs, laboratory changes, and toxicokinetics of brodifacoum in the horse. Can J Vet Res 1991; 55(1):21–27.
Caravallo E Poppinga R, Kinde H, et al. Cluster of cases of massive hemorrhage associated with anticoagulant detection in racehorses. J Vet Diagn Invest 2015; 27(1):112–116.
McConnico R, Copedge K, Bischoff K. Brodifacoum toxicosis in two horses. J Am Vet Med Assoc 1997; 21(7):882–887.
Vrins A, Carlson G, Feldman B. Warfarin: A review with emphasis on its use in the horse. Can J Vet Res 1983; 24:211–213.
Zakain A, Sajad M, Nouri M, et al. Brodifacoum toxicosis in an Arabian mare. Vet Research Forum 2019; 10 (2):173–176.

Author: Ashley Smit, DVM
Consulting Editor: Lynn R. Hovda, RPh, DVM, MS, DACVIM

Bromethalin

DEFINITION/OVERVIEW

- Bromethalin is a rodenticide with marked neurotoxic effects.
- Currently it is available in two different concentrations: 0.01% and 0.025%.
- The LD_{50} is approximately 0.5 and 2.5 mg/kg in cats and dogs, respectively. The minimum lethal dose is approximately 0.25 and 1 mg/kg in cats and dogs, respectively.
- The LD_{50} and minimum lethal dose in horses have not been established. Poisoning is expected to be rare in adult horses due to the low concentration of bromethalin in baits as opposed to the large size of the horse. Foals, weanlings, and miniature horses are more likely to be affected.
- Some websites recommend using 0.1 mg/kg BW as the maximum dose required for treatment.

ETIOLOGY/PATHOPHYSIOLOGY

- Reported poisonings from bromethalin are increasing, in part due to the restrictions placed on the use of anticoagulant rodenticides.

Mechanism of Action

- The presumed mechanism of bromethalin and its active/more toxic metabolite, desmethylbromethalin, is by uncoupling oxidative phosphorylation. This results in insufficient energy available for Na^+- K^+ ion channel pumps and the development of cerebral edema.
- The CNS is the most severely affected, likely because it depends so greatly on oxidative phosphorylation. Myelin edema (cerebral edema) causes increased pressure on nerve axons, decreased nerve conduction, paralysis and death. Increased cerebral lipid peroxidation also occurs and may contribute to clinical signs.

Toxicokinetics

- The following is based primarily on rat studies.
- Absorption:
  - Oral absorption is rapid and complete.

Blackwell's Five-Minute Veterinary Consult Clinical Companion: Equine Toxicology,
First Edition. Edited by Lynn R. Hovda, Dionne Benson, and Robert H. Poppenga.
© 2022 John Wiley & Sons, Inc. Published 2022 by John Wiley & Sons, Inc.
Companion website: www.wiley.com/go/hovda/equine

- Distribution:
  - Peak plasma levels occur within 4–6 hours of exposure.
  - Product is widely distributed to brain, fat, liver, and kidney.
  - Highly lipophilic and crosses the BBB.
- Metabolism:
  - Metabolized in the liver by mixed function oxidases to its active and more toxic metabolite, desmethylbromethalin.
  - Undergoes enterohepatic recirculation which can delay excretion from the body.
- Excretion:
  - Via the biliary system with a small amount excreted via the urine.
  - The half-life of elimination is estimated to be 3–6 days depending on the species.

Toxicity

- There is no truly effective treatment once CNS signs have developed, so decontamination is the best option.

Systems Affected

- Neurological.
- Gastrointestinal.
- Respiratory.
- Ophthalmic.

SIGNALMENT/HISTORY

There is no true breed or sex predilection, but smaller weight animals (foals, weanlings, miniature horses) are expected to be affected more often than adult horses.

Risk Factors

- Small body weight.
- Chronic, repeated ingestion.

Historical Findings

- Evidence of exposure – tan/greenish/brown material in feces.
- Owners report exposure.

Location and Circumstances of Poisoning

- Barns, training centers, indoor riding arenas where horses have ready access.
- Large containers of product accidently left out by pesticide elimination officer – perhaps one of the most common equine routes of exposure.

CLINICAL FEATURES

- Base on limited equine case data, often anecdotal.
- CNS depression, head pressing, muscle tremors, ataxia, seizures (rare).

- Inappetence (backing off food) to total anorexia.
- Nystagmus.
- Respiratory depression.

DIFFERENTIAL DIAGNOSIS

- Primary neurological disease – infectious (viral, bacterial).
- EPM.
- Hepatic encephalopathy.
- Other CNS toxicants.

DIAGNOSTICS

CBC/Serum Chemistry/Urinalysis

- Abnormalities would be secondary to clinical signs (e.g., dehydration, increased CK from tremors, myoglobinuria, etc.) and not helpful with the diagnosis.

Other Diagnostic Tests

- Elevated CSF pressure (rarely measured in veterinary medicine).
- Ante-mortem bromethalin testing – bromethalin/desmethylbromethalin may be detected in serum at several laboratories and used mainly to confirm exposure.
- Postmortem bromethalin testing – bromethalin/desmethylbromethalin can be detected from stomach contents, fat, liver, or brain tissues at necropsy.

Imaging

- MRI may reveal generalized brain edema.

Pathological Findings

- Gross – may be evidence of mild cerebral edema.
- Histopathology – spongy degeneration in the cerebellum, cerebrum, brainstem, and spinal cord due to myelin edema.

THERAPEUTICS

Detoxification

- Gastric lavage with a large-bore stomach tube if early and witnessed ingestion.
- AC 1–3 g/kg PO in a watery slurry, followed by magnesium sulfate (Epsom salts) 250–500 mg/kg PO in 2–4 L of warm water × one dose.
- Two additional doses of AC may be administered every 8 hours.

Appropriate Health Care

- Hospitalize as needed.
- Monitor vitals and mentation q6h.

Antidotes

- There is no specific antidote available.

Drugs of Choice

- Tremors:
  - Methocarbamol 22–55 mg/kg IV slowly for severe conditions; 4.4–22 mg/kg IV for moderate conditions. Do not exceed 330 mg/kg/day.
- Seizures:
  - Diazepam 0.1–0.4 mg/kg IV prn (foal); 25–50 mg IV prn (adult horses).
  - Phenobarbital 16–20 mg/kg IV × one dose.

Alternative Drugs

- Intravenous fat emulsion. Bromethalin and desmethylbromethalin are lipid-soluble based on their logP-values of 6.70 and 4.26, respectively. There is limited clinical support for the use of IV fat thus far and use needs to be considered in terms of amount ingested, ongoing signs, and time since exposure. The greatest benefit is likely shortly after ingestion, before CNS signs have become severe.

COMMENTS

Client Education

- This poisoning primarily affects smaller weight horses such as foals, weanlings, and miniature horses.
- Based on larger body size, adult horses are less likely to be affected.

Prevention/Avoidance

- Prevention is critical. Follow directions for use and place the product appropriately.
- Keep the product, especially large containers, far away from horses.

Possible Complications

- Passage in the milk is likely if the mare ingests a toxic dose due to the lipophilic nature of bromethalin, but there are no data to show if or how much is passed in the milk.

Expected Course and Prognosis

- Dependent upon dose ingested and timing of intervention.

Abbreviations

See Appendix 1 for a complete list.

Suggested Reading

Coppock R. Bromethalin rodenticide – no known antidote. Can Vet J 2013; 54:557–558.

Filigenzi MS, , Bautista AC, Aston LS, Poppenga RH. Method for the detection of desmethylbromethalin in animal tissue samples for the determination of bromethalin exposure. J Agric Food Chem 2015; 63:5146–5151.

Gupta RC. Non-anticoagulant rodenticides. In: Veterinary Toxicology: Basic and Clinical Principles 3rd edn. New York: Elsevier, 2018; pp. 616–616.

Van Lier RB, Cherry LD. The toxicity and mechanism of action of bromethalin: a new single feeding rodenticide. Fundam Appl Toxicol 1988; 11(4):664–672.

Authors: Lynn R. Hovda, RPH, DVM, MS, DACVIM; Sherry Rippel, DVM, DABT, DABVT
Consulting Editors: Lynn R. Hovda, RPH, DVM, MS, DACVIM

Chapter 75

Cholecalciferol

DEFINITION/OVERVIEW

- Cholecalciferol is a form of vitamin D, specifically vitamin D3 (a secrosteroid).
- The most common unit of measure for cholecalciferol is IU (international units) – 40,000 IU is equivalent to 1 mg of cholecalciferol.
- Horses are most commonly exposed to cholecalciferol through grain supplementation:
  - An inappropriate mixture could result in overdose.
  - Exposure to a grain mixed for another species can result in toxicity.
- Cholecalciferol rodenticide is becoming more commonly used and horses are likely to have more exposure when placed in barns and fields.

ETIOLOGY/PATHOPHYSIOLOGY

Mechanism of Action

- Cholecalciferol increases absorption of calcium from the GI tract and the kidneys.
- Cholecalciferol mobilizes calcium and phosphorus from bones to the circulation.
- Acute renal failure develops secondary to hypercalcemia.
- Cardiac arrhythmias occur because of mineralization of the heart or changes in the ratio of intracellular-to-extracellular ion concentrations and an increase in the depolarization threshold.

Toxicokinetics

- Rapidly absorbed from the GI tract.
- Distribution:
  - Very lipid-soluble and distributed in the adipose tissue.
  - Can be present in milk due to lipophilicity.
  - LogP = 9.72; logD (pH 7.4) = 8.65.
- Metabolism:
  - Cholecalciferol is hydroxylated in the liver to 25-hydroxycholecalciferol (calcifediol) by the enzyme 25-hydroxylase.
  - Calcifediol is the primary circulating enzyme.
  - In the kidney, 25-hydroxycholecalciferol is metabolized to 1,25-dihydroxycholecalciferol (calcitriol).

Blackwell's Five-Minute Veterinary Consult Clinical Companion: Equine Toxicology, First Edition. Edited by Lynn R. Hovda, Dionne Benson, and Robert H. Poppenga.
© 2022 John Wiley & Sons, Inc. Published 2022 by John Wiley & Sons, Inc.
Companion website: www.wiley.com/go/hovda/equine

- Calcitriol is the principal active enzyme.
- Undergoes enterohepatic recirculation.
■ Excretion:
  - Elimination half-life is not available for horses.
  - Elimination half-life of plasma cholecalciferol in dogs is 19–25 hours, with a terminal half-life of weeks to months.
■ Toxicity:
  - Daily allowance 6.6 IU/kg.
  - Upper limit 44 IU/kg/day.
  - Toxic dose in two horses 12,000–13,000 IU/kg/day × 30 days – death was reported in one horse.

Systems Affected

- The following is primarily from human and canine data.
- Renal – mineralization of kidney; vasoconstriction of renal afferent arterioles leading to decreases in renal blood flow and GFR, ischemia and acute tubular necrosis.
- Gastrointestinal – mineralization of gastric mucosa, GI stasis, increased gastric acid secretion.
- Cardiovascular – mineralization of the blood vessels and endocardium, cardiac murmurs, bradycardia, tachycardia, EKG changes (shortened Q–T and prolonged P–R intervals).
- Musculoskeletal – limb stiffness, painful flexor tendons.
- Respiratory – mineralization of the lungs, pulmonary edema, pulmonary hemorrhage.

SIGNALMENT/HISTORY

Risk Factors

- Miniature horses.
- Younger animals.
- Nursing foals.
- High dietary calcium and phosphorus.
- Dehydration.
- Underlying medical condition – renal failure.
- Individual variation.

Historical Findings

- Rodenticide on premises.
- Sudden onset of signs in horses may be associated with inappropriate amount in feed.

CLINICAL FEATURES

- Depression.
- Decreased appetite.
- Weight loss.

- Stiffness
- Painful flexor tendons.
- Cardiac murmur.
- Tachycardia.
- Polyuria.
- Hyposthenuria.

 DIFFERENTIAL DIAGNOSIS

- Exposure to cholecalciferol in feed.
- Exposure to vitamin D-containing plants.
- Ethylene glycol.
- Exposure to soluble calcium oxalates.
- Paraneoplastic syndromes.
- Primary hyperparathyroidism.
- Chronic renal failure.
- Hypoadrenocorticism.

 DIAGNOSTICS

CBC/Serum Chemistry/Urinalysis

- Toxicity should be considered with increases in serum calcium and phosphorus. However, acute exposure may not result in immediate hypercalcemia.
- Hyposthenuria and changes in BUN can be noted subsequent to toxicity.

Other Diagnostic Tests

- Measure serum 25-hydroxycholecalciferol (normal 2 ng/mL) for confirmation of exposure (rarely done in veterinary medicine).
- Feed analysis may show a high concentration of cholecalciferol.

Pathological Findings

- May be very wide variation from horse to horse depending on specific product, dose ingested, and time until necropsy performed.
- Gross:
  - Mineralization of the pulmonary valves, the left atrium, leaflets of the AV valve, the left ventricular endocardium, and portions of the aortic and pulmonary artery semilunar valves.
  - Vascular lesions can be seen in, but are not limited to, the cranial thoracic portion of the aorta as well as the trunk and bifurcated pulmonary artery.
  - Mineralization of the peritoneal surface of the diaphragm.
- Histopathology:
  - Kidneys may contain granular, laminated, or large fragmented mineral deposits and sloughed epithelial cells in some distal tubules and collecting ducts.
  - Deposits in the interstitium of the medulla.

- Mineralization of the lamina propria of inner half of the glandular mucosa of the stomach.
- Mineralization of the stroma of the submucosal glands and arterioles of the duodenum, stroma of the tubuloacinar glands of the soft palate, parotid salivary gland, dura mater, and subserosal elastic and collagen fibers of the diaphragm.

THERAPEUTICS

Detoxification

- Activated charcoal 1–3 g/kg as a warm water slurry via NG tube.
- Cathartic – magnesium sulfate 250–500 mg/kg in 2–4 L warm water.

Appropriate Health Care

- Some horses may do well with at home care and daily monitoring of calcium and phosphorous.
- Some will require hospitalization and treatment.
- IV 0.9% NaCl 1.5–2× maintenance rate.
- Monitor calcium and phosphorous daily.
- If no response to IV fluids, consider the use of a bisphosphonate drug.
- If serum calcium or ionized calcium remains elevated, add in furosemide
- Corticosteroids are added to horses non-responsive to other treatments.
- Low-calcium diet

Antidotes

- No known true antidote.
- Many consider a bisphosphonate as an antidote:
  - Clodronate and tiludronate, equine bisphosphonate drugs, are *not* approved for use in cholecalciferol overdoses. Anecdotally, clodronate has been successfully used off-label.
  - Pamidronate is the bisphosphonate of choice in small animal medicine.

Drugs of Choice

- Furosemide – 0.5–2 mg/kg PO or IV q8–12h prn.
- Corticosteroids:
  - Prednisolone – 0.5–2 mg/kg PO q24h.
  - Dexamethasone – 2.5–10 mg (total dose) IV, IM, PO q24h.
- GI protectants:
  - Omeprazole – 4 mg/kg PO q24h.
  - Sucralfate – 20 mg/kg PO q6h.
  - Ranitidine – 6.6–10 mg/kg PO q8h.

Precautions/Interactions

- Furosemide should be administered only after fluid deficits are corrected.
- Corticosteroids should be used very cautiously in horses due to risk of laminitis.
- Use of bisphosphonates as anti-hypercalcemic agent for treatment of cholecalciferol toxicosis is anecdotal in horses.

COMMENTS

Prevention/Avoidance
- Place rodenticide away from barn/pasture and do *not* put them in horse stalls or arenas.
- Monitor vitamin D supplementation in feed.

Expected Course and Prognosis
- Outcome depends on the length of and severity of hypercalcemia.
- The full course of treatment may take from 1 week to several weeks.

Abbreviations
See Appendix 1 for a complete list.

Suggested Reading
Green TG. Hypercalcemia. In: Chew DJC, ed. Small Animal Critical Care Medicine. St Louis, MO: Saunders Elsevier, 2009; pp. 234–238.

Harrington DDH, Page EHP. Acute vitamin D3 toxicosis in horses: Case reports and experimental studies of the comparative toxicity of vitamins D2 and D3. J Am Vet Med Assoc 1983; 182(12):1358–1369.

Jankovsky JM, Newman SJN. Pathology in practice. J Am Vet Assoc 2017; 251(5):531–534.

Rumbeiha WKR. Cholecalciferol. In: Talcott P, Peterson M, eds. Small Animal Toxicology, 3rd edn. St Louis, MC: Elsevier, 2013; pp 489–498.

Author: Dijana Katan, DVM, MPH, DABT
Consulting Editor: Lynn R. Hovda, RPh, DVM, MS, DACVIM

Chapter 76

Phosphides

DEFINITION/OVERVIEW

- Phosphides (zinc, aluminum, magnesium) are rodenticides and grain fumigants that produce phosphine gas when exposed to moisture or acidic environments.
- The gas produced is directly corrosive and rapidly absorbed, causing acute severe GI effects, cardiovascular collapse, pulmonary edema, metabolic acidosis, methemoglobinemia, wide-ranging CNS signs and a hepatic encephalopathy type syndrome.
- Inhalation of phosphine gas may affect barn personnel and veterinary professionals. Nasogastric tubes should only be passed in a very well-ventilated area.

ETIOLOGY/PATHOPHYSIOLOGY

- Phosphides (zinc, aluminum, magnesium) are used as rodenticides and grain fumigants.
  - Horses are most likely to be exposed to treated grain by gaining access to feed storage or accidental feeding.
  - Phosphide rodenticides are typically used underground for management of moles, voles, and gophers. These products come in a variety of formulations and, if used without following label directions, ingestion is possible.
- Initial signs include sweating, ataxia, tachycardia, tachypnea, and fever. Signs progress to muscle fasciculations, hypermetria, tremors, and seizures.
  - Suspicion should be strong if multiple horses in a facility develop clinical signs within hours of one another, as well as horses that may have broken into feed storage areas and non-stall areas of a barn. This should prompt investigation into changes in feed, water sources, and environment.

Mechanism of Action

- Phosphine gas is produced when exposed to moisture. Acidic environments increase gas production.
- The gas is directly corrosive to gastric mucosa and rapidly systemically absorbed. Inhalation exposure is more likely to affect animal owners and veterinary professional staff.

Blackwell's Five-Minute Veterinary Consult Clinical Companion: Equine Toxicology, First Edition. Edited by Lynn R. Hovda, Dionne Benson, and Robert H. Poppenga.
© 2022 John Wiley & Sons, Inc. Published 2022 by John Wiley & Sons, Inc.
Companion website: www.wiley.com/go/hovda/equine

Toxicokinetics

- Poorly understood pharmacokinetic process.
- Rapid onset of systemic signs supports the idea that GI absorption is rapid.

Toxicity

- There is not an established toxic dose in horses.
- Extrapolation from known species and clinical experience indicates signs are possible at 20–40 mg/kg.

Systems Affected

- Cardiovascular – tachycardia, myocardial damage, vascular congestion.
- Endocrine/metabolic – metabolic acidosis.
- Hemic/lymphatic/immune – hyperlactatemia, methemoglobinemia.
- Gastrointestinal – pain, ulceration, anorexia, ileus.
- Hepatobiliary – encephalopathic signs, elevations in hepatic enzymes.
- Nervous – ataxia, hypermetric gait, seizures.
- Neuromuscular – muscle fasciculations.
- Renal/urologic – azotemia, acute renal failure.
- Respiratory – tachypnea, pulmonary edema, pulmonary effusion.

SIGNALMENT/HISTORY

- No know sex or breed predisposition exists.
- Barns and boarding facilities that fumigate large grain stores may put horses at increased risk if caretakers are not well educated on feed withholding times after treatment of stored grain.

Risk Factors

- Lower gastric pH which occurs after feeding increases production of phosphine gas.

Historical Findings

- Recently fumigated feed stores.
- Gaining access to storage areas where rodenticides are stored.
- Owner or care manager suspects and reports colic in multiple horses over an acute period.

Location and Circumstances of Poisoning

- Equine boarding or housing facilities.
- Barns and storage areas.

CLINICAL FEATURES

- Tachycardia, tachypnea, dyspnea.
- Hyperthermia.
- Ataxia.
- Fish or rotten odor breath.

- Cyanotic or brown mucous membranes.
- Muscle fasciculations.
- Looking at or kicking abdomen, rolling.
- Profuse sweating, tremor, seizures.
- Increased bronchovesicular sounds or crackles.
- Stilted gait, dilated pupils.
- Altered mentation.

DIFFERENTIAL DIAGNOSIS

- Colic.
- EEE, WEE, VEE.
- EPM.
- Grain overload.
- Heat stress.
- Hypocalcemic tetany.
- Other toxicants:
  - Compound 1080 (fluoroacetate).
  - Blue-green algae (cyanobacteria).
  - Carbamates.
  - Heavy metals.
  - Metaldehyde.
  - Tremorgenic mycotoxins.
  - Organochloride insecticides.
  - Organophosphates.
  - Strychnine.
- Rabies.
- Trauma.

DIAGNOSTICS

CBC/Serum Chemistry/Urinalysis

- Blood gas analysis – metabolic acidosis.
- Blood glucose – hypoglycemia.
- Variety of other abnormalities specific to each horse.

Pathological Findings

- Widespread petechia and ecchymosis of all major organs.
- Possible vascular congestion and pulmonary edema.

THERAPEUTICS

- The goal of therapy is to neutralize the off gassing of the phosphides, gastric lavage as soon as possible, begin shock fluid support, and transport to a facility able to provide round the clock care.

- Management will include pain control, management of CNS signs, fluid adjustments to correct acidosis and hypoglycemia, and ongoing gastrointestinal support.

Detoxification

- Liquid antacid to raise gastric pH which reduces release of phosphine gas.
- Early gastric lavage with a large-bore stomach tube in a very well-ventilated area.
- AC 1–3 g/kg in a water slurry × 1 dose.
- Smectite di-tri-octahedral (DTO) smectite if activated charcoal unavailable.

Appropriate Health Care

- Health care requires a multi-modal approach with patient(s) transported to a facility in which 24-hour care is available.
- Early decontamination is critical.
- Oxygen support for hypoxemia.
- Crystalloid IVF support with 2.5–5% dextrose in fluids.
- Therapies may include bicarbonate, methocarbamol, anticonvulsants, proton pump inhibitors, antioxidants, hepatic support, and frequent laboratory monitoring.
- Leg wraps and bell boots to mitigate self-trauma if rolling or actively seizing.

Antidotes

- None available.

Drugs of Choice

- Liquid antacid to raise gastric pH:
    - Aluminum hydroxide, 17–30 g per adult horse.
    - Magnesium hydroxide, 15 g per adult horse.
    - Oral 5% sodium bicarbonate, 10–12 g per adult horse.
- Sodium bicarbonate to correct severe acidosis.
- Gastroprotectants:
    - Omeprazole 4 mg/kg PO q24h.
    - Pantoprazole 1 mg/kg IV or IG via NG tube q24h.
    - Misoprostol 5 µg/kg PO q8h.
- Seizure control:
    - Phenobarbital 16–20 mg/kg IV diluted in 0.9% saline.
    - Diazepam 0.02–0.4 mg/kg IV (foal); 25–50 mg (adult).
    - Midazolam 0.02–0.4 mg/kg IV.
- Tremor control:
    - Methocarbamol 4.4–22.2 mg/kg IV; up to 330 mg/kg/day.
- Analgesia:
    - Flunixin 1.1 mg/kg IV or PO q12–24h.
    - Hyoscine N-butylbromide (Buscopan) 0.3 mg/kg slow IV q24hr.

Precautions/Interactions

- Gastric lavage should be performed in a very well-ventilated area after administration of a liquid antacid. The phosphine gas presents a significant respiratory exposure risk to humans.

- Remove any access to feedstuffs as digestive enzymes associated with feeding facilitate phosphine gas production.

COMMENTS

Prognosis is guarded to poor if seizures and metabolic imbalance cannot be controlled. All exposures should be treated early and aggressively.

Patient Monitoring

- Frequent monitoring of vital signs, pulses, abdominal and thoracic auscultation.
- Serum lactate, acid–base status, electrolytes, and glucose q8–12h.
- Serum chemistry – monitor liver and kidney values q24h.

Prevention/Avoidance

- Use only certified pest control operators.
- Adhere to all label directions and withdraw times for fumigated feeds
- Have a redundancy plan to ensure all animal caretakers are aware of any stored feed that has been treated with a phosphide.
- Avoid storage of treated grain and rodenticides in tack or feed rooms.

Possible Complications

- These patients are best managed in a hospital setting which is not always feasible for some horse owners.
- Managing down animal in status epilepticus.
- Development of laminitis after successful treatment.

Expected Course and Prognosis

- Prognosis is guarded to poor once clinical signs develop.
- Patients can rapidly deteriorate due to severe metabolic acidosis, gastric mucosal hemorrhage, hepatic encephalopathy-like signs, tremors, and seizures.

Abbreviations

See Appendix 1 for a complete list.

Suggested Reading

Clark, CK, Merritt, AM, Burrow JA, et al: Effect of aluminum hydroxide/magnesium hydroxide antacid and bismuth subsalicylate on gastric pH in horses. J Am Vet Med Assoc 1996; 208(10):1687–1691,

Easterwood L, Chaffin MK, Marsh PS, et al. Phosphine intoxication following oral exposure of horses to aluminum phosphide-treated feed. J Am Vet Med Assoc 2010; 236(4):446–450.

Gray SL. In: Hovda L, Brutlag A, Poppenga R, Peterson K, eds. Blackwell's Five-Minute Veterinary Consult – Small Animal Toxicology, 2nd edn. Ames, IA: Wiley-Blackwell, 2016; pp. 862–870.

Author: Tabatha Regehr, DVM
Consulting Editor: Lynn R. Hovda, RPH, DVM, MS, DACVIM

Chapter 77

Sodium Fluoroacetate (Compound 1080)

DEFINITION/OVERVIEW

- Compound 1080, a commercially produced form of sodium fluoroacetate, is a pesticide used for controlling rodents and predators.
- Its use began in the United States in the 1940s, but significant limitations were placed on its use in the 1970s due to safety concerns. Compound 1080 is categorized as a toxicity category I, indicating the highest level of toxicity.
- Due to its narrow margin of safety in humans and non-target species, Compound 1080's use as a rodenticide was cancelled by the EPA in 1989.
- It is currently allowed in the United States as a restricted-use pesticide for the control of coyotes and supplied as a livestock protection collar. These collars are placed on the neck of sheep or goats and are intended to poison coyotes that may puncture a collar while attacking livestock.
- Compound 1080 is also used in Australia, New Zealand and other countries around the world.
- Naturally occurring sodium fluoroacetate is present in numerous plants. The most common regions for these plants are Africa, Australia and South America; however, they can be found worldwide.
  - Most sodium fluoroacetate is present in low concentrations within plants.
  - However, certain plants, including those in the *Dichapetalum* genus, can contain large concentrations, with reports of seeds containing up to 8,000 mg/kg sodium fluoroacetate.
  - Australia is home to approximately 40 species of sodium fluoroacetate containing plants.

ETIOLOGY/PATHOPHYSIOLOGY

Mechanism of Action

- Compound 1080 blocks the tricarboxylic acid (TCA) cycle. This results in reduced cellular energy production as well as cellular oxidative metabolism.
- The reduced function of the TCA cycle and reduced cellular oxidative metabolism causes a build-up of citric and lactic acid, leading to lactic acidosis and hypocalcemia.
- There is also a decreased production of acetylcholine and other intermediates that are necessary for proper neurologic function.

Blackwell's Five-Minute Veterinary Consult Clinical Companion: Equine Toxicology, First Edition. Edited by Lynn R. Hovda, Dionne Benson, and Robert H. Poppenga.
© 2022 John Wiley & Sons, Inc. Published 2022 by John Wiley & Sons, Inc.
Companion website: www.wiley.com/go/hovda/equine

Toxicokinetics

- Compound 1080 is absorbed by inhalation and ingestion. Absorption through intact skin is poor, but absorption through cuts or wounds can occur.
- It is well absorbed in the stomach after ingestion or the lungs after inhalation.
- Compound 1080 is distributed to soft tissues and organs, with the brain and heart being the most severely affected organs.
- It is metabolized in the liver and excreted in the urine.

Toxicity

- Horses, along with other mammals, are considered to be highly susceptible to Compound 1080 poisoning. By contrast, birds are considered fairly resistant.
- The LD_{50} in horses has been reported between 0.35 and 1.0 mg/kg body weight.
- The onset of signs is expected within 30 minutes to 4 hours.

Systems Affected

- Cardiovascular – tachycardia, myocardial depression, ventricular arrhythmias, ventricular fibrillation, sudden death due to cardiac failure.
- Neurologic – agitation, disorientation, coma.
- Endocrine/metabolic – lactic acidosis, hypocalcemia, hyperglycemia.
- Gastrointestinal – bruxism, colic.
- Ophthalmic – apparent blindness.
- Neuromuscular – ataxia, weakness, recumbency.

SIGNALMENT/HISTORY

- There are no breed, age or sex predilections.

Risk Factors

- Any animal that has been exposed to Compound 1080 is at risk for toxicity, particularly after ingestion.

Historical Findings

- Signs most frequently noted by owners include ataxia, weakness, recumbency and sudden death.

Location and Circumstances of Poisoning

- Horses that are in the same area in which livestock protection collars are used may be exposed if the product is left out in an open area with access by the animal.

CLINICAL FEATURES

- Horses may show ataxia, be unable to stand, profuse sweating with signs of colic and tachycardia with an irregular rhythm on examination.

- Common clinical signs include:
  - Agitation, disorientation, weakness, ataxia, recumbency.
  - Coma.
  - Bruxism, sweating, signs of colic.
  - Tachycardia.
  - Apparent blindness.

DIFFERENTIAL DIAGNOSIS

- Differentials may include, but are not limited to, conditions associated with neurologic or cardiovascular abnormalities:
  - Strychnine poisoning.
  - Mycotoxin poisoning.
  - Ionophore poisoning.
  - Cardiac glycoside containing plants poisoning:
    - *Taxus* spp.
    - *Nerium* sp.
  - Sodium fluoroacetate containing plants poisoning:
    - *Dichapetalum* spp.
    - *Palicourea margravii.*
    - *Amorimia rigida.*
    - *Gastrolobium* spp.
  - Lead poisoning.
  - Chlorinated hydrocarbon poisoning.
  - Intestinal torsion/impaction.

DIAGNOSTICS

CBC/Serum Chemistry/Urinalysis

- Calcium or ionized calcium.
- Blood glucose.
- Blood gas analysis.

Other Diagnostic Tests

- Stomach contents or suspected bait analysis – GC-MS.

Pathological Findings

- Gross findings:
  - Hydropericardium – pale yellow pericardial fluid.
  - Epicardial hemorrhage – moderate to severe ecchymotic and suffusive hemorrhages.
  - Heart may be flaccid and pale.
  - Hydrothorax.
  - Ascites.

- Histopathologic findings:
  - Myocardial degeneration and necrosis.
  - Suppurative interstitial myocarditis.
  - Perivascular interstitial edema and mixed inflammatory infiltrates of neutrophils and macrophages.
  - Epicardial hemorrhage.
  - Fragmentation of individual and small clusters of myofibers with contraction bands and/or mild vacuolation.
  - Pulmonary edema and congestion.

THERAPEUTICS

Detoxification

- Decontamination with AC (1–3 g/kg in a water slurry) and a cathartic (magnesium sulfate 250–500 mg/kg in 2–4 L of water) may be of benefit in an acute case and initiated prior to onset of signs.

Appropriate Health Care

- Treatment consists of symptomatic and supportive care if the exposure is detected shortly after exposure. Most animals die rapidly before any therapy can be initiated.
- Continuous ECG monitoring for changes in cardiac rhythm will help to determine response to therapy.
- IV fluids; correct acidosis.
- Blood gas monitoring until lactic acidosis resolves.
- Serum calcium (iCa preferred) monitoring until hypocalcemia and/or cardiac signs resolve.
- Improvement in neurologic signs will help to determine likelihood of survival.

Antidotes

- There is no antidote.

Drugs of Choice

- Lidocaine for ventricular arrhythmias:
  - Lidocaine 0.25–0.5 mg/kg IV slowly, repeat in 5–10 minutes if needed.
- Anticonvulsants if seizures occur:
  - Diazepam 25–50 mg IV (adults); 0.1–0.4 mg/kg IV (foals).
  - Phenobarbital 16–20 mg/kg IV × 1 dose.
- Skeletal muscle relaxants:
  - Methocarbamol 4.4–22 mg/kg IV (moderate signs); 22–55 mg/kg IV (severe signs).
- Calcium gluconate 0.2–0.5 mL/kg IV (5% solution) given slowly to treat hypocalcemia.

Precautions/Interactions

- Use of sodium bicarbonate may improve survival; however, it may also contribute to hypocalcemia and hypokalemia. If used, monitoring of calcium and potassium levels is recommended.

COMMENTS

Client Education

- Given the very narrow margin of safety and high likelihood of fatality, it is important to educate owners on the importance of keeping horses away from any possible source of Compound 1080.

Prevention/Avoidance

- Horses should not be allowed access to area where Compound 1080 is stored or used.

Possible Complications

- Most animals will succumb to poisoning and not recover.

Expected Course and Prognosis

- Prognosis is poor to grave, even in animals with early intervention.
- Once signs develop, recovery is not expected.

Abbreviations

See Appendix 1 for a complete list.

Suggested Reading

Adaska, JH, Rimoldi G, et al. Multiple episodes of 1080 (sodium monofluoroacetate) intoxication in a California calf-raising operation. J Vet Diagn Invest 2018; 30(5):747–751.

Dalefield R. Vertebrate pesticides. In: Dalefield R, ed. Veterinary Toxicology for Australia and New Zealand. Masterton: Elsevier, 2017.

Gupta, RC. Non-anticoagulant rodenticides. In: Gupta RC, ed. Veterinary Toxicology, 3rd edn. San Diego: Elsevier 2018; pp. 619–621.

Leong, LE, Khan S, Davis CK, Denman SE, McSweeney CS. Fluoroacetate in plants – a review of its distribution, toxicity to livestock and microbial detoxification. J Anim Sci Biotechnol 2017; 8:55.

Author: Renee Schmid, DVM, DABT, DABVT
Consulting Editor: Lynn R. Hovda, RPh, DVM, MS, DACVIM

Chapter 78

Strychnine

DEFINITION/OVERVIEW

- Strychnine is an indole alkaloid derived from the *Strychnos nux-vomica* tree, particularly the seeds and bark, found in southern Asia and Australia.
- Most commonly known as an active ingredient in pesticide/rodenticide bait, its plant origins were first discovered in 1818.
- Strychnine was first registered as a pesticide in the United States in 1947, although its use occurred for many years prior to this time.
- Currently, strychnine is classified as restricted use by the EPA and only below-ground application as bait to control gophers is allowed.
- As specific medicinal use in horses, strychnine has been given as a SC and IM injection for symptomatic treatment of locomotor deficits of medullary origin.
- In addition to accidental ingestion, exposure as a result of malicious intent is a known concern in veterinary medicine.
- Common signs include muscle rigidity, seizures, and hyperthermia.
- Strychnine has a very narrow margin of safety in the equine patient and fatalities are common.

ETIOLOGY/PATHOPHYSIOLOGY

Mechanism of Action

- Strychnine inhibits glycine, an inhibitory neurotransmitter, by competitive antagonism.
- This results in an increased reflex excitability in the spinal cord, leading to CNS excitation, muscle rigidity, tonic-clonic seizures and respiratory paralysis.

Toxicokinetics

- Strychnine is rapidly absorbed from injection, exposure to mucous membranes of the eyes and mouth, inhalation and ingestion.
- Most strychnine exposures occur by ingestion.
- The majority of absorption takes place in the small intestine after ingestion.

Blackwell's Five-Minute Veterinary Consult Clinical Companion: Equine Toxicology, First Edition. Edited by Lynn R. Hovda, Dionne Benson, and Robert H. Poppenga. © 2022 John Wiley & Sons, Inc. Published 2022 by John Wiley & Sons, Inc. Companion website: www.wiley.com/go/hovda/equine

- Strychnine has wide tissue distribution and low protein binding. The highest concentrations of strychnine are found in the liver, with low levels of strychnine present in the blood and kidney.
- Metabolism takes place in the liver, and elimination is through urine and feces.
- Up to 20% of strychnine is excreted unchanged in the urine and most elimination is complete within 24–48 hours.

Toxicity

- Strychnine has a very narrow margin of safety in mammals, birds, and fish.
- Signs of toxicity may be seen within 10 minutes to 2 hours after exposure.
- The lethal dose for horses is 0.5 mg/kg. Fatalities due to respiratory arrest are common.

Systems Affected

- Musculoskeletal – muscle rigidity, lactic acidosis, contraction of voluntary muscles.
- Neurologic – apprehension, hyperthermia, seizures.
- Respiratory – respiratory paralysis/arrest.
- Gastrointestinal – hypersalivation due to bitter taste.

SIGNALMENT/HISTORY

- There are no specific breed or sex predilections.

Risk Factors

- Horses housed near or allowed access to areas where bait is used or stored are at risk of potential poisoning.
- Horses treated with injectable strychnine formulations by untrained caregivers may inadvertently cause a therapeutic error.

Historical Findings

- Signs and observations are often reported by the owner.
- An owner or handler may find the animal more responsive to sound or stimuli, seizing and in respiratory distress.
- Finding a deceased animal is also common due to the rapid progression of poisoning.

Location and Circumstances of Poisoning

- Horses allowed access to areas where bait is stored is the most common cause of poisoning.
- Ingestion of bait-laced material due to malicious intent may also occur.

CLINICAL FEATURES

- Hyperesthesia, apprehension.
- Hyperthermia, sweating.
- Hypersalivation.
- Stiff/stilted gait.

- Seizures.
- Respiratory distress, shallow breathing.
- Development of lactic acidosis.

DIFFERENTIAL DIAGNOSIS

- Tremorgenic mycotoxin – Penitrem A and roquefortine poisoning.
- Head trauma
- Meningitis, EEE, WEE, WNV.
- Cerebral abscess, vascular event.
- Rabies.
- Other rodenticides - Compound 1080, bromethalin poisoning, phosphides.
- Cyanobacteria poisoning.
- Nitrite poisoning.
- Metaldehyde poisoning.
- *Cicuta maculata* poisoning.
- *Asclepius* spp. poisoning.
- Organophosphate/carbamate poisoning.

DIAGNOSTICS

CBC/Serum Chemistry/Urinalysis

- Elevated CK.
- Myoglobinuria.
- Blood gas analysis – lactic acidosis.

Other Diagnostic Tests

- Identification of bait in stomach contents.
- Chemical analysis of stomach contents, liver, kidney, blood, urine with GC-MS.

Pathological Findings

- Gross findings:
    - Bait in the stomach.
    - Pulmonary edema, cyanosis, possible myocardial hemorrhage, myoglobinuria, rapid rigor mortis.
- Histopathologic findings – no specific findings.

THERAPEUTICS

Detoxification

- AC (1–3 g/kg in a watery slurry) and a cathartic (magnesium sulfate 250–500 mg/kg in 2–4 L of water) can be used successfully in asymptomatic horses to minimize absorption of strychnine.

Appropriate Health Care

- Hospitalize; keep in a dark, quiet stall and avoid stimulation.
- Aggressive care is necessary early after exposure, as signs progress rapidly and fatalities are common.
- Control tremor and seizure activity.
- Oxygenation and respiratory rate/rhythm should be closely monitored for evidence of respiratory distress.
- Provide ventilation support if respiratory arrest occurs.
- IV fluids as needed.
- Correct lactic acidosis if present. Monitoring blood gas for resolution of lactic acidosis in animals that survive the first few hours should be performed as needed based on clinical response to therapy.

Antidote

- No specific antidote is available.

Drugs of Choice

- Anticonvulsants:
  - Diazepam 25–50 mg IV (adults); 0.1–0.4 mg/kg IV prn (foals).
  - Phenobarbital 16–20 mg/kg IV × 1 dose.
- Sedation/tremor control:
  - Detomidine 0.01–0.04 mg/kg IV.
  - Xylazine 1.1 mg/kg IV; 2.2 mg/kg IM.
  - Methocarbamol 4.4–22 mg/kg IV to effect (moderate condition); 22–55 mg/kg IV (severe condition). Do not exceed 330 mg/kg/day.
- Full anesthesia:
  - Pentobarbital, diazepam., and xylazine have been used in combination for full anesthesia with success.

Alternative Drugs

- Choosing standard anticonvulsants or anesthetic agents available to the treating veterinarian can be used.

COMMENTS

Client Education

- Due to the severity of clinical signs and likelihood of respiratory arrest, at-home care is not available.
- Animals may be very difficult to restrain, causing significant risk of harm to caregivers.

Prevention/Avoidance

- Prevent access by horse to storage areas where strychnine bait may be located.
- If injectable strychnine is used, an abundance of caution should be exercised to ensure that the appropriate dose is administered.

Possible Complications

- Fatalities are a common outcome, especially with horses where the exposure has not been witnessed and rapid intervention is not possible.

Expected Course and Prognosis

- The prognosis is poor with therapy and grave if medical intervention is not available.
- Recovery in symptomatic horses has been reported, although rare.

Abbreviations

See Appendix 1 for a complete list.

Suggested Reading

Gupta RC. Non-anticoagulant rodenticides. In: Gupta RC, ed. Veterinary Toxicology, 3rd edn. San Diego: Elsevier, 2018; pp. 633–635.

Khan SA. Overview of strychnine poisoning. In: Line S, ed. Merck Veterinary Manual, 11th edn. Kenilworth: Merck & Co., 2016.

Stoltenow CL, Mostrom M, Stoltenow LR, et al. Treatment of accidental strychnine poisoning in horses. J Eq Vet Sci 2002; 22:507–509.

Author: Renee Schmid, DVM, DABT, DABVT
Consulting Editor: Lynn R. Hovda, RPh, DVM, MS, DACVIM

Toxic Gases

Air Contaminants: CO, NH₃, H₂S

Chapter 79

DEFINITION/OVERVIEW

- Carbon monoxide (CO):
  - CO is an odorless, colorless, tasteless gas that is readily soluble in water.
    - Its solubility allows it to be easily absorbed in the upper respiratory tract of the horse.
    - Common sources include exhaust from motor vehicles and fuel-consuming space heaters within barns, generators and, less commonly, fires.
- Ammonia (NH_3):
  - NH_3 is a colorless gas that has a distinct, sharp, pungent smell.
    - It can be deodorized via reaction with sodium bicarbonate or acetic acid. This reaction forms ammonium salt.
  - It is commonly formed in areas of organic waste build-up (horse stalls, manure pits, etc).
- Hydrogen sulfide (H_2S):
  - H_2S is a colorless gas that has a characteristic "rotten egg smell".
  - It accumulates in wet manure pits and sewage ponds in areas with poor ventilation.

ETIOLOGY/PATHOPHYSIOLOGY

Mechanism of Action

- Carbon monoxide:
  - CO combines with hemoglobin to form carboxyhemoglobin.
  - It binds to the site that oxygen normally binds:
    - CO has 250 times the affinity for binding to hemoglobin when compared with oxygen.
    - Furthermore, CO can displace oxygen that is already bound to hemoglobin.
  - Carboxyhemoglobin also shifts the oxyhemoglobin saturation curve to the left which decreases the release of oxygen in peripheral tissues.
  - Organs with high oxygen demand are most profoundly affected:
    - Brain and heart.
- Ammonia:
  - NH_3 is readily absorbed by the tissues of the upper respiratory tract.

Blackwell's Five-Minute Veterinary Consult Clinical Companion: Equine Toxicology, First Edition. Edited by Lynn R. Hovda, Dionne Benson, and Robert H. Poppenga.
© 2022 John Wiley & Sons, Inc. Published 2022 by John Wiley & Sons, Inc.
Companion website: www.wiley.com/go/hovda/equine

- Here it causes mucosa damage and impairs ciliary activity:
  - This predisposes the horse to secondary infections within the upper respiratory tract and potentially lower respiratory tract infections (though this is relatively rare).
- Because it is highly water-soluble, ammonia is typically absorbed by the mucosal cells of the upper respiratory tract:
  - Here it damages the cilia of the tracheal mucosal cells, which impairs the protective mucociliary apparatus.
- Other poor environmental factors such as dust, fungal spores or poor-quality hay could act opportunistically to cause secondary infection.
- Hydrogen sulfide:
  - H_2S inactivates mitochondrial cytochrome oxidase which impairs cellular respiration.
  - H_2S also induces apoptosis of smooth muscle cells.

Toxicity

- Carbon monoxide:
  - Estimated concentrations by geographic location:
    - Rural areas – 0.02 ppm.
    - Urban areas – 13 ppm.
    - High traffic areas – 40 ppm.
- Ammonia:
  - Low concentrations (occasionally found in horse stables) cause hypersecretion of nasal discharge:
    - Range: 1–10 mg/m^3 (1.44–14.36 ppm).
  - Moderate concentrations cause significant irritation to the mucosa and dermal layer of the airways:
    - Range: 20–25 mg/m^3 (28.71–35.89 ppm).
  - High concentrations irritate the eyes in addition to respiratory mucosa:
    - > 70 mg/m^3 (100 ppm).
- Hydrogen sulfide:
  - The minimum concentration at which humans (and presumably animals) can smell H_2S is 0.025 ppm.
  - At moderate concentrations (50–150 ppm), H_2S causes olfactory fatigue and pulmonary edema.
  - At high concentrations (500–2000 ppm), H_2S severely impairs the respiratory system by paralyzing the muscles of respiration.
  - At concentrations > 500 ppm, severe, non-reversible neurologic damage occurs.

Systems Affected

- Carbon monoxide:
  - Respiratory – tachypnea, respiration with increased abdominal effort, increased lung sounds.
  - Nervous – altered mentation (ranging from confusion to obtundation), ataxia, blindness, deafness and seizures.
  - Cardiovascular – tachycardia, hypotension, brick-red mucus membranes.

- Ammonia:
  - Respiratory – irritation to upper airway mucosa causes dysfunction of and damage to cilia of the cells of the tracheal mucosa.
  - Ocular – at higher concentration, acts as an irritant, conjunctivitis.
  - Hematological – decreased PCV may be observed.
    - Suspected splenic sequestration.
- Hydrogen sulfide:
  - Respiratory – toxicity is dose-dependent.
    - High doses cause immediate respiratory paralysis.
  - Olfactory – even at low concentrations, olfactory fatigue is experienced.
  - Ocular – ocular pain, lacrimation and photophobia.
  - Nervous – nausea, ataxia, dizziness, convulsions.
  - Cardiovascular – arrythmias, hypotension (in situations of chronic, low-dose exposure).

SIGNALMENT/HISTORY

- No species, age or breed predilections exist.

Risk Factors

- Horses stalled in facilities with poor air flow, in stalls that are not regularly cleaned and horses who live in urban areas with high traffic flow are at an increased risk of exposure to air pollutants.

Historical Findings

- Knowledge of where a horse is stabled and the routine husbandry that occurs may provide clues to diagnosing a horse that has been clinically affected by inhalation of a toxic gas.

Location and Circumstances of Poisoning

- Carbon monoxide:
- CO formed from the partial oxidation of carbon-containing compounds.
  - Often associated with exhaust from car engines or generators or space heaters located in poorly ventilated areas.
- Ammonia:
  - Different bedding types have varying abilities to absorb urine (water-binding ability) and produce ammonia.
  - Straw pellets absorb the most water, followed by wheat straw and then wood shavings.
  - One experiment showed that over a 14-day time period, wheat straw contained the highest concentration of ammonia compared with other bedding types:
    - Wheat straw (178 mg/m^3).
    - Wood shavings (155.2 mg/m^3).
    - Straw pellets (60.3 mg/m^3).
  - An accidental spill of ammonia (commonly used to supplement nitrogen for crops) may result in extremely high exposure concentrations.

- Hydrogen sulfide:
  - H$_2$S is often released after the disturbance of a manure pit.
  - Because H$_2$S is highly water-soluble, it is often not emitted from manure pits or sewage ponds until the contents are mixed.

CLINICAL FEATURES

- Carbon monoxide:
  - Because CO displaces oxygen from hemoglobin and decreases delivery of oxygen to peripheral tissues, the following clinical signs of desaturation may be observed:
    - Brick-red mucus membranes.
    - Increased respiratory effort and rate.
    - Increased lung sounds.
    - Tachycardia.
  - Horses may also display neurologic signs, including ataxia, blindness and seizures in severe cases.
- Ammonia:
  - At lower concentrations, mild-to-moderate nasal discharge is seen
  - At moderate concentrations, ocular discharge is seen in addition to nasal discharge
    - No significant changes in vital parameters are observed.
  - Horses who have had longer-term exposure are at risk of developing secondary infections.
    - These horses may cough and/or be tachypneic.
- Hydrogen sulfide:
  - H$_2$S impairs or paralyzes the respiratory system quickly:
    - Exposure to very high concentrations can result in collapse and rapid death secondary to respiratory failure.
    - Exposure to lower doses will cause CNS stimulation, ataxia, tremors, irritation of the epidermis and eyes and tachypnea.
    - Animals experiencing long-term low-dose exposure can also present with a cough, bronchitis, bronchial hemorrhage, or pulmonary edema.
    - Additional clinical signs include hypotension, weight loss, and behavioral changes.

DIFFERENTIAL DIAGNOSIS

- Primary respiratory disease – pneumonia, heaves, pulmonary edema.
- Primary CNS disease – infectious (encephalitis), metabolic.
- Primary hepatic disease – hepatic encephalopathy (in cases of hyperammonemia).
- Other toxins.

DIAGNOSTICS

CBC/Serum Chemistry/Urinalysis

- A complete blood count, serum chemistry panel and urinalysis should be completed to evaluate organ function.

Other Diagnostic Tests

- Carbon monoxide:
    - Ideally, blood COHb should be measured at presentation and checked every 24 hours. Elevated COHb is diagnostic of CO intoxication.
    - Clinical signs are dose-dependent:
        - < 1% COHb is considered normal.
        - At lower percentages, ataxia, confusion and mild-to-moderate respiratory signs are observed.
        - 40–50% causes acute respiratory failure.
        - > 60% is fatal.
    - Serial arterial blood gas analysis may be helpful to analyze PaO_2 concentrations.

Imaging

- Thoracic radiographs and/or computed tomography may be helpful in determining if pulmonary edema or bronchiolitis is present.

THERAPEUTICS

Detoxification

- Removal of the horse from the area containing toxic gas is the first and most important step. The horse should be moved to an area with good, fresh air circulation.

Appropriate Health Care

- If soiled bedding is the source of ammonia or H_2S, complete removal of the soiled bedding and replacement with clean, dry bedding is recommended.
- Supplementation with 100% oxygen may be required.
- In severe cases, hyperbaric oxygen therapy can be considered.
- Activity:
    - These patients should have their activity restricted until recovery.
    - Affected horses should be kept in an area where they will not be subject to stressful situations.

COMMENTS

Patient Monitoring

- Placement of pulse oximetry may or may not be helpful to monitor oxygen saturation:
    - The user should be aware that most pulse oximeter devices with two wavelengths of light may be inaccurate in patients with severe COHb concentrations.
    - Pulse oximeters with eight wavelengths of light are much more accurate when monitoring these horses with high concentrations of COHb.
- Arterial blood samples can also be taken to monitor PaO_2.
- Serial neurologic examinations should be performed.

Prevention/Avoidance

- Stalls should be routinely cleaned, and bedding kept dry.
- If heaters or other machinery that burns fuel are used inside a barn, adequate air flow is essential for removal of toxic gases produced by these devices.

Possible Complications

- Permanent neurologic, pulmonary and/or ocular damage may occur.

Expected Course and Prognosis

- Prognosis is dose-dependent.
- Dependent on COHb concentration and the degree of hypoxic brain damage
- Pulmonary function should be monitored for 2–6 weeks following removal from the toxic environment.

Abbreviations

See Appendix 1 for a complete list.

Suggested Reading

Cope R. Toxic gases and vapors. In: Gupta RC, ed. Veterinary Toxicology: Basic and Clinical Principles, 3rd edn. London: Elsevier, 2018; pp 629–645.

Davis MS, Foster WM. Inhalation toxicology in the equine respiratory tract. In: Lekeux P, ed. Equine Respiratory Diseases. International Veterinary Information Service, 2013.

Fleming K, Hessel EF, Van den Weghe HFA. Evaluation of factors influencing the generation of ammonia in different bedding materials used for horse keeping. J Eq Vet Sci 2008; 28(4):223–231.

Katayama Y, Oikawa Yoshihara T, Kuwano A, Hobo S. Clinico-pathological effects of atmospheric ammonia exposure on horses. J Eq Vet Sci 1995; 6(3):99–104.

Van der Merwe D. Respiratory toxicity. In: Gupta RC, ed. Veterinary Toxicology Basic and Clinical Principles, 3rd edn. London: Elsevier, 2018; pp. 215–226.

Author: Sarah Jacosinski, DVM
Consulting Editor: Lynn R. Hovda, RPh, DVM, MS, DACVIM

Smoke

Chapter 80

DEFINITION/OVERVIEW

- Smoke is a mixture of hot air, solid particulates, gases, fumes, and vapors.
- Smoke composition depends on burning material(s) and fire environment.
- Structural fires and wildfires present different hazards.

ETIOLOGY/PATHOPHYSIOLOGY

Mechanism of Action

- Primary injury mechanisms include direct thermal injury, injury from chemical irritants, injury from toxic gases – carbon monoxide, hydrogen cyanide, and hydrogen sulfide.
  - Heat/flame thermal injury denatures proteins, leading to edema in the upper respiratory tract (URT).
  - Thermal injury also damages cilia, compromising the mucociliary clearance.
  - Thermal burns to the skin are not covered in this book but require attention.
- Chemical burns are caused by irritants in the smoke.
- Carbon monoxide, hydrogen cyanide, and hydrogen sulfide are common asphyxiants:
  - Asphyxiants interfere with tissue oxygenation, leading to hypoxia.
  - Hemoglobin has 200–250× higher affinity for carbon monoxide than oxygen.
  - Cyanide and hydrogen sulfide inhibit cytochrome c oxidase in mitochondria.
  - Water-soluble irritants such as ammonia cause irritation in the URT, leading to epithelial necrosis and edema.
  - Particulates ≤ 5μm cause lung or respiratory tract injury depending on size; particulates ≤ 2.5μm reach lower respiratory tract and alveoli.

Toxicokinetics

- Smoke is a complex mixture of solid particulates, gases, fumes, and vapors, each with unique toxicokinetic properties.

Toxicity

- Acute smoke-inhalation toxicity manifests as an early phase (within 24 hours), intermediate phase (12 hours to 5 days), and late phase (> 5–7 days):

Blackwell's Five-Minute Veterinary Consult Clinical Companion: Equine Toxicology,
First Edition. Edited by Lynn R. Hovda, Dionne Benson, and Robert H. Poppenga.
© 2022 John Wiley & Sons, Inc. Published 2022 by John Wiley & Sons, Inc.
Companion website: www.wiley.com/go/hovda/equine

- Clinical signs of early phase are caused mainly by carbon monoxide and hydrogen cyanide (asphyxiation) gases and by thermal injury to URT.
- Clinical signs of the intermediate phase are caused by pulmonary edema and systemic inflammatory response from thermal and irritant injury.
- Late-phase signs are caused by bronchopneumonia; impaired mucociliary clearance and alveolar macrophage function predispose patients to Gram-negative bacterial infection.
- Post-hypoxic leukoencephalopathy characterized by laminar cortical necrosis and reactive gliosis caused by apoptotic die-off triggered by carbon monoxide is a delayed effect of smoke inhalation.

■ Chronic smoke inhalation may occur following wildfires and may result in weeks of exposure.

Systems Affected

■ Multiple systems are affected, including skin, ocular, respiratory, cardiovascular, nervous, and renal systems.
■ Extent of injury depends on types of burning materials, whether in open or closed space, and duration of exposure.

SIGNALMENT/HISTORY

Risk Factors

■ Fires in confined/enclosed spaces are associated with higher risks of asphyxiation.
■ Proximity to the burning fire; close proximity associated with both thermal injury plus smoke.
■ Wild bush fire smoke carries risk of particulate matter exposure.
■ Pre-existing conditions such as asthma, chronic obstructive pulmonary disease, and cardiovascular, CNS, or renal disease increase the risk of a severe outcome.

Historical Findings

■ Smoke inhalation is associated with a history of fire outbreak.

Location and Circumstances of Poisoning

■ Enclosed structural (e.g., barn) fires are associated with widespread systemic injury because of asphyxiation from carbon monoxide.
■ Plastic, wool, cushion fires in enclosed places generate hydrogen cyanide in smoke.
■ Smoke from wildfires generates risk for particulate matter exposure which affects eyes and respiratory tract.

CLINICAL FEATURES

■ Severity depends on the smoke composition, exposure duration, and presence/absence of predisposing medical conditions.
■ Singed hair, URT inflammation, soot-stained nasal discharge, and the smell of smoke suggest smoke exposure; observe asymptomatic patients closely for 1 week after exposure for delayed respiratory and/or neurologic effects.

- Early-phase clinical signs may reflect carbon monoxide and/or cyanide poisoning: signs of severe hypoxemia, depression, ataxia, irritable behavior, or animal is moribund to comatose. Horses may exhibit tachypnea and tachycardia.
- Heat and chemical injuries may cause tachypnea, dyspnea, cough, drooling, or nasal discharge.
- Cyanosis and dehydration may be observed.
- Severe respiratory distress and signs of shock may be evident in the intermediate phase.
- Upper airway edema may be progressive and lead to airway obstruction.
- Pseudomembranous casts can obstruct airways, causing dyspnea.
- Small airway obstruction leads to emphysema and pneumothorax.
- Thoracic auscultation may reveal decreased lung sounds, crackles, or wheezes.
- Signs of multiple organ failure may be present in severe cases – acute renal failure, cardiac failure, and CNS effects such as ataxia, seizures, and coma.
- In the late phase, clinical findings may be similar to bronchopneumonia.
- In cases of secondary bacterial infection, fever will be present.
- Worsening of clinical signs after initial improvement suggests secondary bacterial bronchopneumonia.

DIFFERENTIAL DIAGNOSIS

- Inflammatory airway diseases – use endoscopy, physical examination, tracheobronchial aspirates or lavage, clinical pathology.
- Heaves (severe equine asthma, recurrent airway obstruction) – seasonal disorder associated with environmental changes, physical examination, endoscopy, radiography, bronchoalveolar lavage fluid cytology.
- Acute respiratory distress syndrome – physical examination, history, radiographs, arterial blood gases.
- Pneumonia (bacterial or fungal) – clinical signs, physical examination, clinical pathology, endoscopy, radiography, tracheobronchial aspirates or lavage, ultrasonography.
- Exposure to poisonous gases or vapors – e.g., ammonia, hydrogen sulfide, chlorine.
  - History of exposure, possible environmental gas measurement.
- Pulmonary neoplasia – endoscopic examination, tracheobronchial aspirates or lavage, radiography, ultrasonography, biopsy.
- Pneumothorax.
- Allergic bronchitis.

DIAGNOSTICS

CBC/Serum Chemistry/Urinalysis

- Leukocytosis and hyperfibrinogenemia indicate an inflammatory process.
- Severe cases may reveal increased creatinine and blood urea nitrogen, suggesting prerenal or renal failure.
- Lactic acidosis.

Other Diagnostic Tests

- Arterial blood gas analysis.
- Decreased oxygen saturation using pulse oximetry.
- Pulmonary function tests.
- Carboxyhemoglobinemia for carbon monoxide.
- Blood cyanide for cyanide poisoning.
- Methemoglobinemia.
- ECGs are recommended for animals with pre-existing cardiovascular disease.

Imaging

- Thoracic radiography:
  - Chest radiographs are a very important diagnostic aid. Expect diffuse bronchial and peribronchial lesions or diffuse, patchy interstitial infiltration, which are suggestive of edema.
  - Radiographic findings indicative of pneumothorax, pneumomediastinum, and emphysema may be found in severe cases.
  - Because the disease is progressive, take serial chest radiographs to monitor presence or lack of disease progression.
  - Radiographic lesions may not correlate with the severity of pulmonary dysfunction.
- Endoscopy, bronchoscopy may reveal airway edema and inflammation, mucosal necrosis, and soot deposits.
- MRI for leukoencephalopathy.

Pathological Findings

- Thermal/chemical burns.
- Ocular and respiratory tract mucosal inflammation.
- Edema of respiratory tract.
- Upper and lower respiratory tract obstructive casts/occlusion.
- Bronchiectasis.
- Sepsis.
- Pneumonia.

THERAPEUTICS

Detoxification

- Remove animals from further smoke exposure.

Appropriate Health Care

- General supportive care should be aimed at providing a patent airway, reversing bronchospasms and hypoxemia, decreasing pulmonary inflammation and edema, and providing ventilatory support.
- Nebulization.
- Supplemental humidified 100% oxygen may be needed if hypoxemia is severe.
- Suction the URT to clear mucus and fluid, soot, and cell debris.

- Perform a tracheotomy if signs suggest upper airway obstruction; patients maintained with tracheal tubes require careful and frequent nursing care to prevent obstruction of the tube by secretions.
- IV fluid administration is indicated in most horses, because dehydration and renal failure are often present. Administer with caution, however, to prevent exacerbation of pulmonary edema and overhydration. Fluid selection is based on serum electrolyte disturbances and acid–base status.
- Antibiotics to treat bronchopneumonia.
- Tender loving care and excellent hygiene.

Antidotes

- Cyanide poisoning – sodium nitrite, sodium thiosulfate, hydroxocobalamin (vitamin B_{12}).
- Carbon monoxide – humidified oxygen.

Drugs of Choice

- NSAIDs (e.g., phenylbutazone 4.4 mg/kg PO or IV daily) may be beneficial in decreasing mediator release and controlling fever.
- Early use of bronchodilators to control bronchospasm and airway obstruction:
    - $Beta_2$-adrenergic agonists (e.g., clenbuterol 0.8–3.2 µg/kg PO q12h or albuterol [salbutamol] by inhalation) may be administered safely to most horses.
    - Aminophylline (5–10 mg/kg PO or IV q12h).
- Furosemide (1–2 mg/kg IM or IV) may be given for treatment of upper airway or pulmonary tract edema.
- Nebulized heparin to reduce airway fibrin cast.
- DMSO (1.0 g/kg in a 20% solution IV [slowly] q12h or q24 h), NAC, vitamin E may be potentially effective antioxidants.
- Antibiotic prophylaxis in affected horses is controversial because it may lead to development of bacterial resistance. In severe cases, however, early antibiotic treatment with broad-spectrum activity may be justified. In cases of confirmed secondary bacterial infection, use specific antibiotics as determined by culture and sensitivity tests.

Precautions/Interactions

- Concurrent treatment with aminophylline may potentiate the diuretic effect of furosemide.
- Aminophylline may be associated with toxic side effects (e.g., tachycardia, hyperesthesia, and excitement).
- Corticosteroid therapy is controversial and associated with increased septic complications (e.g., bacterial bronchopneumonia); avoid such therapy if possible.
- Tracheostomy will prevent animal from coughing – ability to clear respiratory tract.

COMMENTS

Client Education

- Smoke is complex and smoke inhalation can be a difficult disease to treat; some affected animals may heal without complication while others develop permanent respiratory tract injury.

- Extensive follow-up diagnostics is recommended to determine residual lung function.
- Restrict activity when air quality index is > 100.

Prevention/Avoidance

- Use smoke alarms and fire sprinkler systems.
- Remove from smoke-filled environment; this may best be done by firefighters
- Have fire extinguishers close by.
- Use less combustible construction and furnishing materials.

Possible Complications

- Bronchopneumonia from secondary bacterial infections.
- Chronic hypersensitive airways leading to wheezing, chronic cough.
- Chronic inflammation of airways and lung fibrosis.

Expected Course and Prognosis

- Quite variable depending on duration, severity of exposure, and smoke composition
- Some surviving animals may not manifest any symptoms, while others will develop permanent lesions.

Abbreviations

See Appendix 1 for a complete list.

Internet Resources

Magdesian G. Treatment of smoke inhalation in horses. Available at: https://www.vetmed.ucdavis.edu sites/g/files/dgvnsk491/files/inline-files/smoke-inhalation-DVM-reference.pdf.

Suggested Reading

Geor RJ, Ames TR. Smoke inhalation injury in horses. Compend Contin Educ Prac Vet 1991; 13:1162–1169.
Kemper T, Spiers S, Barratt-Boyes SM, et al. Treatment of smoke inhalation in five horses. J Am Vet Med Assoc 1993; 202:91–94.
McFarlane D. Smoke inhalation injury in the horse. J Eq Vet Science 1995; 15(4):159–162.
Marsh PS. Fire and smoke inhalation injuries in horses. Vet Clin North Am Equine Pract 2007; 23:19–30.

Author: Wilson K. Rumbeiha, DVM, PhD, DABT, DABVT, ATS
Consulting Editor: Lynn R. Hovda, RPh, DVM, MS, DACVIM

Trees

Chapter 81

Black Locust (*Robinia pseudoacacia*)

DEFINITION/OVERVIEW

- *Robinia pseudoacacia* (black locust) toxicosis results from an unknown toxin found in all portions of the plant except the flowers.
- A glycoprotein called robin is the putative toxin, although other biologically active components might contribute (glycoside robitin, alkaloid robinine, and other glycoproteins [lectins or toxalbumens] such as ricin and phasin).
- Signs relate to GI, cardiovascular and neurologic effects of the toxin.
- Among domestic livestock species, horses appear to be the most susceptible.

ETIOLOGY/PATHOPHYSIOLOGY

- The tree is widely distributed east of the Mississippi River but can be found throughout the U.S.
- Reported cases are limited.

Mechanism of Action

- Unknown; several plant constituents have biological activity.

Toxicity

- Most intoxications in horses are believed to be due to ingestion of bark.
- An aqueous suspension of 1,250 g of bark has been reported to cause clinical signs.
- Also, clinical signs have been reported in horses ingesting as little as 70 g of bark.

Systems Affected

- Gastrointestinal – colic and diarrhea due to unknown mechanism; constipation.
- Cardiovascular – congestion of oral mucous membranes, weak pulse, arrhythmias, cold extremities due to unknown mechanism.
- Respiratory – dyspnea.

Blackwell's Five-Minute Veterinary Consult Clinical Companion: Equine Toxicology, First Edition. Edited by Lynn R. Hovda, Dionne Benson, and Robert H. Poppenga.
© 2022 John Wiley & Sons, Inc. Published 2022 by John Wiley & Sons, Inc.
Companion website: www.wiley.com/go/hovda/equine

SIGNALMENT/HISTORY

- No known breed, age, or genetic susceptibilities.

Risk Factors

- Presence of the tree in the environment of the horse.
- Poor-quality diet predisposing to ingestion of the plant.
- Leaves are palatable and will be eaten if other forage is of poor quality or unavailable.
- Boredom.

CLINICAL FEATURES

- Depression.
- Colic.
- Diarrhea or constipation.
- Decreased intestinal peristalsis.
- Weakness.
- Cardiac dysrhythmias.
- Hyperexcitability.
- Signs consistent with hyperammonemia (enteral encephalopathy).
- Dyspnea.
- Laminitis.

DIFFERENTIAL DIAGNOSIS

- Ionophore intoxication – differentiated by detection of an ionophore in feed or tissues.
- *Eupatorium rugosum* (white snakeroot) intoxication – evidence of plant consumption.
- Other causes of colic – appropriate physical examination and diagnostics such as imaging (e.g., ultrasonography, radiography)

DIAGNOSTICS

CBC/Serum Chemistry/Urinalysis

- Hypocalcemia was noted in two ill horses after leaf ingestion.
- Recumbent horses have increased serum CK concentrations.
- Hyperammonemia has been repored; hypothesized to be secondary to GI dysfunction.

Other Diagnostic Tests

- ECG may demonstrate cardiac dysrhythmias, but the types of dysrhytmias are not well documented.

Pathological Findings

- Gross findings:
  - Plant material (e.g., bark, leaves, pods) in stomach contents.
  - Watery and hemorrhagic intestinal contents.
- Histopathologic findings:
  - Enteritis characterized by diffuse villus-tip necrosis and hemorrhage.

THERAPEUTICS

- Treat dysrhythmias as needed.
- Analgesics for abdominal discomfort.
- Balanced electrolyte fluids.
- Hyperammonemia – lactulose to decrease ammonia absorption and increase ammonium ion excretion via feces.

Detoxification

- AC (1–4 g/kg PO in water slurry [1 g of AC in 5 mL of water]).
- One dose of cathartic PO with AC if no diarrhea or ileus – 70% sorbitol (3 mL/kg) or sodium or magnesium sulfate (250 mg/kg), with the latter two in a water slurry.

Antidotes

- None currently available.

Drugs of Choice

- NSAIDs – flunixin meglumine (1.1 mg/kg IV or IM q12h).
- Lactulose – 0.5 mL/kg BW, PO, q6h.

Precautions/Interactions

- Use NSAIDs with caution in dehydrated patients.
- Do not give mineral oil concurrently with AC because of potentially impaired binding ability of AC.

Alternative Drugs

- Many other analgesic options to control colic pain.

COMMENTS

Client Education

- Make client aware of the toxicity of the plant.

Patient Monitoring

- Regular assessment of cardiac rate and rhythm.

Prevention/Avoidance

- Prevent access to black locust; if not practical, provide good-quality diet in adequate amounts.
- Do not confine a horse near the tree.

Possible Complications

- Laminitis is a reported sequela.

Expected Course and Prognosis

- Guarded prognosis in symptomatic animals, although symptomatic and supportive care has resulted in recovery in reported cases.
- Recovery can take several weeks.
- No long-term sequelae are expected in recovered animals.

Abbreviations

See Appendix 1 for a complete list.

Suggested Reading

Burrows GE, Tyrl RJ. Toxic Plants of North America, 2nd edn, Ames: John Wiley and Sons, 2013; p. 595.
Vanschandevijl K, van Loon G, Lefere L, Deprez, P. Black locust (*Robinia pseudoacacic*) intoxication as a suspected cause of transient hyperammonaemia and enteral encephalopathy in a pony. Equine Vet Edu 2010; 22:336–339.

Author: Robert H. Poppenga, DVM, PhD, DABVT
Consulting Editor: Robert H. Poppenga, DVM, PhD, DABVT

Chapter 82

Black Walnut (*Juglans nigra*) Toxicosis

DEFINITION/OVERVIEW

- *Juglans nigra* (black walnut) is a large tree (15–30 m, 50–100 ft) native to the eastern USA and Canada whose wood is prized for furniture and gun stocks.
- When fresh black walnut shavings are used as bedding, horses can develop laminitis and pyrexia within 12–18 hours.
- Bedding containing 20% fresh black walnut shavings made from old or new wood is associated with the onset of clinical signs.
- Black walnut shavings can be identified by their dark brown color (with a hint of purple).
- Black walnut can also induce laminitis if ingested and, while this is not a common means of toxicosis, it should be considered if there is a history of exposure.

ETIOLOGY/PATHOPHYSIOLOGY

Mechanism of Action

- Similar to other causes of laminitis.
- Changes in hemodynamics of blood flow to the foot and hoof with decreased perfusion to the hoof.

Toxicokinetics

- Absorbed through coronary band and skin; also absorbed orally from ingestion of shavings, sawdust, or tree bark.
- Onset of action in 12–18 hours.
- Mild-to-moderate cases of laminitis typically resolve within 48 hours with supportive care.

Toxicity

- Generally, a stable-wide problem that occurs after black walnut shavings, sawdust or other salvage are used as bedding. Most agree that as little as 20% results in toxicosis; a few suggest anywhere from 5% to 20%.
- Toxicity of shavings decreases with exposure to light and air.

Blackwell's Five-Minute Veterinary Consult Clinical Companion: Equine Toxicology,
First Edition. Edited by Lynn R. Hovda, Dionne Benson, and Robert H. Poppenga.
© 2022 John Wiley & Sons, Inc. Published 2022 by John Wiley & Sons, Inc.
Companion website: www.wiley.com/go/hovda/equine

- Juglone was once proposed as toxin, but aqueous solutions of juglone do not result in toxicosis.
- The current theory is that an unknown aqueous toxin other than juglone is responsible for signs.

Systems Affected

- Cardiovascular – tachycardia (pain response).
- Endocrine – pyrexia.
- Gastrointestinal – colic.
- Musculoskeletal – laminitis, pitting edema of distal limbs.
- Respiratory – increased respiratory rate (pain response).

SIGNALMENT/HISTORY

- No breed, age, or sex predilection.

Risk Factors

- Introduction of fresh black walnut shavings.
- Presence of black walnut trees in pasture, paddock or turn-out areas.

Historical Findings

- Use of new shavings identified as black walnut.
- Location and Circumstances of Poisoning
- Multiple horses within the facility developing laminitis simultaneously.

CLINICAL FEATURES

- Early signs:
  - Acute laminitis – warm hooves, digital pulses, stiff gait, reluctance to move, shifting weight from limb to limb.
  - Pitting edema of distal limbs (stocking up).
  - Depression.
- Later signs as toxicity progresses:
  - Tachypnea and tachycardia.
  - Pyrexia.
  - Colic.
  - Laminitis progressing to coffin bone rotation in severe cases.

DIFFERENTIAL DIAGNOSIS

- Other causes of laminitis – carbohydrate overload, exposure to lush pasture, endotoxemia.
- *Berteroa incana* (hoary alyssum) ingestion – evidence of exposure.

DIAGNOSTICS

CBC/Serum Chemistry/Urinalysis

- Largely non-specific.
- The typical hematologic changes seen with other forms of laminitis (shock and hemoconcentration, colic, or severe electrolyte derangements) have not been seen with black walnut-induced laminitis.
- CBC:
  - Transient neutropenia prior to onset, followed by rebound neutrophilia with left shift.
  - Mild to minimal reductions in hematocrit, red blood cell count, and hemoglobin after 12 hours of exposure have been seen in research settings but these do not amount to a significant finding.
- Chemistry:
  - Elevations in serum bilirubin and creatinine have occurred in a research setting.

Other Diagnostic Tests

- Elevated plasma cortisol in severe cases.
- Samples of shavings can be submitted to diagnostic laboratories or forestry departments for positive identification by microscopy.

Imaging

- Radiographic evidence of laminitis (rotation of third phalanx) mirrors severity of clinical signs.

Pathological Findings

- Histopathologic changes correspond with severity of clinical illness.
- Loss of normal architecture and development of necrotic epidermal laminae in severe cases.
- Vacuolation and congestion of the dorsal laminar vessels.
- Evidence of disorganized regenerative hyperplastic epithelial cells within necrotic foci.

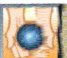
THERAPEUTICS

Detoxification

- If recent ingestion, oral AC at 1–3 g/kg body weight in a water slurry × 1 dose.
- Follow with a cathartic such as epsom salts (250–500 mg/kg in 2–4 L of warm water).

Appropriate Health Care

- Remove all bedding and replace with fresh pine shavings.
- Decontaminate exposed skin with mild soap and water.
- Supportive therapy for laminitis including but not limited to anti-inflammatories, IV fluids, NSAIDs for pain and endotoxemia, and corrective shoeing if warranted.

Antidotes

- There is no specific antidote.

Drugs of Choice

- NSAIDs:
  - Flunixin 1.1 mg/kg IV or PO q12–24h.
  - Phenylbutazone 2.2–4.4 mg/kg IV or PO q12–24h.
  - Ketoprofen 2.2 mg/kg IV q24h.
- Butorphanol for severe pain:
  - 0.05–0.1 mg/kg IV q3–4h.

COMMENTS

Client Education

- Purchase shavings from a reputable source and avoid those from furniture manufacturers.
- Do not plant black walnut trees in pastures, paddocks, or turn-out areas.

Prevention/Avoidance

- Inspect bedding deliveries for black walnut contamination.

Possible Complications

- Ventral rotation or sinking of the third phalanx.
- Secondary colic and dehydration if severe or left untreated.

Expected Course and Prognosis

- Good with no complications for most cases.
- Radiographic evidence of third phalanx rotation or sinking complicates recovery.

Abbreviations

See Appendix 1 for a complete list.

Suggested Reading

Belknap JK. Black walnut extract: an inflammatory model. Vet Clin North Am: Equine Pract 2010; 26(1):95–101.

Burrows GE, Tyrl RJ. Toxic Plants of North America. Ames, IA: Iowa State University Press, 2001, pp. 725–728.

Galey FD, Whitely HE, Goetz TE, et al. Black walnut (*Juglans nigra*) toxicosis: a model for equine laminitis. J Comp Path 1991; 104:313–326.

Uhlinger C. Black walnut toxicosis in ten horses. J Am Vet Med Assoc 1989; 195:343–344.

Acknowledgment The author and editors acknowledge the prior contribution of Larry Thompson.

Author: Tyne K. Hovda, DVM
Consulting Editor: Lynn R. Hovda, RPh, DVM, MS, DACVIM

Chapter 83

Boxelder (*Acer negundo*)

DEFINITION/OVERVIEW

- Ingestion of seeds may cause a highly fatal non-exertional rhabdomyolysis of horses at pasture, termed seasonal pasture myopathy (SPM) in North America. Atypical myopathy (AM) is a similar disease in Europe and New Zealand caused by *Acer pseudoplatanus* (sycamore maple).
- Boxelder trees grow in low, moist areas throughout the Midwest and eastern United States and Canada.
- The winged seeds, similar to other maple trees, grow in clusters and fall in September to March (see Fig. 83.1).
- Both SPM and AM are characterized by early signs of stiffness, dark urine, and difficulty walking, followed by recumbency and inability to rise.
- In North America only a few horses on a given pasture are affected. Larger outbreaks have occurred in Europe.
- Highly fatal, mortality rate of 75–90%.
- Toxin is hypoglycin A, a toxic amino acid present in boxelder seeds, which blocks muscle lipid metabolism.
- Currently there is no commercially available test for hypoglycin A in blood.

ETIOLOGY/PATHOPHYSIOLOGY

Mechanism of Action

- MCPA (methylenecyclopropylacetic acid), the toxic metabolite of hypoglycin A, inhibits various mitochondrial dehydrogenases, resulting in acquired multiple acyl-CoA dehydrogenase deficiency (MADD).
- MADD causes disruption of fatty acid beta-oxidation and subsequent lipid accumulation and degeneration in muscle with high oxidative capacity, such as postural, respiratory, and cardiac muscles.

Toxicokinetics

- Onset of 12–24 hours after ingestion of toxic amount.
- Death occurs within 72 hours of clinical onset.

Blackwell's Five-Minute Veterinary Consult Clinical Companion: Equine Toxicology, First Edition. Edited by Lynn R. Hovda, Dionne Benson, and Robert H. Poppenga.
© 2022 John Wiley & Sons, Inc. Published 2022 by John Wiley & Sons, Inc.
Companion website: www.wiley.com/go/hovda/equine

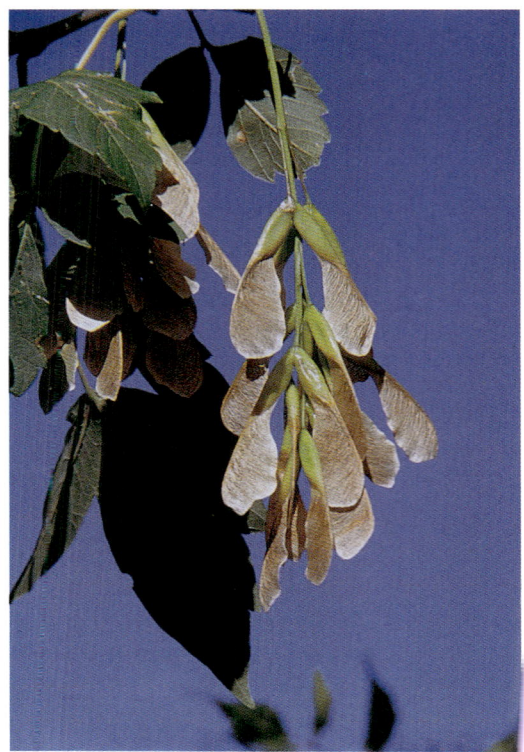

■ **Fig. 83.1.** Boxelder tree (*Acer negundo*) and seeds. The seeds (fruit) are closely paired, winged samaras that create an inverted or upside down V-shape. Seeds mature in the late summer and many remain attached to the tree throughout the winter. *Source:* USDA photo/Wikimedia Commons.

Toxicity

- Highly fatal.
- Morality rate of 75–90%.

Systems Affected

- Musculoskeletal – primarily.
- Respiratory – primarily.
- Cardiovascular.
- Gastrointestinal.
- Urinary.

 # SIGNALMENT/HISTORY

- No breed, sex, or gender predilection.

Risk Factors

- Young horses recently introduced to the pasture.
- Poor-quality pasture or lack of forage, so consumption of seeds increases.
- Cold weather which may lead to a negative energy balance and strong winds that disperse seeds.
- Stressors such as transport and weather changes.

Historical Findings

- Presence of boxelder trees and seeds on pasture.

Location and Circumstances of Poisoning

- Typically occurs in the fall when seeds are abundant and pasture grass is sparse. Fewer cases in the spring.

CLINICAL FEATURES

- Musculoskeletal – lethargy, acute muscular weakness, muscle tremor, stiffness, reluctance to move, rapidly progressing to recumbency and inability to rise are common features.
- Respiratory – tachypnea and dyspnea are common.
- Cardiovascular – mild tachycardia and heart murmurs.
- Urinary – myoglobinuria, dysuria, distended bladder.
- Gastrointestinal – sweating, colic signs, esophageal obstruction, dysphagia.

DIFFERENTIAL DIAGNOSIS

- *Eupatorium rugosum* (white snake root) or ionophore (monensin, lasalocid, etc.) toxicosis.
- Exertional rhabdomyolysis.
- Nutritional myopathies.
- Laminitis.
- Colic.

DIAGNOSTICS

CBC/Serum Chemistry/Urinalysis

- CBC:
    - Elevated PCV.
    - Leukocytosis/neutrophilia.
- Chemistry:
    - Marked increase in CK and AST.
    - Increased liver enzymes.
    - Elevation in BUN and creatinine.
    - Hyperglycemia.
    - Lactic acidemia.
    - Hyperlipemia.
- Urinalysis:
    - Myoglobinuria.

Other Diagnostic Tests

- Elevated cTnI possible.
- Elevated acylcarnitine in serum/organic acids in urine.

- Elevated hypoglycin A and MCPA carnitine in serum.
- Muscle biopsy of postural or intercostal muscle shows Zenker's necrosis and neutral lipid accumulation (Oil red O or Sudan III stain) in type 1 muscle fibers.

Pathological Findings

- Multifocal areas of pallor or hemorrhage in postural and respiratory muscles and less frequently in myocardium.
- Histopathology – severe acute myonecrosis and lipid storage myopathy.

THERAPEUTICS

Detoxification

- The use of AC or cathartics is not recommended unless there is a single, acute witnessed ingestion.

Appropriate Health Care

- Care is supportive, typically requiring immediate referral.
- Goals are to limit further muscle damage, restore circulating blood volume, correct metabolic disturbances (acid–base, electrolyte), provide analgesia as needed.
- IV fluid therapy for diuresis to prevent pigment nephropathy.
- Frequent carbohydrate-rich meals or IV glucose supplementation (1–4 mg/kg) to supply muscle energy from carbohydrate metabolism.
- Monitor electrolyte derangements, renal, respiratory, and cardiac function.

Antidotes

- There is no specific antidote.

Drugs of Choice

- Insulin to combat hyperglycemia and stimulate insulin-mediated lipogenesis.
- Riboflavin (vitamin B2) is a precursor of flavin adenine dinucleotide, a cofactor of all acyl-CoA dehydrogenases affected in MADD, and supplementation may enhance residual enzyme activity.
- Antioxidants:
  - Ascorbic acid 30–50 mg/kg q12h in IV fluids.
  - Vitamin E 20 IU/kg PO.
- NSAID – use judiciously and monitor BUN and creatinine:
  - Flunixin 1.1 mg/kg IV or PO q12–24h.
  - Phenylbutazone 2.2–4.4 mg/kg IV or PO q12–24h.
  - Ketoprofen 2.2 mg/kg IV q24h.
- Butorphanol for severe pain:
  - 0.05–0.1 mg/kg IV q3–4h.

Precautions/Interactions

- Oral carnitine – lack of evidence of beneficial effects and possibly arrhythmogenic side effects in human MADD patients.

COMMENTS

Client Education

- Identify boxelder trees in or around the pasture, paddock or horse turn-out area. Cut down or otherwise remove female boxelder trees.
- If removal is not possible, trim low-hanging branches and vacuum or rake seeds in the fall.

Prevention/Avoidance

- Provide adequate nutrition for horses prior to turn-out and provide access to hay while on fall pastures.
- Keep young or newer horses off pastures with boxelder trees in the fall.
- Do not use overgrazed pastures if there are boxelder trees present.
- Reduce turn-out time to less than 12 hours/day or avoid using the pasture.

Possible Complications

- Recovered horses may not regain prior physical fitness.

Expected Course and Prognosis

- Case fatality rate is high (75–90%).
- Severely elevated PCV associated with poor outcome.
- Rapid progression with death or euthanasia within 72 hours of onset of clinical signs.

Abbreviations

See Appendix 1 for a complete list.

Internet Resources

University of Minnesota Extension. Boxelder seeds cause seasonal pasture myopathy. Available at: https://extension.umn.edu/horse-pastures-and-facilities/seasonal-pasture-myopathy

Suggested Reading

McKenzie RK, Hill FI, Habyarimana JA, et al. Detection of hypoglycin A in the seeds of sycamore (*Acer pseudoplatanus*) and box elder (*Acer negundo*) in New Zealand; the toxin associated with cases of equine atypical myopathy. New Zeal Vet J 2016; 64(3):182–187.

Sander J, Cavalleri JMV, Terhardt M, et al. Rapid diagnosis of hypoglycin A intoxication in atypical myopathy of horses. J Vet Diagn Invest 2016; 28:98–104.

Valberg S. Review of the discovery of the basis for a seasonal pasture myopathy/atypical myopathy. In: Proceedings of the 60th Annual Convention of the American Association of Equine Practitioners, Salt Lake City, Utah, USA, December 6–10, 2014; pp. 184–187.

Valberg S, Sponseller BT, Hegeman AD, et al. Seasonal pasture myopathy/atypical myopathy in North America associated with ingestion of hypoglycin A within seeds of the box elder tree. Equine Vet J 2013; 45(4) 419–426.

Acknowledgement: The author and editors acknowledge the prior contribution of Beatrice T. Sponseller.

Author: Tyne K Hovda, DVM
Consulting Editor: Lynn R. Hovda, RPh, DVM, MS, DACVIM

Chapter 84

Oak (Quercus spp.)

DEFINITION/OVERVIEW

- This genus of plants contains a variety of species, including trees and shrubs.
- All *Quercus* spp. should be considered toxic.
- Species more commonly associated with poisoning include Gambel's oak (*Quercus gambelii*), Havard or shinnery oak (*Quercus havardii*), and white shin oak (*Quercus sinuata* var. *breviloba*). Other species implicated in poisonings include wavyleaf oak (*Quercus undulata*), Emory oak (*Quercus emoryi*), shrub live oak (*Quercus turbinella*), and silverleaf oak (*Quercus hypoleucoides*).
- Ingestion of large quantities of leaves, leaf buds, or acorns results in a severe gastroenteritis/nephrotoxic syndrome.
- Poisoning is most commonly associated with ingestion of acorns (especially green acorns) or new leaf buds, hence the common name "oak-bud poisoning".

ETIOLOGY/PATHOPHYSIOLOGY

Mechanism of Action

- Exact mechanism of action is not completely understood.
- Tannins – gallotannins and metabolites are the suspected toxins.
- Ingested tannins bind with peptide linkages and precipitate in the GI tract, resulting in mucosal damage, ischemia, and necrosis.

Toxicokinetics

- Toxicosis generally occurs when oak forms > 50% of the diet.
- Onset may be peracute or acute with death in 12–36 hours.
- Duration of signs in those horses that recover is 72 hours to several weeks.

Toxicity

- Poisoning is uncommon in horses.
- Occurs in the early spring with ingestion of new leaf buds or in late fall with ingestion of acorns.

Blackwell's Five-Minute Veterinary Consult Clinical Companion: Equine Toxicology,
First Edition. Edited by Lynn R. Hovda, Dionne Benson, and Robert H. Poppenga.
© 2022 John Wiley & Sons, Inc. Published 2022 by John Wiley & Sons, Inc.
Companion website: www.wiley.com/go/hovda/equine

Systems Affected

- Gastrointestinal – primarily.
- Renal – primarily.
- Cardiovascular/circulatory.
- Respiratory.
- Hepatic – rarely.

SIGNALMENT/HISTORY

- No particular breed, age or sex predilection.

Risk Factors

- Lack of available forage or dietary supplementation.
- Drought or conditions that inhibit other forages from growing predispose to ingestion of oak.

Location and Circumstances of Poisoning

- Access to oak trees in pastures, paddocks, and turn-out areas.
- Season of year – spring and fall.

CLINICAL FEATURES

- Inappetence, abdominal pain, depression, tenesmus, constipation (early) followed by mucoid hemorrhagic diarrhea.
- Colic.
- Peripheral edema, weakness, icterus (rare).
- Polydipsia, polyuria, brownish-colored urine.
- Tachycardia, hyperpnea.

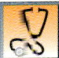

DIFFERENTIAL DIAGNOSIS

- *Amaranthus* spp. (pigweed), aminoglycoside, and oxalate toxicosis.
- Infectious disease (*Salmonella*, *Clostridium difficile*, others).
- Other causes of colic or colitis.

DIAGNOSTICS

CBC/Serum Chemistry/Urinalysis

- Markedly elevated PCV; hypoproteinemia.
- Increased BUN and creatinine, hypocalcemia, hypomagnesemia, increased AST.
- Metabolic acidosis
- Hyposthenuria, proteinuria, hematuria

Other Diagnostic Tests

- Abdominocentesis – increased total protein; normal nucleated cell count.

Imaging

- Abdominal Ultrasound – ± thickening of the small intestine and colon walls.

Pathological Findings

- Gross:
    - Subcutaneous edema, mucoid and/or hemorrhagic enteritis, pseudomembranous enteritis, edema of mesenteric lymph nodes, hydropericardium, perirenal edema, swollen and pale kidneys, ascites, petechial hemorrhage of kidneys, and hepatic congestion.
- Histopathology:
    - Kidney – numerous pink to brown casts in the proximal tubules, proximal tubular necrosis, medullary congestion.
    - GI – pseudomembranous, submucosal edema; necrotizing enteritis with hemorrhage and ulceration.
    - Other – vascular congestion of the liver and lungs, generalized tissue congestion.

THERAPEUTICS

Detoxification

- Activated charcoal 1–3g/kg PO once in a water slurry, epsom salts (magnesium sulfate) 250–500 mg/kg in 2–4 L of warm water.

Appropriate Health Care

- Minimize further GI and renal damage with general decontamination and supportive care.
- IV crystalloids for dehydration, hypovolemia, and diuresis
- Fresh or fresh frozen plasma as needed for hypoproteinemia.
- Correct metabolic acidosis with IV fluids (acetated or lactated Ringer's) or sodium bicarbonate.
- IV colloids as needed.
- Antibiotic therapy as needed, based on CBC.
- Monitor urine output and renal function daily.

Antidotes

- There is no specific antidote available.

Drugs of Choice

- Pain medications:
    - Flunixin meglumine 1.1 mg/kg IV or PO q12–24h.
    - Phenylbutazone 2.2–4.4 mg/kg IV or PO q12–24h.
    - Butorphanol for severe pain 0.05–0.1 mg/kg IV q3–4h.
- GI protectants:
    - Sucralfate 10–20 mg/kg PO q6–8h.
    - Omeprazole 4 mg/kg PO q24h.

Alternative Drugs

- Supplementation with calcium hydroxide (15% pellet) as a *prophylactic* agent to inactivate tannins has been beneficial in other species, but its effectiveness in horses is unknown.

COMMENTS

Client Education

- There is no need to cut down mature oak trees, but keep branches trimmed and out of reach.
- Securely fence immature oaks.
- Rake or vacuum acorns in the fall.

Prevention/Avoidance

- Avoid pasturing horses in areas containing oaks unless other adequate forage is unavailable.

Possible Complications

- With severe GI ulceration and necrosis, scarring and strictures are possible.

Expected Course and Prognosis

- Recovery may require 2–3 weeks of intense care.

Abbreviations

See Appendix 1 for a complete list.

Internet Resources

Oak Buds and Green Acorns Can Harm Horses. 1888 Available at: https://extension.umn.edu/horse-pastures-and-facilities/oak-buds-and-green-acorns-can-harm-horses.

Suggested Reading

Anderson GA, Mount ME, Vrins AA, et al. Fatal acorn poisoning in a horse: pathologic findings and diagnostic considerations. J Am Vet Med Assoc 1983; 182(10):1105–1110.
Harper KT, Ruyle GB, Rittenhouse LR. Toxicity problems associated with the grazing of oak in the intermountain and southwestern USA. In: James LF, Ralphs MH, Nielsen DB, eds. The Ecology and Economic Impact of Poisonous Plants on Livestock Production. Boulder, CO: Westview Press, 1988; pp. 197–206.
Smith S, Naylor RJ, Knowles EJ, et al. Suspected acorn toxicity in nine horses. Eq Vet J 2015; 47(5):568–572.

Acknowledgement: The author and editors acknowledge the prior contribution of Jeffery O. Hall.

Author: Lynn R. Hovda, RPh, DVM, MS, DACVIM
Consulting Editor: Lynn R. Hovda, RPh, DVM, MS, DACVIM; Dionne Benson, DVM, JD

Chapter 85

Red Maple (*Acer rubrum*)

DEFINITION/OVERVIEW

- Toxicosis is associated with ingestion of wilted or dried *Acer rubrum* (red maple) leaves, although some related hybrids, including the sugar maple (*Acer saccharum*) may result in similar signs if ingested.
- Commonly referred to as Carolina maple, swamp maple, soft maple, scarlet maple.
- Red maple leaves are palmate with three to five lobes and a serrated or jagged leaf margin. The underside is a silver grey and the leaves green until fall when they become a vibrant red and, less often, orange or yellow.
- Toxicosis is typically seen in the fall, but may occur in the spring or summer when horses have access to wilted or dried leaves from fallen branches.
- Most frequently reported in the eastern United States and Canada.
- Diagnosis is typically presumptive and based on history and exposure.
- Clinical findings are consistent with oxidative injury to RBC and tissue hypoxia.

ETIOLOGY/PATHOPHYSIOLOGY

Mechanism of Action

- The specific toxin has not been identified.
  - Proposed toxins are pyrogallol and gallic acid.
  - These metabolites have been isolated in diagnosed cases and are formed from intestinal bacterial metabolism of tannic acid (found in wilted or dry leaves).
- Toxin causes oxidative damage to the RBC membrane and hemoglobin, resulting in intra- and extravascular anemia, Heinz body formation and/or methemoglobinemia.
- Two syndromes:
  - Hemolytic anemia:
    - Hemoglobin – protein is precipitated, resulting in Heinz body formation and ultimately intravascular anemia.
    - RBC – changes in cell membrane formability, removal by spleen, and extravascular anemia.
  - Methemoglobinemia, resulting in tissue hypoxia.

Blackwell's Five-Minute Veterinary Consult Clinical Companion: Equine Toxicology,
First Edition. Edited by Lynn R. Hovda, Dionne Benson, and Robert H. Poppenga.
© 2022 John Wiley & Sons, Inc. Published 2022 by John Wiley & Sons, Inc.
Companion website: www.wiley.com/go/hovda/equine

Toxicokinetics

- Onset of action is 12–48 hours, may be delayed up to 5 days.
- Death occurs in 3–6 days; may also be peracute.

Toxicity

- 0.7 kg (1.5 lb) wilted or dried leaves/mature horse may result in clinical signs.
- 1.4 kg (3 lb) of wilted or dried leaves/mature horse generally results in death.
- Leaves remain toxic for several weeks.
- Mortality rate, even in treated horses, is approximately 60%.

Systems Affected

- Cardiovascular – tachycardia secondary to anemia; cyanosis and brown discoloration of the blood due to methemoglobin, Heinz bodies, DIC.
- Musculoskeletal – laminitis.
- Nervous – depression.
- Renal – pigmenturia, hematuria, and proteinuria; kidney failure secondary to hemoglobin deposition in the kidney.
- Reproductive – abortion secondary to fetal hypoxia.
- Respiratory – increased respirator rate secondary to anemia.

SIGNALMENT/HISTORY

- No breed, gender, or age predilections.

Risk Factors

- Presence of red maple leaves on pasture or in areas where horses have access.
- Poor management of pruned or fallen limbs and branches in pastures and turn-out areas.

Location and Circumstances of Poisoning

- Spring and summer months, generally after storms when branches or limbs fall in pasture.
- Fall months when fallen leaves are not removed from pasture or turn-out.

CLINICAL FEATURES

- Common exam findings include red or brown urine, pyrexia, tachycardia, lethargy, depression, weakness, and muddy or cyanotic mucous membranes.
- Additional findings include polypnea, dehydration, and signs consistent with systemic inflammation. Colic and laminitis have also been reported.
- Acute death (within 18 hours) can result from rapid formation of methemoglobin.
- Alternatively, hemolytic crisis can develop over several days as the hemolysis and methemoglobinemia progressively worsen.

DIFFERENTIAL DIAGNOSIS

- Anemia – immune-mediated hemolytic anemias – drug-induced, idiopathic, infecticus (equine infectious anemia, piroplasmosis); snake envenomation, hepatic failure hypertonic or hypotonic solutions, neoplasia, and DMSO.
- Methemoglobinemia – congenital, onions (*Allium* spp.), phenothiazine toxicosis, and nitrates.

DIAGNOSTICS

CBC/Serum Chemistry/Urinalysis

- CBC:
    - Interpretation may be difficult due to hemolysis.
    - Decreased PCV, hemoglobin, and erythrocyte count confirm anemia, whereas increased mean corpuscular hemoglobin concentration and mean corpuscular hemoglobin support intravascular hemolysis with hemoglobinemia.
    - PCV may fall to 8–10% and hemoglobin concentration to 50 g/L.
    - Possible inflammatory leukogram (most commonly leucocytosis with left shift).
    - Cell morphology:
        - Heinz bodies are not present in all cases, and are more readily apparent in new methylene blue-stained smears.
        - Eccentrocytes and ghost cells have been reported.
- Chemistry
    - Elevated serum bilirubin.
    - Increased albumin and total protein secondary to dehydration.
    - Elevated BUN and creatinine in cases of nephropathy and acute kidney failure.
    - Elevated liver enzymes and CPK may occur, likely secondary to cell damage caused by anemia-induced hypoxia.
- Urinalysis – proteinuria and hemoglobinuria, with few or no intact erythrocytes.

Other Diagnostic Tests

- Percentage of methemoglobin in the blood often is elevated.

Pathological Findings

- Gross:
    - Generalized icterus, enlarged spleen, and discolored kidneys.
    - Petechiae and ecchymoses may be present.
- Histopathology:
    - Erythrophagocytosis by macrophages, renal pigment casts and sloughed epithelial cells, splenic and hepatic hemosiderin, and centrilobular hepatic lipidosis.
    - Pulmonary thrombosis possible.

THERAPEUTICS

Detoxification

- Prevent toxin absorption with AC 1–3 g/kg BW or cathartic such as magnesium sulfate 250–500 mg/kg dissolved in 2–4 L of warm water.

Appropriate Health Care

- In-patient or outpatient according to severity. The goals are to improve tissue oxygenation and perfusion, reduce inflammation, provide analgesia, and minimize potential complications.
- Continuous nasal oxygen administration may be helpful.
- Whole blood or packed RBC transfusion if PCV is low or falling rapidly.
- IV crystalloids to maintain renal perfusion, expand volume, and promote diuresis, but PCV must be corrected prior to use.
- IV colloids as needed.
- Monitor methemoglobinemia and anemia and adjust therapy as indicated.
- Monitor BUN and creatinine and adjust IV fluids and medications as needed.

Antidotes

- No specific antidote available.

Drugs of Choice

- Ascorbic acid for antioxidant effects:
    - 30–50 mg/kg q12h, add to IV fluids or 50–100 g IV every day.
- NSAIDS for inflammation and pain control:
    - Phenylbutazone 2.2–4.4 mg/kg IV or PO q12–24h.
    - Flunixin meglumine 1.1 mg/kg IV q12–24h.
- Butorphanol for severe pain:
    - 0.05–0.1 mg/kg IV q3–4h.
- Transdermal fentanyl may be an effective alternative for pain control.

Precautions/Interactions

- Use NSAIDS cautiously due to potential renal toxicity.
- Corticosteroids and DMSO are thought to be contraindicated.
- The use of methylene blue to treat methemoglobinemia is controversial due to poor efficacy and possible increase in Heinz body formation.

Alternative Drugs

- Alpha-tocopherol has been suggested as a preventative.

COMMENTS

Client Education

- Keep maple trees outside of pastures, paddocks, and turn-out areas and fence and manage those that are adjacent.

- Remove fallen branches and limbs and rake and destroy fallen leaves before they wilt or dry.

Prevention/Avoidance

- Provide horses year-round a good-quality, palatable forage.

Possible Complications

- Laminitis can occur during or after the course of the disease.
- Anemia and methemoglobinemia may result in fetal hypoxia, followed by abortion.

Expected Course and Prognosis

- Prognosis depends on the quantity of leaves ingested, but is poor even in treated horses
- Death is attributed to severe methemoglobinemia, anemia, or acute kidney failure.
- Severity of decreased PCV has not been shown to be a negative prognostic indicator.

Abbreviations

See Appendix 1 for a complete list.

Suggested Reading

Agrawal K, Ebel JG, Altier C, et al. Identification of protoxins and a microbial basis for red maple (*Acer rubrum*) toxicosis in equines. J Vet Diagn Invest 2013; 25(1):112–119.

Alward A, Corriher CA, Barton MH, et al. Red maple (*Acer rubrum*) leaf toxicosis in horses: A retrospective study of 32 cases. J Vet Int Med 2006; 20:1197–1201.

O'Callaghan DK, Schall SA, Birmingham SS, et al. Protective effects of ascorbic acid and α-tocopherol on the in vitro oxidation of equine erythrocytes caused by extracts of wilted red maple leaves. J Eq Vet Sci 2015; 35(11–12):940–946.

Acknowledgement: The author and editors acknowledge the prior contribution of Scott L. Radke.

Author: Tyne K. Hovda, DVM
Consulting Editor: Lynn R. Hovda, RPh, DVM, MS, DACVIM

Zootoxins

Blister Beetles (*Epicauta* spp. and *Pyrota* spp.)

Chapter 86

DEFINITION/OVERVIEW

- Blister beetles (*Epicauta* spp. and *Pyrota* spp.) are flower-feeding insects that contain cantharidin, a toxic vesicant agent that blisters tissue on contact. Three-striped blister beetles (*E. occidentalis* and *E. temexa*) account for most cases of equine toxicosis (see Fig. 86.1).
- Swarms of beetles tend to congregate in alfalfa fields of the south, central, and eastern United States (see Fig. 86.2). When alfalfa is simultaneously crimped and cut, beetles and toxin are crushed into the hay, posing a serious hazard to horses that later consume it.
- Cantharidin remains stable in stored hay for prolonged periods.
- Toxicosis is most common in Oklahoma, Texas, and surrounding states but can occur anywhere that affected alfalfa products are shipped.
- Clinical signs appear within minutes to hours of ingestion and reflect vesicant effects on the GI and urinary tracts, hypocalcemia, and myocardial necrosis in severe cases.

ETIOLOGY/PATHOPHYSIOLOGY

Mechanism of Action

- In addition to direct vesicant effects, cantharidin inhibits protein phosphatases 1 and 2A, disrupting membrane permeability, signal transduction, and cellular metabolism.
- Dose-dependent effects occur at three main target sites:
  - Ulceration of GI mucosa.
  - Renal tubular dysfunction and mucosal ulceration of the ureters, bladder, and urethra.
  - Myocardial necrosis.

Toxicokinetics

- Cantharidin is rapidly absorbed and distributed, then excreted unchanged through the urinary tract.

Toxicity

- Estimated minimum lethal dose of cantharidin is 0.5–1 mg/kg.
- Beetles contain variable amounts of toxin (approximately 1–5% of dry weight), but as little as 5 g of dried beetles may be sufficient to kill a 450-kg (1,000 lb) horse.

Blackwell's Five-Minute Veterinary Consult Clinical Companion: Equine Toxicology, First Edition. Edited by Lynn R. Hovda, Dionne Benson, and Robert H. Poppenga.
© 2022 John Wiley & Sons, Inc. Published 2022 by John Wiley & Sons, Inc.
Companion website: www.wiley.com/go/hovda/equine

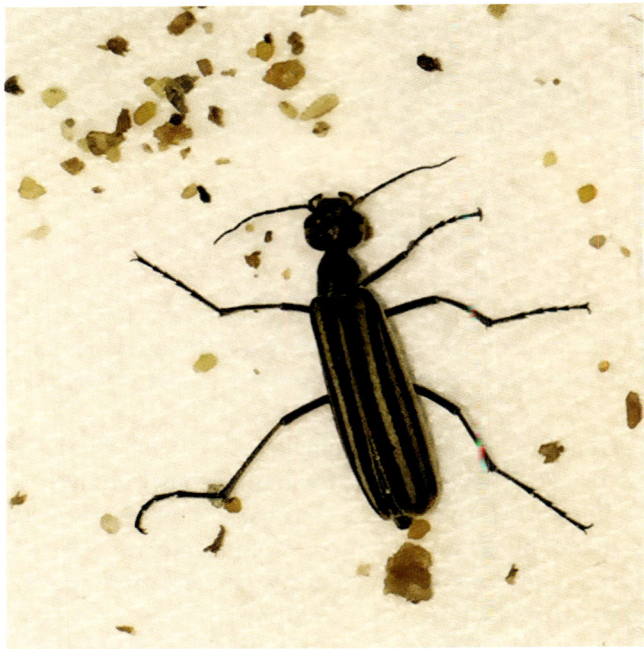

■ **Fig. 86.1.** Three striped blister beetle. *Source:* Photo courtesy of Dr Elizabeth Davis, Kansas State University.

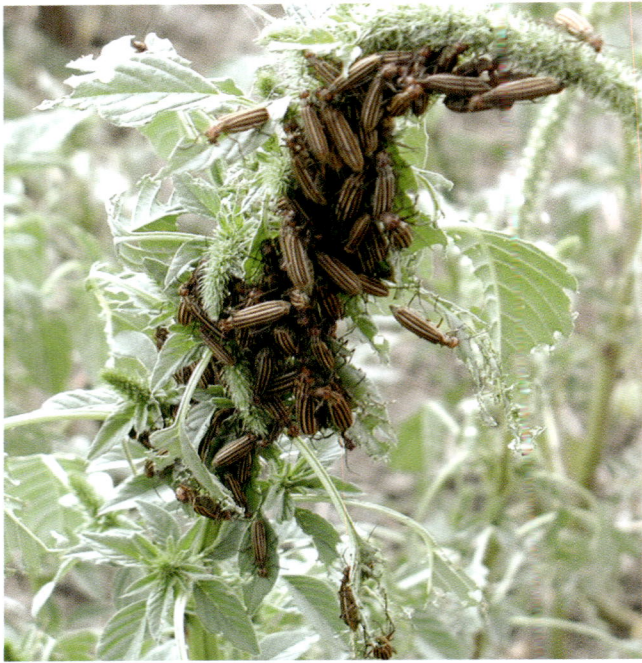

■ **Fig. 86.2.** Swarms of blister beetles in an alfalfa field. *Source:* Photo courtesy of Dr Elizabeth Davis, Kansas State University.

Systems Affected

- Cardiovascular – tachycardia, hypovolemic and/or endotoxemic shock, myocardial necrosis rare instances of severe myocardial dysfunction.
- Endocrine/metabolic – hypocalcemia (muscle tremors, stiff gait, synchronous diaphragmatic flutter), hypomagnesemia.
- Gastrointestinal – inflammation and ulceration, ptyalism, anorexia, bruxism, colic, diarrhea, fever.
- Musculoskeletal – laminitis, rare rhabdomyolysis.
- Renal/urologic – hyposthenuria, hemorrhagic cystitis and urethritis, dysuria, pollakiuria or polyuria, possible progression to acute renal failure.

SIGNALMENT

- One or more horses of any age, breed, or sex may be affected.

History/Location

- History of being fed alfalfa hay.
- Toxicosis from infested alfalfa cubes and pellets is possible but much less common.

CLINICAL FEATURES

- Clinical signs are dose-dependent and range from lethargy and inappetance to shock and death within several hours of ingestion.
- The most consistent clinical signs at presentation are colic, fever, and dysuria.
- Variable signs include depression, ptyalism, bruxism, splashing in the water bucket without drinking, pollakiuria or polyuria, hematuria, signs of ionized hypocalcemia (muscle tremors, stiff gait, synchronous diaphragmatic flutter), diarrhea, and hypovolemic or endotoxemic shock.

DIFFERENTIAL DIAGNOSIS

- Colic differential diagnosis guided by severity and concurrent findings.
- Causes of acute diarrhea, fever, and endotoxemia:
    - Infectious enterocolitis (*Salmonella* spp., *Clostridium* spp., *Neorickettsia risticii*, coronavirus).
    - Anterior enteritis.
    - Septic peritonitis.
    - Grain overload.
    - Sand enteropathy.
    - Toxic agents (ionophores, NSAID toxicity, hoary alyssum).
- Causes of dysuria, pollakiuria, and hematuria:
    - Bacterial cystitis, urolithiasis, urethral trauma, bladder or urethral neoplasia.

DIAGNOSTICS

- Presumptive diagnosis is based on compatible clinical and laboratory findings and identification of beetles in hay; failure to find beetles does not exclude diagnosis.
- Definitive diagnosis is by GC-MS (preferred) or HPLC demonstration of cantharidin in urine, stomach contents, serum, or kidney. Urine and GI contents are specimens of choice.

CBC/Serum Chemistry/Urinalysis

- Serum chemistry – hypocalcemia is a consistent feature, but absence does not exclude diagnosis. Hypomagnesemia is also common and aggravates hypocalcemia if not addressed.
- Urinalysis – hyposthenuria (USG 1.004–1.007) regardless of hydration status; microscopic hematuria.
- Common nonspecific findings include hemoconcentration, azotemia, hyperglycemia and hypokalemia.
- Many affected horses exhibit elevated serum cTnI, but clinically significant cardiac dysfunction is uncommon.

Pathological Findings

- With massive exposure and sudden death, gross pathology may be absent.
- Hyperemia and erosions of the GI tract (oral cavity, esophagus, stomach, and intestine) and urinary tract (bladder, urethra) are typical.
- Microscopic lesions include acantholysis of the GI and urinary mucosae and vasculature, renal tubular necrosis, and myocardial necrosis and inflammation.

THERAPEUTICS

- Treatment is symptomatic and supportive.
- Goals of therapy are to halt toxin ingestion, decontaminate the gut, hasten toxin elimination, control abdominal pain, correct hypocalcemia and hypomagnesemia, and maintain hydration, blood pressure, and tissue perfusion.

Detoxification

- Administer AC (1–3 g/kg) by nasogastric tube as a slurry in water or Epsom salts (500 mg/kg to 1 g/kg dissolved in 4 L of warm water).
- Consider repeating AC treatment (no further Epsom salts) in 12 hours.
- If AC is unavailable, administer DTO smectite (BioSponge®; 3 g/kg) by NG tube as a slurry in water or Epsom salts.
- Do not administer Epsom salts to diarrheic patients.

Appropriate Health Care

- Immediate hospitalization for IV fluid therapy, supportive care, and monitoring.
- Balanced polyionic IV fluids (e.g., lactated Ringer's solution) as needed to correct dehydration and maintain blood pressure and tissue perfusion.

- Monitor ionized calcium, electrolytes, and acid–base status several times daily to guide adjustment of therapy.

Antidotes

- No specific antidote.

Drugs of Choice

- Correct hypocalcemia:
  - Give up to 1 mL/kg 23% calcium gluconate by slow IV injection, preferably diluted at least 1:4 in isotonic fluids and administered over 30 minutes or more.
  - When administering undiluted calcium to patients in distress, monitor heart rate and rhythm during injection and discontinue if sudden changes occur.
  - To address ongoing losses, add 250–500 mL 23% calcium gluconate per 5 L bag of fluids administered at maintenance rate.
- Correct hypomagnesemia. For a full-sized horse receiving 30 L of IV fluids per day, add 25 mL of 50% magnesium sulfate solution to each 5 L bag.
- Consider low-dose flunixin (0.25 mg/kg IV q6–8h) and polymyxin B (1,000–2,000 U/kg IV q8–12h) for endotoxemic patients.
- Manage abdominal pain:
  - Flunixin (1.1 mg/kg IV q12h). Minimize dose and duration of therapy, as this medication impedes intestinal healing.
  - If NSAIDs alone are insufficient to control pain, or if renal compromise precludes their use, consider detomidine, opioids, and lidocaine:
  - Detomidine (0.01–0.04 mg/kg IV).
  - Butorphanol (0.01–0.04 mg/kg IV or IM as needed).
  - Butorphanol CRI – 0.02 mg/kg IV loading dose followed by continuous rate infusion at 13–22 µg/kg/hour IV.
  - Lidocaine (1.3 mg/kg slow IV injection loading dose followed by 0.05 mg/kg/min CRI). Avoid in horses with marked ionized hypocalcemia and exercise caution in horses with myocardial dysfunction.
- GI protectants:
  - Omeprazole (4 mg/kg PO q24h).
  - Sucralfate (22 mg/kg PO q6–8h).
- Patients with severe GI injury and neutropenia may benefit from broad-spectrum antimicrobial therapy.
- Consider altrenogest (0.044 mg/kg PO q24h) for pregnant mares.

Precautions/Interactions

- Use caution with nephrotoxic drugs (NSAIDs, polymyxin B) as these patients are at risk of acute kidney injury and renal failure. Do not use aminoglycoside antibiotics.
- Do not mix calcium and sodium bicarbonate in IV fluids.

COMMENTS

- Other livestock species (ruminants, camelids) are also susceptible to cantharidin, so affected hay should be discarded.

Patient Monitoring

- Frequent monitoring of electrolytes, azotemia, and acid–base status
- Because cantharidin induces hyposthenuria, USG is an unreliable indicator of hydration status in these patients; physical parameters, serum chemistry, and blood gas analysis are particularly important for assessment of hydration and tissue perfusion.
- Monitor for laminitis, which occurs in up to 10% of patients. Consider continuous cryotherapy and sand bedding or hoof pads.

Prevention/Avoidance

- Recommendations for hay producers.
    - Learn to recognize blister beetles and implement harvesting methods that reduce the risk of hay contamination.
    - Cutting hay without simultaneous crimping allows beetles to survive and depart the field before hay is baled, but also lengthens drying time.
    - Manage harvest intervals to minimize flowering, which attracts beetles.
    - From July through September, scout hay fields before cutting and postpone harvesting if beetles are present.
    - If swarms are noted during harvesting, stop to allow dispersal before proceeding.
- Recommendations for horse owners:
    - Feed small square bales and inspect each flake of hay for beetles before feeding it. Note that the absence of visible beetles does not ensure safety, as the toxin is released when beetles are crushed during harvest.
    - First-cutting hay is generally considered safe because beetles do not become active until later in the season.
    - Develop a good working relationship with local hay producers so you can be confident of their harvesting practices and hay quality.
    - If possible, grow your own alfalfa to control production and minimize risk.

Possible Complications

- Acute renal failure.
- Laminitis.
- Rare cases of myocardial dysfunction and severe rhabdomyolysis.

Expected Course and Prognosis

- Prognosis is guarded and dose-dependent, but with early diagnosis and aggressive therapy many patients recover.
- Survival beyond 2 days is a good prognostic indicator.
- Complications may reduce the likelihood of survival.

Abbreviations

See Appendix 1 for a complete list.

Suggested Reading

Gwaltney-Brant SM, Dunayer E, Youssef H. Terrestrial zootoxins. In: Gupta RC, ed. Veterinary Toxicology: Basic and Clinical Principles, 3rd edn. San Diego, CA: Academic Press, 2018; pp. 786–789.

Helman RG, Edwards WC. Clinical features of blister beetle poisoning in equids: 70 cases (1983–1996). J Am Vet Med Assoc 1997; 211:1018–1021.
Holbrook TC. Treating cantharidin toxicosis. Comp Equine Contin Educ Vet 2009; 4:353–357.
Stair EL, Plumlee KH. Insects, blister beetles. In: Plumlee KH, ed. Clinical Veterinary Toxicology. St Louis, MO: Mosby, 2004; pp. 101–103.

Author: Christie Ward, DVM, MVSc, PhD, DACVIM
Consulting Editor: Lynn R. Hovda, RPh, DVM, MS, DACVIM

Chapter 87

Snakes – Crotalids (Pit Vipers)

DEFINITION/OVERVIEW

- Pit vipers are a subfamily of vipers with over 200 species including rattlesnakes, cottonmouths (water moccasins), and copperheads.
- Of the pit vipers, rattlesnakes make up the majority of reports of equine envenomation with reported cases having a mortality rate between 9% and 25% (see Figs 87.1–87.3).
- However, many horses are likely bitten by rattlesnakes and show only mild signs that are never reported to a veterinarian.

ETIOLOGY/PATHOPHYSIOLOGY

- In North America, rattlesnake bites are primarily reported between March and October and are an unlikely cause of observed clinical signs outside of this time period.
- The bites have been described in horses housed outside in paddock/pasture but have also occurred while being ridden on the trail.
- In areas where rattlesnakes are endemic, practicing equine veterinarians may see multiple cases per month.

Mechanism of Action

- Rattlesnake venom contains numerous enzymes, proteins, and polypeptides that can result in coagulopathy, neurotoxicity, and tissue necrosis.
- Envenomation causes a release of inflammatory mediators that can have effects on multiple organ systems.
- The components of venom and the associated toxicity tend to vary between the subspecies of rattlesnake.

Systems Affected

- Respiratory – the majority of rattlesnake bites take place on the face and can result in extreme swelling that obstructs the upper airway. Respiratory distress or even death may occur. Less commonly, an aspiration pneumonia has also been observed that is likely due to problems with swallowing water or feed following envenomation.
- Hematological – severe thrombocytopenia as well as prolongation of clotting times are common findings following rattlesnake envenomation. In severe cases, animals may

---

Blackwell's Five-Minute Veterinary Consult Clinical Companion: Equine Toxicology,
First Edition. Edited by Lynn R. Hovda, Dionne Benson, and Robert H. Poppenga.
© 2022 John Wiley & Sons, Inc. Published 2022 by John Wiley & Sons, Inc.
Companion website: www.wiley.com/go/hovda/equine

have spontaneous bleeding from the nose or around the eyes. If bleeding is severe, a moderate to marked anemia may be present.
- Musculoskeletal – in cases where the bite occurs on the leg, severe lameness may be present. Swelling may extend from the foot up the entire leg. Some horses may be reluctant to walk, which can make transport to a veterinary hospital challenging.
- Cardiovascular – myocardial damage has been reported in horses with rattlesnake envenomation. Up to 70% of horses may have a cardiac arrhythmia following rattlesnake envenomation. The degree of myocardial involvement may depend on the species or subspecies of snake.

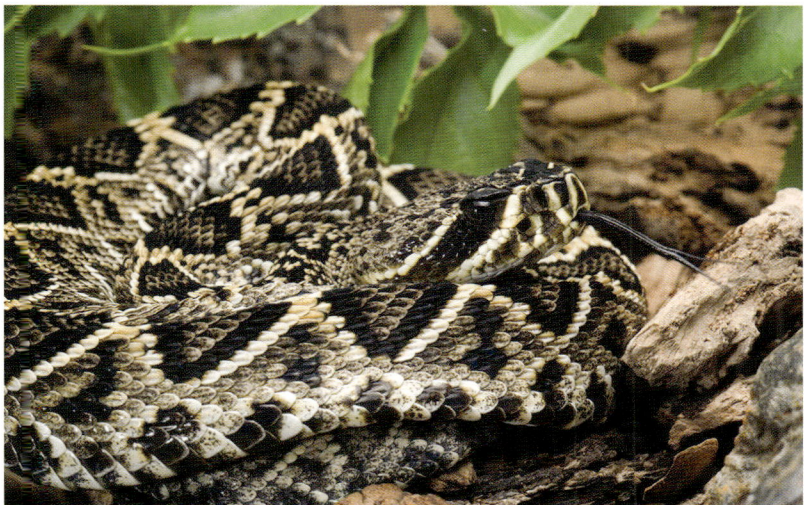

■ Fig. 87.1 Eastern diamondback rattlesnake (*Crotalus adamanteus*). *Source*: Photo courtesy of Barney Oldfield.

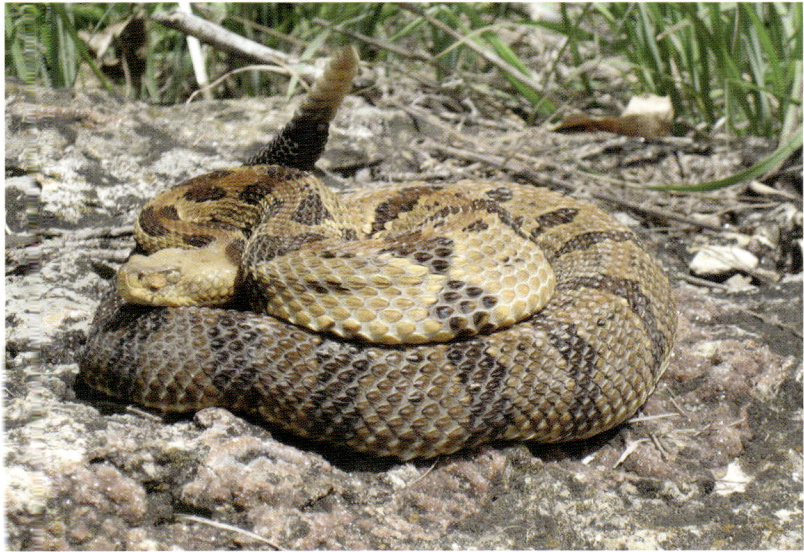

■ Fig. 87.2. Timber rattlesnake (*Crotalus horridus*). *Source*: Photo courtesy of Trevor Keyler.

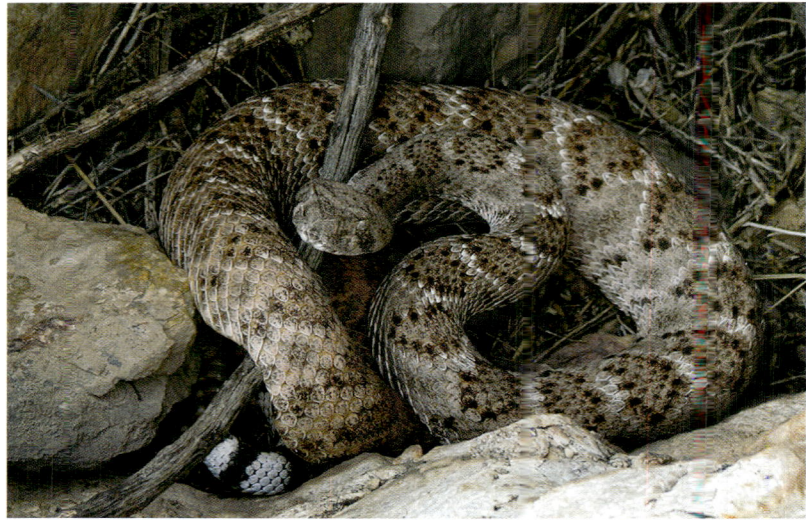

■ **Fig. 87.3.** Western diamondback rattlesnake (*Crotalus atrox*). *Source*: Photo courtesy of Dan Keyler.

- Integument (skin) – swelling, pain, and skin discoloration are common. The fang marks can often be identified but are not always evident. Regions of tissue necrosis are possible but not present in all cases.
- Nervous system – neurologic deficits have been observed following rattlesnake bites and have included facial nerve paralysis, ataxia, and bladder dysfunction. However, many cases of envenomation do not have any evidence of neurologic abnormalities.

 ## SIGNALMENT/HISTORY

Horses of any age, sex, or breed can be bitten by rattlesnakes. However, miniature horses appear to present more commonly for veterinary treatment and may have more severe clinical signs.

History/Location

- In a small number of cases, the bite is observed, but most commonly the horse is found with rapidly progressive swelling.
- Typically, the owners of the animal have reported seeing snakes in the area prior to the incident.

 ## CLINICAL FEATURES

- The most common clinical finding in horses following rattlesnake envenomation is the acute onset of swelling on the muzzle (see Fig. 87.4). Less commonly the swelling may be present on the leg. If the head is involved, loud breathing sounds affecting inspiration

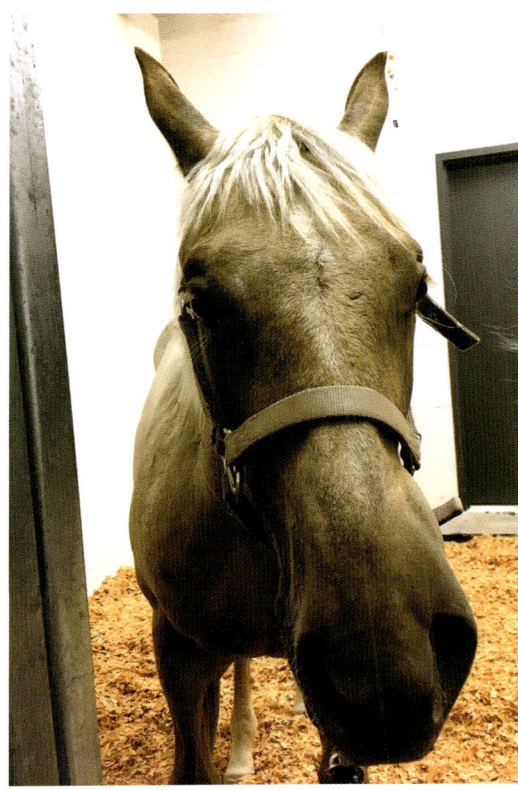

■ **Fg. 87.4** Rattlesnake bite to nose and muzzle with diffuse swelling. *Source*: Photo courtesy of Langdon Fielding.

and/or expiration will be present. Depending on the degree of respiratory obstruction, the animal may appear distressed (see Fig. 87.5).
- Careful examination of the swelling will often reveal two small puncture wounds which support the diagnosis of rattlesnake bite. In some cases, bleeding may be observed from the nose or bite wound.

 DIFFERENTIAL DIAGNOSIS

- Other causes of acute onset of swelling include local infections, allergic reactions, and heart failure. Local infections and allergic reactions can often have a similar appearance, with focal pain over the swelling and respiratory obstruction if the condition is severe.

 DIAGNOSTICS

- While laboratory tests exist to detect the presence of some types of snake venom, a test for rattlesnake venom is not readily available in clinical practice.
- The clinical signs, time of year, geographical location (endemic area for rattlesnakes), and the presence of prolonged clotting times and/or decreased platelet counts can all support the diagnosis.

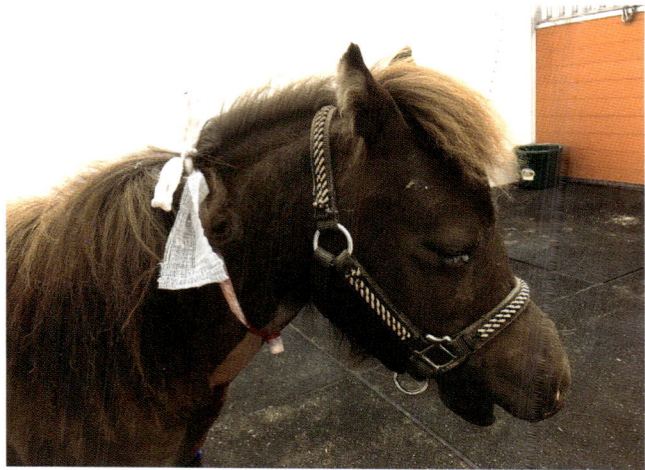

■ **Fig. 87.5.** Horse in respiratory distress after snakebite. Note the tracheotomy tube. *Source*: Photo courtesy of Langdon Fielding.

CBC/Biochemistry/Urinalysis

- Mild-to-moderate anemia.
- CK may be elevated.
- Hemoglobinuria or myoglobinuria secondary to rhabdomyolysis.

Other Diagnostic Tests

- Thrombocytopenia.
- Prolongation in clotting times.
- Elevated cTnI.

Diagnostic imaging

- Not usually required, but ultrasound can be used to help evaluate the swelling for the presence of an abscess.

 THERAPEUTICS

- The two cornerstones of treatment are:
  - Protect the airway:
    - A tracheotomy can be performed in the standing horse which can be life-saving for many patients with snake bite. However, some horses can be difficult to handle if they are in extreme distress and heavy sedation can make the situation more dangerous. If the horse collapses, it may be necessary to anesthetize the horse and quickly perform the tracheotomy. Complications following tracheotomy are uncommon and the procedure is essential if the animal is unable to breathe.
    - In some cases, if the swelling has not progressed, a piece of plastic tubing can be inserted into one or both nostrils to help protect the airway as further swelling develops. The tubing must be long enough to extend past the

swollen tissue into the pharynx. Many horses will not allow the tubing to be placed due to the discomfort of the procedure. Horse owners may attempt this procedure while waiting for veterinary help to arrive. Securing the tubing in place can also be challenging and the tubing may become displaced during transport to a veterinary hospital.
- Administer antivenin as needed to mitigate clinical and laboratory derangements:
  □ The use of equine-derived antivenin has been described in horses and appears to be effective in stopping the progression of swelling as well as improving platelet counts and clotting times.
  □ Antivenin (Crotalidae) Polyvalent, IgG (equine) – Boehringer-Ingelheim. Administration of one vial may be adequate for many cases, but three or more vials may be required in more severe envenomations.
  □ Rattler Antivenin (Crotalidae), Polyvalent, Equine Origin – Mg Biologics. 50 mL; do not dilute.
  □ A recombinant product is available but use in horses is not well described.

Appropriate Health Care

- If swelling from the bite is severe, IV fluids may be needed to maintain hydration while the swelling subsides. Fluids can be supplemented with dextrose at a rate of 1 mg/kg/min if the animal is unable to eat for a prolonged period of time
- The use of broad-spectrum antibiotics has been described as a treatment for snakebite in horses but may not be needed in uncomplicated cases.

Antidotes

- See "Antivenin" above (see also Chapter 4).

Drugs of Choice

- NSAID such as flunixin meglumine (1 mg/kg IV or PO BID) is often given for the first few days following a bite.

Precautions/Interactions

- Corticosteroids should be avoided.
- There is also little evidence that antihistamines are effective in reducing the swelling or pain associated with the bite.
- Verify the tetanus vaccination status of the animal.

 COMMENTS

Client Education

- Clients should be educated about the risk of airway obstruction following a snakebite. They should seek veterinary care immediately if the bite takes place on the face and the airway is being compromised. Waiting too long to seek veterinary care can result in the death of the animal.
- A rattlesnake vaccine is available, but clients should still seek veterinary attention for a horse bitten by a rattlesnake, regardless of vaccination status.

Patient Monitoring

- Monitoring of the clinical signs, platelet count, and clotting times can be useful after each dose of antivenom.
- If improvement is not noticed within 4 hours of administration, an additional vial of antivenom should be considered.

Possible Complications

- Long-term cardiac complications and neurologic deficits have been reported with some patients.
- However, many animals return to normal without long-term abnormalities.

Expected Course and Prognosis

- With the protection of the airway and the administration of antivenom, the prognosis is considered excellent. Swelling typically subsides over 48–72 hours.
- Supportive care is needed until the animal can eat and drink an adequate amount without assistance.

Abbreviations

See Appendix 1 for a complete list.

Suggested Reading

Dickinson CE, Traub-Dargatz JL, Dargatz DA, et al. 1996. Rattlesnake venom poisoning in horses: 32 cases (1973–1993). J Am Vet Med Assoc 1996; 208:1866–1871.

Fielding CL, Pusterla N, Magdesian KG, et al. 2011. Rattlesnake envenomation in horses: 53 cases (1992–2009). J Am Vet Med Assoc 2011; 238:631–635.

Gilliam LL, Holbrook TC, Ownby CL, et al. Cardiotoxicity, inflammation, and immune response after rattlesnake envenomation in the horse. J Vet Intern Med 2012; 26:1457–1463.

Lawler JB, Frye MA, Bera MM, et al. 2008. Third-degree atrioventricular block in a horse secondary to rattlesnake envenomation. J Vet Intern Med 2008; 22:486–490.

Author: Langdon Fielding, DVM, MBA, DACVECC, DACVSMR
Consulting Editor: Lynn R. Hovda, RPh, DVM, MS, DACVIM

Snakes – Elapids (Coral Snakes)

Chapter 88

DEFINITION/OVERVIEW

- Elapidae family – frontal maxillary fixed fangs.
- Snakes use a chewing motion to inject venom.
- Reclusive, non-aggressive snake; bites usually occur secondary to harassment.
- Reports of equine envenomation from coral snakes are very rare. Typically, coral snakes with their small mouth size do not pose a problem for adult horses. Foals, weanlings, and miniature horses would be more susceptible.
- Anecdotally, bites to the tongue, lips, and the soft tissue around the mouth are the most common areas associated with envenomation.
- Two genera in the United States (*Micrurus* and *Micruroides*).
- North American coral snakes – three species range across the southern USA:
  - Eastern coral snake (*Micrurus fulvius*) (see Fig. 88.1):
    - Florida, Georgia, Alabama, Mississippi, North and South Carolina, and Louisiana (frequently associated with border wetlands).
  - Texas coral snake (*Micrurus tener*) (see Fig. 88.2):
    - Texas, Louisiana (western), and Arkansas (southern).
  - Arizona coral snake (*Micruroides euryxanthus*) (see Fig. 88.3):
    - Arizona and southwestern New Mexico.
- Bright, glossy-colored snake with a black head followed by fully encircling bands of yellow (caution) and red (danger). The yellow and red bands will be touching each other; black bands do not make contact with red bands.
- Same sequence for Arizona coral snake except the colors red, white, and black (or very, very dark bluish).
- Coral snakes are often confused with several non-venomous species that have overlapping geographic distribution ranges with the eastern and Texas coral snakes.
- Several "look-alike" species exist. Eastern and Texas coral snakes are similarly colored to the scarlet kingsnake (*Lampropeltis elapsoides*) and scarlet snake (*Cemopohora coccinea*) except the yellow bands do not touch the red bands. In the western USA the longnose snake (*Rhinocheilus leconti*) and Sonoran mountain kingsnake (*Lampropeltis pyromelana*) have been confused with the Arizona/Sonoran coral snake.
- Veterinarians are encouraged to know the differences in coloration so they can assist with accurate identification.

Blackwell's Five-Minute Veterinary Consult Clinical Companion: Equine Toxicology,
First Edition. Edited by Lynn R. Hovda, Dionne Benson, and Robert H. Poppenga.
© 2022 John Wiley & Sons, Inc. Published 2022 by John Wiley & Sons, Inc.
Companion website: www.wiley.com/go/hovda/equine

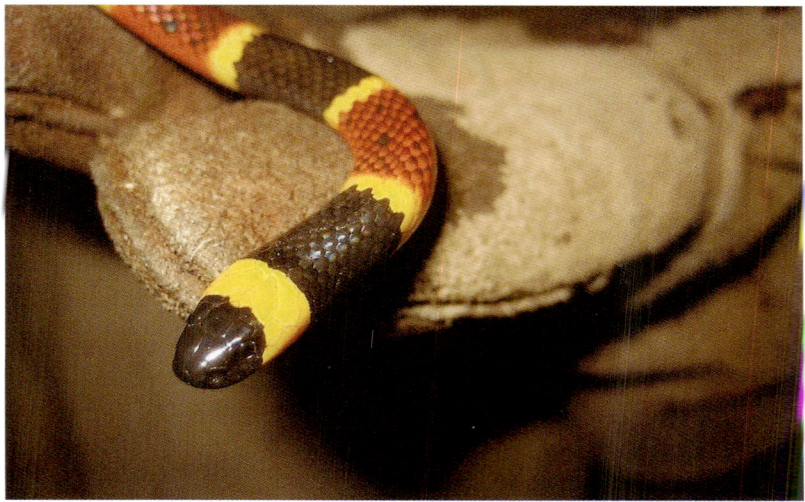

■ **Fig. 88.1.** Eastern coral snake (*Micrurus fulvius*); red and yellow bands touch each other; head is small with a black snout. *Source*: Photo courtesy of David Seerveld, AAAnimal Control, Orlando.

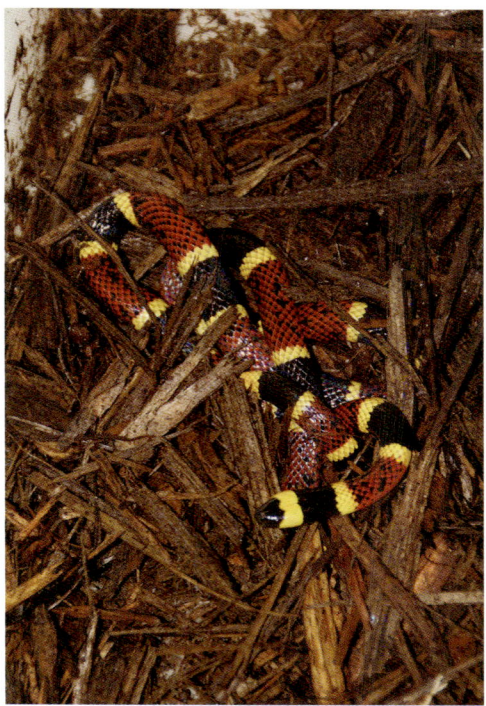

■ **Fig. 88.2.** Texas coral snake (*Micrurus tener*); red bands have more speckling as compared with the Eastern coral snake. *Source*: Photo courtesy of Dan Keyler.

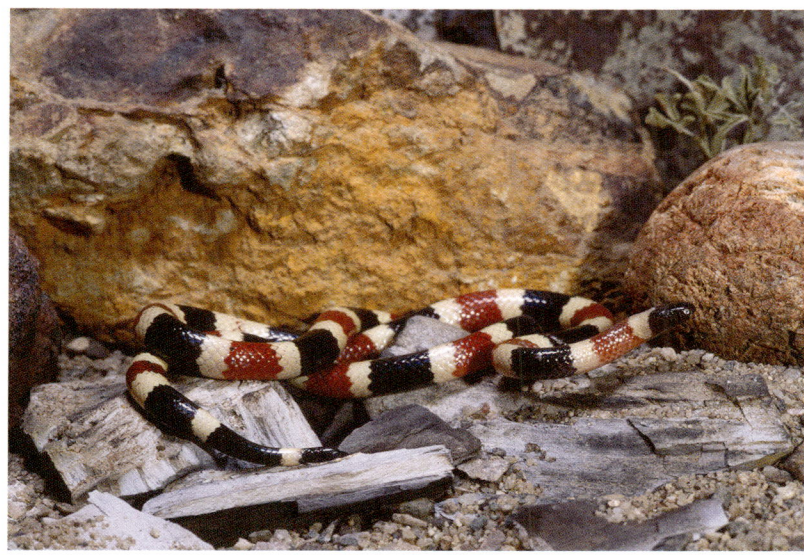

■ **Fig. 88.3.** Arizona coral snake (*Micruroides euryxanthus*); red and white bands touch each other; head is small with a black snout. *Source*: Photo courtesy of Barney Oldfield.

 # ETIOLOGY/PATHOPHYSIOLOGY

- Coral snakes are usually timid and non-aggressive in nature.
- Small, fixed fangs and need to "chew" or hold onto tissue when injecting venom.
- Bite wounds in horses primarily soft tissue – lips, tongue, nose. Typical picture is that of a coral snake hanging onto the lips or tongue while the horse is swinging its head from side to side to dislodge the snake.
- Fang marks may or may not be present, or bites may appear as scratches.

Mechanism of Action

- Pre- and postsynaptic neurotoxic venom components block nicotinic acetylcholine receptors at neuromuscular junctions.
- Cardiotoxicity due to venom's antagonism of acetylcholine receptors.
- Venous injection of the venom causes dramatic hypotension.

Toxicokinetics

- Onset of clinical signs may be delayed for 12–18 hours.
- Duration of clinical signs may be up to 14 days.

Toxicity

- Bites in horses are rare due to the coral snake's small mouth size and non-aggressive nature.
- Eastern coral envenomations are typically more severe and neurological than those of the Texas coral snake.
- Arizona coral snake bites are very rare in all species, including horses.

Systems Affected

- Neuromuscular – muscle fiber depolarization.
- Respiratory – depression.
- Cardiovascular – primarily related to venom interacting with muscarinic receptors on vasculature.

SIGNALMENT/HISTORY

- No specific breed, age, or species predilection. Foals and miniature horses are more susceptible due to smaller body size/amount of venom injected and inquisitive nature.

Risk Factors

- Size of animal – foals and miniature horses.
- Species and size of snake.
- Amount of venom injected, especially as it relates to body size.
- The longer the snake is attached with the bite, the greater the degree of envenoming.

Historical Findings

- May see snake still attached to soft tissue of horse's tongue or mouth area.
- May see snake stomped on and found dead in stalls, paddocks, or pastures.

Location and Circumstances of Poisoning

- South central and southeastern USA where coral snakes are located.
- Typically, coral snakes are non-aggressive but will bite when disturbed.

CLINICAL FEATURES

- Anecdotal
- Vary depending on size of horse and coral snake and amount of venom injected/size of horse, and duration of bite attachment.
- Typically, no local swelling or discoloration at bite site.
- CNS depression, potentially decreased spinal reflexes, altered balance and potential ataxia.
- Respiratory depression – usual cause of death.
- ± hypotension and cardiac effects.

DIFFERENTIAL DIAGNOSIS

- Trauma.
- Puncture wounds.
- Black widow spider envenomation (respiratory distress).

DIAGNOSTICS

- Examine the potentially bitten area thoroughly to look for even the slightest scratch or tissue insult. There have been cases of coral snake envenomation without visible fang or tooth punctures. There may be minimal swelling with no discoloration.
- Look for pin-prick marks on the lips, tongues, and other soft tissue areas of animals as coral snakes have short needle-like fangs, and bites may also appear like scratches on the lips, tongue, and even the ears.
- If the snake bites a horse, it will tend to hang on; the snake has a chewing nature with its bite – the fangs can get hung-up in soft tissue.
- Confirm the snake identity – check if bite was witnessed, look at the dead snake, or take a photo of the snake.

CBC/Serum Chemistry/Urinalysis

- = elevated CK and AST.
- = hemoglobinuria, myoglobinuria.

THERAPEUTICS

Detoxification

- Clip and clean bite with soap and water as soon as possible.

Appropriate Health Care

- Foals and miniature horse with witnessed envenomations will need to be hospitalized for at least 48 hours.
- Most of these bites are in the soft tissue around the tongue, mouth, or nose so monitor these areas for swelling.
- Keep the patient quiet and calm.
- Treat signs/symptoms as they develop.
- Monitor for respiratory depression and cardiac abnormalities.
- Severely envenomated horse may require intubation.
- IV fluids as needed for dehydration and renal perfusion.
- Broad-spectrum antibiotics not usually needed and should only be used if local tissue damage with infection has occurred.

Antidotes (see Chapter 4)

- Use only to treat systemic effects (cardiovascular and neurological signs).
- North American Coral Snake Antivenin (LLC [subsidiary of Pfizer Inc.] has a new product, Lot Y 03625 [3-year shelf life]) available. Product is prescription only. Contact for new in-date antivenin: [844] 646-4398). However, cost is considerable, and as such veterinary use may be difficult.
- Mexican, Costa Rican, and Australian antivenoms have been shown to be effective in neutralizing North American coral snake venoms. (Coralmyn™, Instituto Bioclon,

Mexico; and Anticoral antivenom, Instituto Clodomiro Picado, Costa Rica; Australian ANG Polyvalent Snake Antivenom [CSL Limited, Australia]). These antivenoms may be available through some zoos or by contacting a regional poison center with Antivenom Index access.
- Neostigmine (acetylcholinesterase inhibitor) has been used in animals and humans to successfully reverse *Micrurus* venom-induced cholinesterase actions. In the absence of antivenom this may be considered for rescue and short-term use.

Drugs of Choice

- NSAIDS for inflammation and pain control:
  - Flunixin 1.1 mg/kg IV or PO q12–24h.
  - Phenylbutazone 2.2–4.4 mg/kg IV or PO q12–24h.
  - Ketoprofen 2.2 mg/kg IV q24h.
- Butorphanol for severe pain 0.05–0.1 mg/kg IV q3–4h

Precautions/Interactions

- Be prepared if antivenom used:
  - Anaphylaxis – treat with fluids and epinephrine.
  - Anaphylactoid reactions – treat by stopping the antivenom administration, administering diphenhydramine, waiting 5 minutes, then resuming the antivenom administration more slowly.
  - Serum sickness may occur 1–4 weeks after infusion and may be treated with corticosteroids and antihistamines.

 COMMENTS

Client Education

- Accurate identification of snake is vitally important as there are several "look-alike" snakes that may bite but are not venomous. Photos of the snake are useful.

Expected Course and Prognosis

- Good with early intervention.
- Marked signs may last for up to 14 days with several months needed for a full recovery.

Abbreviations

See Appendix 1 for a complete list.

Suggested Reading

Brazil OV. Coral snake venoms; mode of action and pathophysiology of experimental envenomation. Rev Inst Med, Trop Sao Paulo 1987; 29:199–126.
McAninch SA, Morrissey RP, Rosen P, et al. Snake eyes: coral snake neurotoxicity associated with ocular absorption of venom and successful treatment with exotic antivenom. J Emerg Med 2019; 56:519–522.
Morgan DL et al. Texas coral snake (*Micrurus tener*) bites. Southern Med J 2007; 100:152–156.

Sanchez EE, et al. Neutralization of two North American coral snake venoms with United States and Mexican Antivenoms. Toxicon 2008; 51:297–303.

Vital Brazil, Vieira RJ. Neostigmine in the treatment of snake accidents caused by *Micrurus frontinalis*: report of two cases. Rev Inst Med Trop Sao Paulo 1996; 38:61–67.

Tang DC, Dobson J, Chochran C, et al. The bold and the beautiful: a neurotoxicity comparison of new world coral snakes in the *Micruroides* and *Micrurus* genera and relative neutralization by antivenom. Neurotox Res 2017; 32:487–495.

Authors: Daniel E. Keyler, BS, PharmD, FAACT; Lynn R. Hovda, RPh, DVM, MS, DACVIM
Consulting Editor: Lynn R. Hovda, RPh, DVM, MS, DACVIM

Chapter 89

Spiders – Brown Recluse and Black Widow

DEFINITION/OVERVIEW

- The two most common venomous spiders native in the USA are the brown recluse (*Loxosceles reclusa* and 11 *Loxosceles* spp., and two non-native species), and black widow spiders (*Latrodectus mactans* and four other *Latrodectus* spp., and a single non-native species, *L. geometricus*).
- Brown recluse spiders, also known as the fiddleback or violin spiders, are brown with a dark brown violin shape on their back (cephalothorax). They have delicate legs that span 2–3 cm as adults. A unique feature for identifying *Loxosceles* spp. is their three pairs of eyes (dyads) for a total of six eyes, which is in contrast to other spider species that have eight eyes. They are nocturnal and are often found in undisturbed areas of barns and closets in the southwest and south central regions of the USA (see Fig. 89.1).
- Black widow spiders (females mostly responsible for envenomation and much larger than males) are glossy black (or brown) with a red hourglass or other red shape on the ventral abdomen. They prefer to live outside under old woodpiles or in dark places, and geographically range across the USA. Their adult leg span is approximately 2–2.5 cm (see Fig. 89.2).
- Diagnosis (in the absence of having the offending spider) is difficult because of a lack of specific biomarkers.
- Toxicosis is uncommon in horses. Bites from brown recluse spiders tend to be in folds of the axilla or groin. Those of the black widow spider can occur anywhere on the body.

ETIOLOGY/PATHOPHYSIOLOGY

Mechanism of Action

- Brown recluse (*Loxosceles* spp.):
  - Venom is a mixture of cytotoxic enzymes, proteases and phospholipases that induce local and systemic signs.
  - Sphingomyelinase D in the venom causes platelet aggregation, and other effects inducing inflammation, leading to dermonecrosis.
  - Interspecies venom variability can influence the degree of severity of dermonecrotic lesions.

Blackwell's Five-Minute Veterinary Consult Clinical Companion: Equine Toxicology,
First Edition. Edited by Lynn R. Hovda, Dionne Benson, and Robert H. Poppenga.
© 2022 John Wiley & Sons, Inc. Published 2022 by John Wiley & Sons, Inc.
Companion website: www.wiley.com/go/hovda/equine

CHAPTER 89   SPIDERS – BROWN RECLUSE AND BLACK WIDOW   **475**

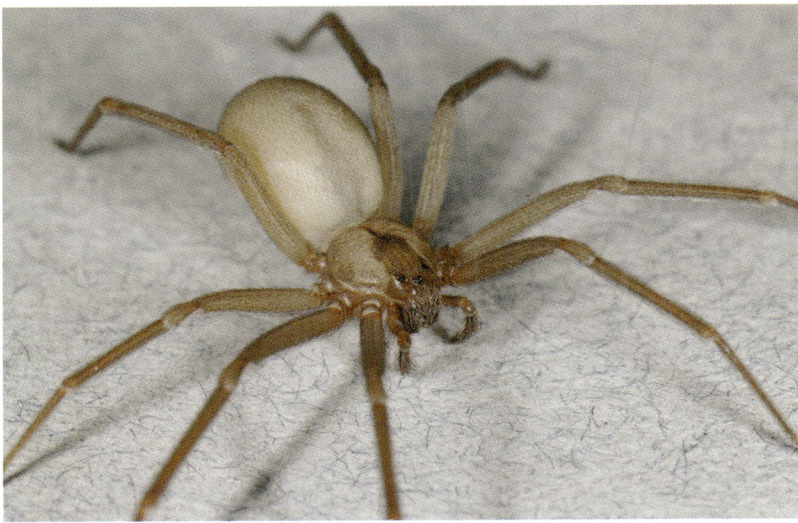

■ **Fig. 89.1.** Brown recluse spider (*Loxosceles reclusa*). Note the violin mark on the dorsal cephalothorax. It is often poorly demarcated in immature spiders or other species. *Source*: Photo courtesy of Richard Vetter, Department of Entomology, University of California.

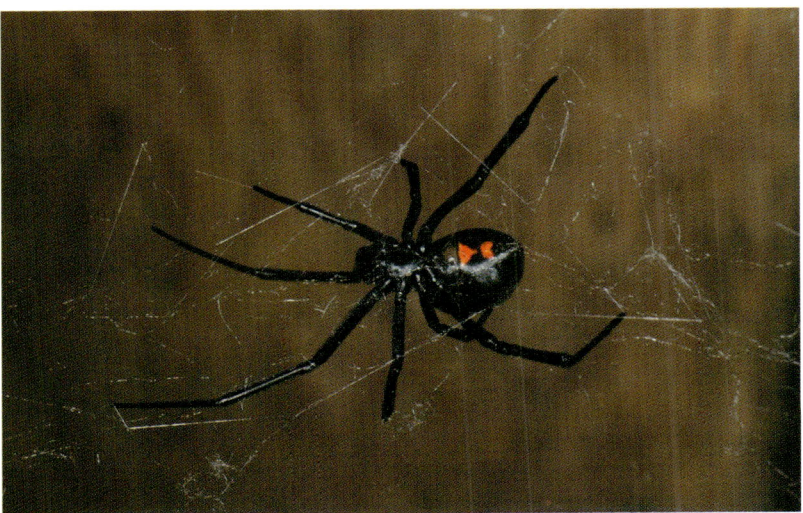

■ **Fig. 89.2.** Black widow spider (*Latrodectus* spp.). *Source*: Photo courtesy of Richard Vetter, Department of Entomology, University of California.

- Black widow (*Latrodectus* spp.):
    - Venom contains neuroactive proteins and proteolytic enzymes and is neurotoxic.
    - The principal toxin is α-latrotoxin, which causes an initial large release of acetylcholine and norepinephrine at postganglionic sympathetic synapses followed by depletion of the neurotransmitters.

Toxicokinetics

- Brown recluse (*Loxosceles* spp.) spider:
  - Rapid symptom onset; dermonecrotic signs develop within 15 minutes to 8 hours of envenomation.
  - Systemic signs within 72 hours.
  - Tissue around bite wound may slough after 3–5 weeks.
- Black widow (*Latrodectus* spp.) spider:
  - Rapid symptom onset with pain at the bite site within 30 minutes to 2 hours.
  - Muscle cramping in 2–3 hours.
  - Acute signs resolve in 1–2 days but lethargy and weakness may continue for weeks.

Toxicity

- Brown recluse (*Loxosceles* spp.) spider:
  - Varies from species to species and individual horse to individual horse.
  - Bites to fatty areas are more severe.
  - Very little scientific data available in the horse. Anecdotally, a classic clinical sign of envenomation observed is an erythematous to violaceous lesion (bull's eye lesion, eschar, deep ulcer).
  - Tissue necrosis at the site of the bite is caused by ischemia due to coagulation and occlusion of local circulation.
- Black widow (*Latrodectus* spp.) spider:
  - Very little scientific data available in the horse.
  - Only the female black widow spider has fangs long enough to penetrate horse skin.
  - As observed in other animal species, agitation, muscle pain, spasms, and rigidity, tachypnea, tachycardia, and potential cardiotoxicity should be anticipated.

Systems Affected

- Brown recluse (*Loxosceles* spp.) spider:
  - Integument – little initial pain with localized swelling, pruritus, later mild-to-moderate pain with target lesion characterized by scabbing and ulceration with eschar formation and very slow healing.
  - Hemic/lymph/immune – hemolytic anemia, thrombocytopenia, prolonged coagulation.
  - Hepatobiliary.
  - Renal.
  - Endocrine – increased body temperature.
  - Gastrointestinal.
- Black widow (*Latrodectus* spp.) spider:
  - Musculoskeletal – muscle pain and cramping.
  - Nervous – tremors, seizures.
  - Respiratory.
  - Gastrointestinal – colic.

 # SIGNALMENT/HISTORY

- Brown recluse (*Loxosceles* spp.) spider:
  - No sex, breed, or gender predilection.

- Black widow (*Latrodectus* spp.) spider:
  - No sex, breed, or age predilection, although the small body weight of neonates and foals and miniature horses would allow more toxin/kg than a mature horse.

Risk Factors

- Brown recluse (*Loxosceles* spp.) spider:
  - Presence in environment.
- Black widow (*Latrodectus* spp.) spider:
  - Presence in environment.

Historical Findings

- Brown recluse (*Loxosceles* spp.) spider:
  - Diagnosis in horses is based primarily on clinical signs (bull's eye lesion with eschar), direct observation of spider, and geographical location (southwest and southern USA).
- Black widow (*Latrodectus* spp.) spider:
  - Some owners have reported seeing spiders in the barn or stalls. Direct observation of spider.

Location and Circumstances of Poisoning

- Brown recluse (*Loxosceles* spp.) spider:
  - Shy, nocturnal spider that lies in dark areas under leaves, rocks, and other areas. In barns, it hides under piles of horse blankets, behind boards, towels, and other clothing.
  - Many modern barns have problems with brown recluse spider infestation.
- Black widow (*Latrodectus* spp.) spider:
  - Shy spider found outside under leaves and old hay piles. In barns it hides in corners of stalls and under storage cabinets. Webs with female are often made in window areas.

CLINICAL FEATURES

- Brown recluse (*Loxosceles* spp.) spider:
  - Two distinct forms (at least in humans):
    - Local (dermonecrotic) – bite wound begins as edema and erythema, slowly becoming necrotic. Eschar forms with a deep ulcer and tissue sloughing that takes weeks to heal. Secondary infections may occur.
    - Systemic – uncommon. Severe hemolytic anemia with coagulation abnormalities and thrombocytopenia. Hypotension, fever, renal failure.
- Black widow (*Latrodectus* spp.) spider:
  - Most sensitive to *L. mactans* or *L. hesperus*.
  - Muscle tremors, spasms, cramping, and rigidity are major presentations.
  - Flaccid paralysis progressing to ascending paralysis possible.
  - Ataxia.
  - Agitation, seizures.

- Colic.
- Dyspnea possible.
- Cardiotoxicity (rare).

DIFFERENTIAL DIAGNOSIS

- Diagnosis of spider bite is usually presumptive and based on clinical presentation, recent activity in geographical areas where the spider is known to occur, circumstance of the apparent bite (ie. spiders are observed on the stable floor at night, and bites to the head and neck may have occurred while down and sleeping), visualization of small puncta at the apparent bite site, or actual identification of the responsible spider.
- Brown recluse (*Loxosceles* spp.):
  - Puncture injury, trauma.
  - Hemolytic anemia.
  - Chemical burns.
  - Immune-mediated disease.
  - Infectious – fungal, parasitic, bacterial, viral.
  - Lyme disease.
  - Exudative dermatitis.
  - Neoplasia.
  - Vascular disease.
  - Venomous snakebite (rattlesnake, copperhead, and cottonmouth species).
- Black widow (*Latrodectus* spp.) spider:
  - Trauma or injury.
  - Tremorgenic mycotoxin.
  - Acute abdomen.
  - Scorpion sting.
  - Bee and hornet stings.
  - Venomous snakebite (coral snakes).
  - Pesticide toxicity (organophosphate).

DIAGNOSTICS

CBC/Serum Chemistry/Urinalysis

- Brown recluse (*Loxosceles* spp.) spider:
  - CBC/serum chemistry may show evidence of a Coomb's negative hemolytic anemia.
  - Hemolytic anemia with hemoglobinuria.
  - BUN.
  - PT.
  - Serum creatinine.
- Black widow (*Latrodectus* spp.) spider:
  - Elevated CK.

Pathological Findings

- Brown recluse (*Loxosceles* spp.) spider:
  - Tissue necrosis and ulceration resulting in targetoid lesions is the primary lesion (sore to touch).
  - May have evidence of secondary infection.
- Black widow (*Latrodectus* spp.) spider:
  - Swelling, erythema and bullseye lesion around the bite may be the only pathology noted.

THERAPEUTICS

Detoxification

- Brown recluse (*Loxosceles* spp.) spider:
  - None other than good wound care.
- Black widow (*Latrodectus* spp.) spider:
  - None.

Appropriate Health Care

- Brown recluse (*Loxosceles* spp.) spider:
  - Clean bite area well with soap or dilute chlorhexidine and water.
  - Cool compresses as needed, no heat.
  - Meticulous daily wound care.
  - IV crystalloids as needed for dehydration.
  - Blood products as needed.
  - Monitored at least twice a day to determine severity and presence of secondary complications.
  - Antibiotics if there is evidence of secondary infection (not needed prophylactically).
- Black widow (*Latrodectus* spp.) spider:
  - Supportive care.
  - Symptomatic treatment.
  - Judicious used of IV crystalloids, especially if CK is elevated.

Antidotes

- Brown recluse (*Loxosceles* spp.) spider:
  - No specific antidote or antivenom is available.
- Black widow (*Latrodectus* spp.) spider:
  - Antivenin (*Latrodectus mactans*) (Black Widow Spider Antivenin, Equine Origin) – is a biologic drug for use in humans; there is no scientific information on the use in horses. A single 2.5 mL vial diluted to 100 mL and administered IV may be successful in reversing signs (in humans signs begin to subside in 1–2 hours).

Drugs of Choice

- Brown recluse (*Loxosceles* spp.) spider:

- NSAID S for inflammation and pain control
    - Phenylbutazone 2.2–4.4 mg/kg IV or PO q12–24h.
    - Flunixin meglumine 1.1 mg/kg IV or PO q12–24h.
  - Butorphanol for severe pain:
    - 0.05–0.1 mg/kg IV q3–4h.
  - Omeprazole 4 mg/kg PO q24h for GI distress.
  - Broad-spectrum antibiotics should wound become infected.
- Black widow (*Latrodectus* spp.) spider:
  - NSAIDS for inflammation and pain control
    - Phenylbutazone 2.2–4.4 mg/kg IV or PO q12–24h.
    - Flunixin meglumine 1.1 mg/kg IV or PO q12–24h.
  - Butorphanol for severe pain:
    - 0.05–0.1 mg/kg IV q3–4h.
  - Omeprazole 4 mg/kg PO q24h for GI distress.
  - Methocarbamol for muscle tremors and rigidity:
    - 4.4–22 mg/kg IV or PO prn.
    - Diazepam 25–50 mg IV prn (adult horse).

Precautions/Interactions

- Brown recluse (*Loxosceles* spp.) spider:
  - Avoid the use of heat as this may exacerbate signs.
- Black widow (*Latrodectus* spp.) spider:
  - Observe the animal closely for signs of anaphylaxis if antivenin is administered.

Surgical Considerations

- Brown recluse (*Loxosceles* spp.) spider:
  - Wound debridement, at least in human medicine, has fallen from favor It may be necessary in horses for non-healing wounds that have developed exuberant granulation tissue.

COMMENTS

Prevention/Avoidance

- Brown recluse (*Loxosceles* spp.) spider – maintain clean pest-free stalls, sheds, outbuildings, and barns. Regular shampooing with appropriate products per direction of equine specialty DVM.
- Black widow (*Latrodectus* spp.) spider – maintain clean pest-free stalls, sheds, outbuildings, and barns. Regular shampooing with appropriate products per direction of equine specialty DVM.

Possible Complications

- Brown recluse (*Loxosceles* spp.) spider:
  - Secondary wound infection may follow brown recluse bites.
  - Secondary renal failure due to hemolytic products.

Expected Course and Prognosis

- Brown recluse (*Loxosceles* spp.) spider:
  - It will likely take several weeks (rarely months) for the bite wound and ulcer to heal, but the prognosis is good if daily wound care is established.
- Black widow (*Latrodectus* spp.) spider:
  - The prognosis for a full recovery is generally good to excellent. Recovery is generally complete within 7–10 days, and potentially as short as 2 hours following antivenom treatment.

Abbreviations

See Appendix 1 for a complete list.

Suggested Reading

Bush SP, Veeran D. Troponin elevation after black widow spider envenomation. Can J Emerg Med 2015; 17:571–575.

Gwaltney–Brant SM, Dunayer EK, Youssef HY. Terrestrial zootoxins. In: Gupta RC, ed. Veterinary Toxicology: Basic and Clinical Principles, 3rd edn. New York: Elsevier 2018; pp. 781–799.

Shackelford R, Veillon D, Maxwell N, et al. The black widow spider bite: differential diagnosis, clinical manifestations, and treatment options. J La State Med Soc 2015; 167:74–78.

Vetter RS. The Brown Recluse Spider. Ithaca NY: Cornell University Press, 2015.

Vetter RS. Clinical consequences of toxic envenomation by spiders. Toxicon 2018; 152:65–70.

Acknowledgment: The authors and editors acknowledge the prior contribution of Wilson Rumbeiha.

Authors: Daniel E. Keyler, BS. PharmD, FAACT; Lynn R. Hovda, RPh, DVM, MS, DACVIM
Consulting Editor: Lynn R. Hovda, RPh, DVM, MS, DACVIM

Reference Information

section 3

appendix 1

Abbreviations

ABG	arterial blood gas
AC	activated charcoal
ACE	angiotensin-converting enzyme
ACEi	angiotensin-converting enzyme inhibitor
AChE	acetylcholinesterase
ACT	activated clotting time
ADH	alcohol dehydrogenase; antidiuretic hormone
ADP	adenosine diphosphate
AKI	acute kidney injury
ALI	acute lung injury
ALP	alkaline phosphatase
AM	atypical myopathy
AMDUCA	Animal Medicinal Drug Use Clarification Act
AMP	adenosine monophosphate
ANS	autonomic nervous system
aPTT	activated partial thromboplastin time
AQHA	American Quarter Horse Association
ARCI	Association of Racing Commissioners International
ARDS	acute respiratory distress syndrome
ARF	acute renal failure
AST	aspartate aminotransferase/transaminase
ATN	acute tubular necrosis
ATP	adenosine triphosphate
AV	atrioventricular
BBB	blood–brain barrier
BE	base excess
BG	blood glucose
BID	twice a day
BMBT	buccal mucosal bleeding time
BoNT	botulism neurotoxin
BP	blood pressures
Bpm	breaths per minute, beats per minute
BSP	bisphosphonates
BUN	blood urea nitrogen
BW	body weight
cAMP	cyclic adenosine monophosphate
CBC	complete blood count
CBD	cannabidiol
CCA	chromated copper arsenate

Blackwell's Five-Minute Veterinary Consult Clinical Companion: Equine Toxicology,
First Edition. Edited by Lynn R. Hovda, Dionne Benson, and Robert H. Poppenga.
© 2022 John Wiley & Sons, Inc. Published 2022 by John Wiley & Sons, Inc.
Companion website: www.wiley.com/go/hovda/equine

CCB	calcium channel blocker
CG	cyanogenic glycosides
cGMP	cyclic guanosine monophosphate
CK	creatine kinase
CNS	central nervous system
CO	carbon monoxide
CO2	carbon dioxide
CoA	coenzyme A
COHb	carboxyhemoglobin
COX	cyclooxygenase
CPK	creatine phosphokinase
CRI	continuous rate infusion
CRT	capillary refill time
CSF	cerebrospinal fluid
cTnI	cardiac troponin I
CV	cardiovascular
CVP	central venous pressure
CYP	cytochrome P450 enzyme
DAP	diastolic arterial pressure
DEA	Drug Enforcement Agency
DHPA	dehydro-pyrrolizidine alkaloids
DIC	disseminated intravascular coagulation
DMSA	2,3-dimercaptosuccinic acid, succimer
DMSO	dimethylsulfoxide
DNA	deoxyribonucleic acid
ECG	electrocardiogram
EDTA	ethylenediaminetetraacetic acid
EEE	Eastern equine encephalitis
EHV-1	equine herpes myeloencephalopathy
ELEM	equine leukoencephalomalacia
ELISA	enzyme-linked immunosorbent assay
EMS	equine metabolic syndrome
EPA	Environmental Protection Agency
EPM	equine protozoal myeloencephalitis
EPS	extrapyramidal syndrome
ETC	electron transport chain
FDA	Food and Drug Administration
FDP	fibrin degradation product
FEI	Federation Equine International
FGAR	first-generation anti-coagulant rodenticides
FOI	freedom of information
GABA	gamma-aminobutyric acid
GC-MS	gas chromatography-mass spectrometry
GFR	glomerular filtration rate
GGT	gamma glutamyl transferase
GH	growth hormone
GI	gastrointestinal
GSH	glutathione
HAB	harmful algal bloom
Hb	hemoglobin
HbO2	oxyhemoglobin
HCN	hydrogen cyanide

HDL	high-density lipoprotein
Hg	mercury
Hgb	hemoglobin
HGE	hemorrhage gastroenteritis
HPLC	high-pressure/performance liquid chromatography
HR	heart rate
HYPP	hyperkalemic periodic paralysis disease
ICP-MS	inductively coupled plasma mass spectrometry
IgG	immuoglobulin G
IM	intramuscular
IP	intraperitoneal
IU	international units
IV	intravenous
K	potassium
LAAC	long-acting anticoagulant
LC_{50}	median lethal concentration
LC-MS	liquid chromatography-mass spectrometry
LD	lethal dose
LD_{50}	median lethal dose
LDH	lactate dehydrogenase
LOX	lipoxygenase
LRS	lactated Ringer's solution
MADD	multiple acyl-CoA dehydrogenase deficiency
MAP	mean arterial pressure
MCPA	methylenecyclopropylacetic acid
Mg	magnesium
MPA	medroxyprogesterone acetate
MRI	magnetic resonance imaging
NE	norepinephrine
NAC	N-acetylcysteine
NG	nasogastric
NPO	nil per os (nothing by mouth)
NSAIDs	non-steroidal anti-inflammatory drugs
O_2	oxygen
OP	organophosphate
PA	pyrrolizidine alkaloid
PaO_2	partial pressure of oxygen
PCDD	dibenzo-p-dioxin isomers
PCDF	dibenzofuran isomers
PCO	pesticide control officer
PCO_2	partial pressure of carbon dioxide
PCP	pentachlorophenol
PCR	polymerase chain reaction
PCV	packed cell volume
PD	polydipsia
$PGE2$	prostaglandin E2
PIVKA	proteins induced by vitamin K antagonism
PLR	pupillary light reflex/response
plt	platelet
PO	per os (by mouth)
ppb	parts per billion
ppm	parts per million

pRBC	packed red blood cells
PRN	pro re nata (as needed)
PT	prothrombin
PTT	partial thromboplastin time
PU	polyuria
q (q24h, q4–6h)	every (every 24 hours, every 4–6 hours)
RBC	red blood cell
RDC	right dorsal colon
RLP	regional limb perfusion
RNA	ribonucleic acid
RR	respiratory rate
Rx	prescription
SA	sinoatrial
SAM-e	S-adenosyl-L-methionine
SaO2	arterial oxyhemoglobin saturation
SAP	systolic arterial pressure
SARMs	selective androgen receptor modulators
SC	subcutaneous
SDH	sorbitol dehydrogenase
SE	serotonin
SERMs	selective estrogen receptor modulators
SGAR	second-generation anticoagulant rodenticides
SI	small intestine
SNARE	soluble n-ethylmaleimide sensitive factor attachment protein receptor
SNRI	serotonin and norepinephrine reuptake inhibitor
SPM	seasonal pasture myopathy
SVT	supraventricular tachycardia
$T_{1/2}$	half-life
T_3	triiodothyronine
T_4	thyroxine
THC	tetrahydrocannabinol
TIBC	total iron-binding capacity
TID	three times a day
TLC	thin-layer chromatography
TP	total protein
TPR	temperature, pulse, respiration
TSH	thyroid-stimulating hormone
UA	urinalysis
µg/kg	microgram/kilogram
UOP	urine output
USEF	United States Equestrian Federation
USG	urine specific gravity
UTI	urinary tract infection
VBP	venous blood gas
VEE	Venezuelan equine encephalitis
VMAT	vesicular monoamine transporter
VPC	ventricular premature complex/contraction
WB	whole blood
WBC	white blood cell
WNV	West Nile virus
WEE	Western equine encephalitis
Zn	zinc

Herbicides

appendix 2

Limited information is available pertaining to herbicide poisoning in horses. The LD_{50} values and clinical effects listed for rabbits and guinea pigs are provided to serve as a basis for comparison as these species are also hindgut fermenters. In the event of exposure, caution should be used in comparing LD_{50} values and clinical effects due to the variation in species sensitivity and toxicokinetics of the listed compounds. The provided table is not all-inclusive and does not contain all herbicide compounds.

Blackwell's Five-Minute Veterinary Consult Clinical Companion: Equine Toxicology, First Edition. Edited by Lynn R. Hovda, Dionne Benson, and Robert H. Poppenga.
© 2022 John Wiley & Sons, Inc. Published 2022 by John Wiley & Sons, Inc.
Companion website: www.wiley.com/go/hovda/equine

Herbicide Class	Compound	Route of Administration	LD50 (mg/kg)	Non-Equine Species	Clinical Signs	Equine Toxic Dose (mg/kg)	Clinical Signs
Acetamides, amides, and anilides							
	Clomeprop	Dermal	> 5000	Rat			
		Oral	> 5000	Rat		Unknown	Unknown
	Dimethenamid-p	Dermal	> 2000	Rabbit	Eye, skin irritation		
	Propanil	Dermal	4830	Rabbit	Eye, skin irritation		
Arsenicals							
	Monosodium methanearsonate	Oral	102	Rabbit	Weakness, diarrhea	1–25 mg/kg	Tremors, ataxia, derpression, colic, diarrhea
Dipyridyls							
	Diquat	Oral	101	Rabbit	Depressed, dyspnea	Unknown	Unknown
		Dermal	> 400	Rabbit			
	Paraquat	Oral	30	Guinea Pig	Anorexia, dyspnea, GI Liver kidney necrosis, lung hemorrhage and fibrosis, death		Dyspnea, lethargy, seizures
		Derrnal	236	Rabbit	Skin irritation		
Carbamates							
	Asulam	Oral	> 2000	Rabbit	Eye irritation		
	Barban	Oral	600	Rabbit			
		Skin	23 000	Rabbit			
		Oral	240	Guinea pig	Skin sensitization		

Herbicide Class	Compound	Route of Administration	LD50 (mg/kg)	Non-Equine Species	Clinical Signs	Equine Toxic Dose (mg/kg)	Clinical Signs
	Chlorbufam	Oral	2380	Rat		Unknown	Unknown
		Dermal		Rabbit	Erythema		
	Chlorpropham	Oral	5000	Rabbit			
		Oral	1200	Rat	Ataxia, hemorrhage		
	Karbutilate	Oral	3000	Rat			
Thiocarbamates							
	Cycloate	Oral	1600	Guinea pig	Depressed activity		
		Dermal	3000	Rabbit	Eye irritation		
Diallate		Dermal	2000	Rabbit	Eye, skin irritation		
		Oral	420	Guinea pig	Eye, skin irritation	Unknown	Unknown
	EPTC	Oral	2640	Rabbit			
		Dermal	1460	Rabbit	Eye irritation		
	Molinate	Dermal	3536	Rabbit	Eye irritation		
	Triallate	Dermal	8200	Rabbit	Eye, skin irritation		
Aromatic/benzoic acids							
	Chloramben	Dermal	> 3160	Rabbit	Eye, skin irritation		
	Dicamba	Dermal	2000	Rabbit	Eye, skin irritation		
		Oral	2000	Rabbit	Eye, skin irritation	Unknown	Unknown
		Oral	3000	Guinea pig	Eye, skin irritation		
	Naptalam	Dermal	2000	Rabbit	Eye, skin irritation		

(Continued)

Herbicide Class	Compound	Route of Administration	LD50 (mg/kg)	Non-Equine Species	Clinical Signs	Equine Toxic Dose (mg/kg)	Clinical Signs
Phenoxy derivatives							
	2,4-D	Dermal	2000	Rabbit	Eye, skin irritation		
		Oral	800	Rabbit			
	2,4-DB	Dermal	10 000	Rabbit			
	Dalapon	Dermal	5000	Rat	Eye, respiratory, skin irritation		
	Dichlorprop	Oral	620	Guinea pig	Muscle spasms, coma		
		Dermal	4500	Rabbit	Eye, skin irritation	Unknown	Unknown
	MCPA	Dermal	> 2000	Rabbit	Erythema, loss of skin elasticity, weight loss Oral		
			700	Guinea pig			
	MCPB	Dermal	> 10 000	Rabbit	MCPB		
	Mecoprop	Dermal	900	Rabbit	Eye, skin irritation		
	Silvex	Dermal	> 3200	Rabbit	Silvex		
Dinitrophenolics							
	Dinoseb	Oral	20	Guinea pig	Convulsions, seizures, respiratory distress		
		Dermal	500	Guinea pig			
		Dermal	80	Rabbit	Eye, skin irritation		
	DNOC	Oral	24.6	Rabbit		Unknown	Unknown
		Oral	24.6	Guinea pig			
		Dermal	1000	Rabbit	Eye, skin irritation, edema, embryotoxic		

Herbicide Class	Compound	Route of Administration	LD50 (mg/kg)	Non-Equine Species	Clinical Signs	Equine Toxic Dose (mg/kg)	Clinical Signs
	2,4-DB	Dermal	10 000	Rabbit			
Organophosphates							
		Dermal		500	Guinea pig		
	Bensulide	Dermal	2000	Rabbit	Eye irritation		
	Glufosinate	Oral	1620	Rat	Convulsions		
	Glyphosate	Oral	3800	Rabbit		Unknown	Unknown
		Dermal	5000	Rabbit	Eye irritation		
Triazolopyrimidines							
	Cloransulam-methyl	Dermal	> 2000	Rabbit	Irritation		
	Florasulam	Dermal	> 2000	Rabbit	Irritation	Unknown	Unknown
	Flumetsulam	Oral	> 5000	Rat	Eye irritation		
		Dermal	> 2000	Rabbit			
Ureas and thioureas							
	Buturon	Oral	1791	Rat	Developmental complications		
		Dermal	> 500	Rabbit			
	Chlorbromuron	Dermal	> 10 000	Rabbit	Skin irritation		
	Chloroxuron	Dermal	> 10 000	Rabbit	Eye, skin irritation		
	Chlortoluron	Oral	5800	Rat	Fetotoxic		
	Diuron	Oral	3400	Rat	Eye irritation		
	Fenuron	Oral	4700	Rabbit			
		Oral	3200	Guinea pig	Structural defects		
	Flumeturon	Oral	2500	Rabbit	Flumeturon		
		Oral	810	Guinea pig	Depression, coma, death		

(Continued)

Herbicide Class	Compound	Route of Administration	LD50 (mg/kg)	Non-Equine Species	Clinical Signs	Equine Toxic Dose (mg/kg)	Clinical Signs
	2,4-DB	Dermal	10 000	Rabbit			
	Linuron	Oral	2250	Rabbit	Eye, skin irritation	Unknown	Unknown
		Dermal	> 5000	Rabbit	Eye, skin irritation		
	Monuron	Oral	670	Guinea pig	Monuron		
		Dermal	> 2500	Rabbit	Dermal		
	Metobromuron	Dermal	> 10 200	Rabbit	Eye, skin irritation		
	Metoxuron	Oral	2300	Rabbit			
	Siduron	Dermal	> 5500	Rabbit	Eye, skin irritation		
	Tebuthiuron	Oral	286	Rabbit	Eye, skin irritation, diarrhea, emaciation		
	Thidiazuron	Oral	7100	Rabbit	Excitement		
		Oral	2813	Guinea pig	Excitement		
Triazines and triazoles							
	Atrazine	Dermal	7500	Rabbit	Eye, skin irritation		
	Ametryn	Dermal	2020	Rabbit	Eye, skin irritation		
	Cyanazine	Dermal	> 2000	Rabbit	Reproductive effects		
		Oral	141	Rabbit			
	Metribuzin	Dermal	> 20 000	Rabbit			
		Oral	250	Guinea pig		Unknown	Unknown
	Prometryn	Dermal	3100	Rabbit	Eye irritation		
	Prometon	Dermal	2200	Rabbit	Eye, skin irritation		
	Propazine	Dermal	> 10 200	Rabbit	Reproductive effects		
	Simazine	Oral	> 5000	Rabbit	Reproductive effects		
	Terbuthylazine	Dermal	> 3000	Rabbit	Skin irritation		

Herbicide Class	Compound	Route of Administration	LD50 (mg/kg)	Non-Equine Species	Clinical Signs	Equine Toxic Dose (mg/kg)	Clinical Signs
	2,4-DB	Dermal	10 000	Rabbit	Eye, skin irritation, convulsions		
Inhibitors	Terbutryn	Dermal	> 10 200	Rabbit	Skin necrosis		
	Nitrofen	Dermal	> 5000	Rabbit		Unknown	Unknown
	Oxadiazon	Oral	1620	Rabbit	Oxadiazon		
Substituted anilines	Alachlor	Dermal	> 2000	Rabbit	Skin irritation		
	Acetochlor	Oral	13 300	Rabbit			
		Oral	1740	Rabbit	Depression		
		Dermal	3667	Rabbit		Unknown	Unknown
	Butachlor	Oral	600	Rabbit	Eye irritation		
	Propachlor	Dermal	3470	Rabbit	Paralysis, convulsions, dyspnea		
		Oral	392	Rabbit	Skin irritation, ataxia		
Imidazolines	Imazamox	Dermal	380	Rabbit	Eye, skin irritation		
	Imazapic	Dermal	> 4000	Rabbit	Imazapic		
	Imazapyr	Dermal	> 2000	Rabbit	Skin irritation		
	Imazaquin	Dermal	> 2000	Rabbit		Unknown	Unknown
	Imazethapyr	Dermal	> 2000	Rabbit			
		Dermal	> 2001	Rabbit			

Source: Gupta PK. Overview of herbicide poisoning. In: Aiello SE, Moses MA, eds. Merck Veterinary Manual, 11th edn. Kenilworth, NJ: Merck Sharp & Dohme Corp., 2016. PubChem. https://pubchem.ncbi.nlm.nih.gov/

Author: Scott L. Radke DVM, MS

appendix 3

Information Resources for Toxicology

OVERVIEW

- The tens of thousands of metals, minerals, natural products, and synthetic chemicals used in modern civilization provide numerous opportunities for exposure of horses to potentially toxic materials.
- Horses can be exposed to toxic plants or a variety of pesticides (e.g., insecticides, herbicides, or rodenticides) used on fields/pastures or around buildings, providing ample opportunity for a significant exposure to a toxic substance.
- Veterinarians receive questions and calls daily about the safety of a variety of products to which horses are exposed.
- Beyond the personal experience and knowledge gained from frequent encounters with the most familiar products, veterinarians need resources to bolster their personal knowledge when less frequently known exposures or questions occur.
- This appendix presents several sources of information that can help veterinarians extend their service to clients by effectively using toxicology information resources.
- Principal categories of assistance include the following:
  - Animal poison control centers that maintain a staff of skilled and knowledgeable veterinary specialists for consultation when veterinary toxicology questions arise.
  - Persons with in-depth experience relevant to specific toxicants or circumstances. Examples are agronomists, botanists, chemists, limnologists, mycologists, pest control specialists, pharmacists, pharmacologists, pathologists, veterinary extension faculty, wildlife specialists, state and federal regulatory professionals, and many others. Often, veterinary toxicologists are the initial experts consulted and many have developed a network of additional experts to consult if needed.
  - Textbooks and reference books prepared by knowledgeable experts and provided by reliable publishers.
  - Selected peer-reviewed, scientific veterinary journals that routinely accept original reports of toxicology clinical cases or toxicology research.
  - Government agencies with emphasis on toxicology scientific, regulatory or educational services.
  - Reliable internet resources for quick and easy access to useful toxicology information on a 24/7 basis. The key to using internet resources is whether the information is reliable and based upon the best available evidence.

Blackwell's Five-Minute Veterinary Consult Clinical Companion: Equine Toxicology,
First Edition. Edited by Lynn R. Hovda, Dionne Benson, and Robert H. Poppenga.
© 2022 John Wiley & Sons, Inc. Published 2022 by John Wiley & Sons, Inc.
Companion website: www.wiley.com/go/hovda/equine

VETERINARY AND TOXICOLOGY INFORMATION RESOURCES

- As with all professional services, critical evaluation of resources available is essential to gathering reliable information for toxicology support.
- Sources that are well documented and subject to some form of peer review are usually the most reliable.
- If regulatory or legal aspects of toxicology are important for a given situation, official government sources often provide that aspect of information.
- As with all critical information for patient care, the veterinarian must carefully and critically determine how the information applies to their individual practice needs.

Specialists with In-depth Expertise Relevant to Veterinary Toxicology

- Examples are agronomists, botanists, chemists, limnologists, mycologists, pest control specialists, pharmacists, pharmacologists, pathologists, veterinary extension faculty, veterinary toxicologists, wildlife specialists, state and federal regulatory professionals, and many others.
- Knowing about these highly skilled and focused individuals can be invaluable when an infrequently encountered question or exposure demands special knowledge at short notice.
- Prior contact or arrangements with experts that one already knows is often invaluable when a quick and thorough response is required to support a toxicology incident in small animals.

Principal Reference Books and Textbooks

- Many popular textbooks are updated on a regular basis and new information is incorporated for many toxicologic topics. The use of the most current textbook is recommended for this reason, although for many toxicants there is little new information available from prior editions.
- While many textbooks are devoted exclusively to toxicology, other textbooks devoted to other topics such as pharmacology or internal medicine also contain useful information related to toxicology.
- The following textbooks or series of textbooks are useful for veterinarians:
    - Burrows GE, Tyrl RJ, eds. Handbook of Toxic Plants of North America, 2nd edn. Wiley-Blackwell, 2013.
    - Constable PD, Hinchcliff KD, eds. Veterinary Medicine, 11th edn. Elsevier, 2017.
    - Gupta RC, ed. Veterinary Toxicology: Basic and Clinical Principles, 3rd edn. Elsevier, 2018.
    - Knight AP, ed. A Guide to Poisonous House and Garden Plants. Teton New Media, 2005.
    - Plumlee KH, ed. Clinical Veterinary Toxicology. Mosby-Elsevier, 2004.
    - Riet-Correa F. Poisoning by Plants, Mycotoxins, and Related Toxins. CABI, 2011.
    - Southwood LL and Wilkins PA, eds. Equine Emergency and Critical Care Medicine. CRC Press, 2015.
    - Veterinary Clinics of North America Equine Practice, periodic issues related to equine toxicology.

Supportive Reference Books and Textbooks

- Papich MG, ed. Saunders Handbook of Veterinary Drugs, 3rd edn. Saunders Elsevier, 2011.
- Plumb DC, ed. Plumb's Veterinary Drug Handbook, 9th edn. Wiley-Blackwell, 2018 (see also online resource at https://www.plumbsveterinarydrugs.com/home2/).
- Riviere JE, Papich MG, eds. Veterinary Pharmacology and Therapeutics, 10th edn. Wiley-Blackwell, 2017.

Selected Veterinary Journals as References in Toxicology

Advances in Veterinary Medicine
American Journal of Veterinary Research
Australian Veterinary Journal
Canadian Journal of Veterinary Research
Equine Veterinary Journal
Journal of the American Veterinary Medical Association
Journal of Medical Toxicology
Journal of Veterinary Diagnostic Investigation
Journal of Veterinary Emergency and Critical Care
Journal of Veterinary Internal Medicine
Journal of Veterinary Pharmacology and Therapeutics
Research in Veterinary Science
The Veterinary Journal
Veterinary Clinics of North America Equine Practice
Veterinary Quarterly
Veterinary Record

Animal Poison Control Centers

- ASPCA Animal Poison Control Center
    - https://www.aspca.org/pet-care/animal-poison-control
    - +1 (888) 426-4435
    - Fee-based.
- Pet Poison Helpline (animal poison control hotline)
    - http://www.petpoisonhelpline.com/
    - +1 (855) 764-7661
    - Fee-based.

Internet-based Toxicology Resources

- Agency for Toxic Substances and Disease Registry (ATSDR):
    - http://www.atsdr.cdc.gov
    - http://www.atsdr.cdc.gov/toxfaqs/index.asp
- American Association of Poison Control Centers (AAPCC):
    - http://www.aapcc.org/
    - American Association of Poison Control Centers assists 55 poison centers in the United States on a 24/7 basis.
    - Poison Help hotline at 1-800-222-1222 can be dialed from anywhere in the United States and will be automatically routed to an appropriate center.

- Certifies poison control center personnel and owns and maintains the National Poison Data System (NPDS).
- Consultant:
  - https://consultant.vet.cornell.edu
  - Consultant is a diagnostic support system to assist in possible differential diagnoses or causes based on clinical signs entered. When clinical signs are entered, it enables a wide selection of potential differential toxicology diagnoses.
  - Consultant is free of charge, but monetary support is welcome to help defray expenses. It is species specific, provides a brief synopsis of a selected diagnosis/cause, and is supported by three to six recent references pertinent to the diagnosis selected.
  - Supported by a database of approximately 500 signs/symptoms, 7,000 diagnoses/causes, and 18,000 literature references, of which 3,000 are Web sources.
- Cornell University Poisonous Plants:
  - http://www.ansci.cornell.edu/plants/
  - Maintained by the Animal Science Department at Cornell University as a reference only.
  - Includes plant images, pictures of affected animals, and presentations concerning botany, chemistry, toxicology, diagnosis, and prevention of poisoning of animals by plants and other natural flora.
  - The images are copyrighted but may be printed, downloaded, or copied, provided it is in an educational setting and proper attribution is provided.
- Drug Compounding – FDA:
  - http://www.fda.gov/Drugs/GuidanceComplianceRegulatoryInformation/PharmacyCompounding/ucm339764.htm
- FDA-approved Animal Drugs:
  - FDA Approved Animal Drug Products (Green Book)
  - http://www.fda.gov/AnimalVeterinary/Products/ApprovedAnimalDrugProducts/default.htm
- FDA Center for Veterinary Medicine (FDA-CVM)
  - http://www.fda.gov/animalveterinary/default.htm
  - Official Web site for the Center for Veterinary Medicine.
  - Provides information on approved and animal drugs.
  - Monitors and establishes standard for animal feed contaminants and approves safe food additives for animal use.
  - Manages the FDA medicated feed and pet food programs.
  - Reporting problems with horse feeds: https://www.fda.gov/animal-veterinary/report-problem/reporting-problems-horse-or-other-livestock-feedfood
- Consumer Product Information Database:
  - https://www.whatsinproducts.com/
  - Provides a wealth of information about household products including ingredients, potential health risks, and appropriate safety and handling information.
  - This database links over 23,000 consumer brands to health effects from Material Safety Data Sheets (MSDS) provided by manufacturers and allows scientists and consumers to research products based on chemical ingredients. The database is designed to help answer the following typical questions:

- What are the chemical ingredients and their percentage in specific brands?
- Which products contain specific chemical ingredients?
- Who manufactures a specific brand? How can the manufacturer be contacted?
- What are the acute and chronic effects of chemical ingredients in a specific brand?
- What other information is available about chemicals in the toxicology-related databases of the National Library of Medicine?

- IPCS InChem (International Programme on Chemical Safety)
  - http://www.inchem.org/#/search
  - Rapid access to internationally peer-reviewed information on chemicals, including contaminants in the environment and food.
  - Primarily human- and environment-oriented.
  - Consolidates information from a number of intergovernmental organizations to assist in sound management of chemicals.
  - Includes environmental health criteria as well as health and safety guidelines.
  - Provides poison information monographs.
- Medline:
  - https://medlineplus.gov/
  - Service provided by the National Library of Medicine and National Institutes of Health.
  - Updated daily.
  - Human-focused, but can be a good source of information about human drugs encountered by animals.
  - Also a source of information about human antidotes useful in veterinary medicine.
  - Public access is allowed, as information is supported by two well-known federal agencies.
- MSDS Search:
  - There are several Material Safety Data Sheet (MSDS) databases accessible online.
  - These services specialize in providing digital sources of MSDS required by many commercial, business, and manufacturing companies.
  - MSDS sheets contain information about the characteristics and nature of thousands of chemicals to which animals could be exposed.
  - The information is often not assembled consistently in standard references.
  - The MSDS provides a relatively consistent and detailed documentation of composition, use, and potential adverse effects.
  - In many cases, MSDS information for a given product can be located through a search on the product.
- National Institute for Environmental Health Sciences (NIEHS):
  - http://www.niehs.nih.gov/
  - The NIEHS mission is to reduce the burden of human illness and disability by understanding how the environment influences the development and progression of human disease. Some of the NIEHS activities include:
    - Rigorous research in environmental health sciences, and communicating the results of this research to the public.

- Alphabetical listing of major health topics that are related to or affected by environmental exposures.
  - Access to materials and guidance for use by health professionals in educating, diagnosing, and treating patients with conditions and diseases influenced by environmental agents.
- National Pesticide Information Center (NPIC):
  - http://www.npic.orst.edu/
  - +1 (800)-858-7378
  - NPIC provides objective, science-based information about pesticides and pesticide-related topics to enable people to make informed decisions about pesticides and their use. NPIC is a cooperative agreement between Oregon State University and the U.S. Environmental Protection Agency.
- Pub Med:
  - https://pubmed.ncbi.nlm.nih.gov/
  - Pub Med is a search service of the United States National Library of Medicine.
  - It comprises more than 19 million citations for biomedical articles from Medline and life science journals.
  - Citations include links to full-text articles from Pub Med Central or publisher Web sites.
  - Numerous major scientific and applied veterinary journals can be reliably accessed through Pub Med.
- Veterinary Clinical Drug Information Monographs:
  - https://www.aavpt.org/page/43
  - The monographs were initially developed under the auspices of the U.S. Pharmacopeia (USP) through the use of expert panels.
  - The USP is a scientific non-profit organization that sets standards for the identity, strength, quality, and purity of medicines, food ingredients, and dietary supplements manufactured, distributed and consumed worldwide.
- Veterinary Information Network:
  - https://www.vin.com/vin/
  - A veterinary organization and system of education and databases to help busy veterinary professionals be the best clinicians they can be, providing features to include:
  - Bringing veterinarians together worldwide as colleagues.
  - Bringing instant access to vast amounts of up-to-date veterinary information to colleagues.
  - Bringing instant access to "breaking news" that affects veterinarians, their patients, and their practice.
  - Bringing easy access to colleagues who have specialized knowledge and skills.
  - Making continuing education available every day.
- American Board of Veterinary Toxicology:
  - https://www.abvt.org/
  - Website for board-certified veterinary toxicologists.
- American Association of Veterinary Laboratory Diagnosticians:
  - https://www.aavld.org/

- Website for accredited veterinary laboratories; provides links to state laboratories accredited by the AAVLD, many of which have veterinary toxicology experts and toxicology testing capabilities.

Acknowledgement: The authors acknowledge the many contributions of Gary Osweiler to this and many, many other toxicology documents.

Authors: Robert H. Poppenga, DVM, PhD, DABVT; Lynn R. Hovda, RPh, DVM, MS, DACVIM
Consulting Editors: Robert H. Poppenga, DVM, PhD, DABVT; Lynn R. Hovda, RPh, DVM, MS, DACVIM

Index by Toxins and Toxicants

Entries in **bold** refer to chapter topics., Page numbers followed by "f" refer to figures; those followed by "t" refer to tables.

Acer negundo see **Boxelder (*Acer negundo*)**
Acer rubrum see **Red maple (*Acer rubrum*)**
Acroption repens see **Russian knapweed (*Acroption repens*)**
Adonis aestavalis see **Cardiotoxic plants**
Aflatoxins, 215–218
   diagnostics, 217
   pathophysiology, 205–206
   therapeutics, 218
Ageratina altissima see **White snakeroot (*Ageratina altissima*)**
Albuterol, 88–91
  see also **Beta2 agonists**
Algal blooms see **Blue-green algae (Cyanobacteria)**
Alsike clover (*Trifolium hybridum*), 261–264
   diagnostics, 263
   pathophysiology, 261–262
   therapeutics, 263–264
Amitraz, 131–136
   antidotes, 135
   diagnostics, 134
   pathophysiology, 131–133
   therapeutics 135
Ammonia (NH3), 415–420
   diagnostics, 418–419
   pathophysiology, 415–417
   therapeutics, 419
vAmphetamine see **Methamphetamine/Amphetamine**
Andarine see **Selective androgen receptor modulators (SARMs)**

Anticoagulants, 383–387
   antidote, 386
   diagnostics, 385
   pathophysiology, 383–384
   therapeutics, 386
Antipsychotic agents, 78–82
   antidotes, 81
   pathophysiology, 79–80
   therapeutics, 81–82
Apocynum spp. see **Cardiotoxic plants**
Arsenic, 189–192
   antidotes, 191–192
   chelating agents, 24, 154, 191–192
   diagnostics, 191
   pathophysiology, 189–190
   therapeutics, 191–192
   see also **Herbicides**
Asclepias spp. see **Cardiotoxic plants**; **Narrowleaf milkweed (*Asclepias fascicularis*)**
Aspergillus, 215
  see also **Aflatoxins**
Astragalus see **Locoweed (*Astragalus* and *Oxytropis*)**
Avocado (*Persea* spp.) see **Cardiotoxic plants**

Benzodiazepines, 84–87
   antidote, 86
   diazepam, 84
   midazolam, 84
   pathophysiology, 84–85
   therapeutics, 86

Blackwell's Five-Minute Veterinary Consult Clinical Companion: Equine Toxicology, First Edition. Edited by Lynn R. Hovda, Dionne Benson, and Robert H. Poppenga. © 2022 John Wiley & Sons, Inc. Published 2022 by John Wiley & Sons, Inc. Companion website: www.wiley.com/go/hovda/equine

Berteroa incana see **Hoary alyssum (*Berteroa incana*)**
Beta2 agonists, 88–91
 diagnostics, 89–90
 pathophysiology, 88–89
 therapeutics, 90
Bisphosphonates, 92–95
 nitrogenous, 92
 non-nitrogenous, 92
 pathophysiology, 92–93
 therapeutics, 94–95
Black locust (*Robinia pseudoacacia*), 429–432
 diagnostics, 430–431
 pathophysiology, 429
 therapeutics, 431
Black walnut (*Juglans nigra*), 433–436
 diagnostics, 435
 pathophysiology, 433–434
 therapeutics, 435–436
Black widow spider (*Latrodectus* spp.), 475f
 see also **Spiders (brown recluse and black widow)**
Blister beetles (*Epicauta* spp. and *Pyrota* spp.), 453–458, 454f
 diagnostics, 456
 pathophysiology, 453–455
 therapeutics, 456–457
Blue-green algae (Cyanobacteria), 265–270
 cyanotoxins, 265
 diagnostics, 268
 pathophysiology, 265–266
 therapeutics, 268–269
Botulism neurotoxin see ***Clostridium botulinum* toxin**
Boxelder (*Acer negundo*), 437–441, 438f
 diagnostics, 439–440
 pathophysiology, 437–438
 seasonal pasture myopathy (SPM), 437
 therapeutics, 440
Bromethalin, 388–391
 diagnostics, 390
 pathophysiology, 388–389
 therapeutics, 390–391
Brown recluse spider (*Loxosceles* spp.), 475f
 see also **Spiders (brown recluse and black widow)**
Buprenorphine see **Opioids**
Butorphanol see **Opioids**

Caffeine, 110, 112–113
 see also **Methylxanthine**
Calciferol see **Vitamin D (Calciferol)**
Cannabis sativa see **Marijuana**
Carbamate pesticides, 137–141, 490–491t
 diagnostics, 139
 pathophysiology, 137–138
 therapeutics, 140
Carbon monoxide (CO), 415–420, 421–423
 diagnostics, 418–419
 pathophysiology, 415–416
 therapeutics, 419
Cardiotoxic plants, 271–275
 cardiac glycosides, 271
 diagnostics, 273–274
 grayanotoxins, 271
 pathophysiology, 271–272
 taxine alkaloids, 271
 therapeutics, 274–275
Cascabela thevetia, 330, 332f
 see also **Oleander (*Nerium oleander* and *Cascabela thevetia*)**
Centaurea solstitialis see **Yellow star thistle (*Centaurea solstitialis*)**
Cestrum diurnum see **Day blooming jessamine (*Cestrum diurnum*)**
Cheeseweed mallow (*Malva parviflora*) see **Cardiotoxic plants**
Cholecalciferol, 393–397
 antidote, 396
 diagnostics, 395–396
 pathophysiology, 393–394
 therapeutics, 396
Cicuta spp. see Water hemlock (*Cicuta* spp.)
Clenbuterol, 88–91
 see also **Beta2 agonists**
***Clostridium botulinum* toxin**, 245–249
 antidotes, 248–249
 diagnostics, 247–248
 pathophysiology, 245–246
 therapeutics, 248–249
Cobalt, 37–40
 diagnostics, 39
 pathophysiology, 37–38
 therapeutics, 39–40
Cocaine, 41–44
 crack cocaine, 41

diagnostics, 43
pathophysiology, 41–42
therapeutics, 43–44
Cocoa, 110, 111f
see also Methylxanthine
Coffee, 110, 111f
see also Methylxanthine
Compound 1080 see Sodium fluoroacetate (Compound 1080)
Compounded medication, 29–32, 30f, 31f
Conium maculatum see Poison hemlock (Conium maculatum)
Convallaria majalis see Cardiotoxic plants
Copperheads see Crotalids (Pit vipers)
Coral snakes see Elapids (Coral snakes)
Cottonmouths see Crotalids (Pit vipers)
Crotalids (Pit vipers), 460–466, 461f, 462f
   antivenin, 22–23, 465
   diagnostics, 463–464
   pathophysiology, 460–462
   therapeutics, 464–465
Cyanide, 250–253, 421–423
   diagnostics, 252
   pathophysiology, 250–251
   therapeutics, 252–253
Cyanobacteria see Blue-green algae (Cyanobacteria)
Cypermethrin, 166
   see also Pyrethrins and pyrethroid insecticides

Datura stramonium see Jimsonweed (Datura stramonium)
Day blooming jessamine (Cestrum diurnum), 277–280
   diagnostics, 278–279
   pathophysiology, 277–278
   therapeutics, 279–280
Death camas (Zigadenus spp.), 282–285
   diagnostics, 284
   pathophysiology, 282–283
   therapeutics, 284–285
Dermorphin, 45–48
   diagnostics, 47
   pathophysiology, 45–46
Detoxication, 25–26
   activated charcoal, 25
   cathartics, 25

cholestyramine, 25
diuretics, 25–26
Diazepam see Benzodiazepines
Digitalis purpurea see Cardiotoxic plants
Diquat, 156–160
   diagnostics, 158
   pathophysiology, 156–157
   therapeutics, 149
   see also Herbicides
Dogbane (Apocynum spp.) see Cardiotoxic plants

Elapids (Coral snakes), 467–472, 468f, 469f
   antivenin, 22, 471–472
   diagnostics, 471
   pathophysiology, 469–470
   therapeutics, 471–472
Endophyte-infected tall fescue see Fescue
Endosarm see Selective androgen receptor modulators (SARMs)
Epicauta spp. see Blister beetles (Epicauta spp. and Pyrota spp.)
Ergot alkaloids, 220, 221
   see also Fescue

Fentanyl see Opioids
Fertilizers, 147–150
   antidote, 149
   diagnostics, 149
   nitrates, 147–149
   pathophysiology, 147–148
   phosphates, 147
   therapeutics, 149–150
   urea, 147, 149
Fescue, 220–225
   antidote, 224
   diagnostics, 223
   ergovaline, 220
   pathophysiology, 220–221
   therapeutics, 224
Fluoride, 193–196
   diagnostics, 195–196
   fluorosis, 194–196
   pathophysiology, 193–194
   therapeutics, 196
Fluphenazine, 78–82
   antidotes, 81
   pathophysiology, 79–80
   therapeutics, 81–82

Foxglove (*Digitalis purpurea*) *see* **Cardiotoxic plants**
Fumonisins, 227–230
   diagnostics, 229
   pathophysiology, 227
   therapeutics, 229–230
Fusaria, 231–234
   diagnostics, 233
   pathophysiology, 231–232
   therapeutics, 233
   trichothecenes, 231, 232
   zearalenone, 231, 232
   see also **Fumonisins**
Fusarium, 227, 231
   see also **Fumonisins; Fusaria**

Gabapentin, 97–99
   pathophysiology, 97
   therapeutics, 99
Growth hormone and secretagogues, 49–52
   antidote, 52
   diagnostics, 51
   GH-releasing peptides, 50
   interactions, 52
   natural production, 49
   pathophysiology, 49–50
   recombinant GH, 49
   therapeutics, 51–52

Hemlock, 287–293
   diagnostics, 291–292
   pathophysiology, 287–290
   poison hemlock (*Conium maculatum*), 288f
   therapeutics, 292
   water hemlock (*Cicuta* spp.), 289f
Herbicides, 151–155, 490–495t
   antidote, 154
   arsenicals, 151–154
   diagnostics, 153
   pathophysiology, 151–152
   therapeutics, 153–154
   see also Diquat; Paraquat
Hoary alyssum (*Berteroa incana*), 294–299, 295f, 296f
   diagnostics, 297
   pathophysiology, 294–295
   therapeutics, 297–298
Hydrogen sulfide (H2S), 415–420, 421
   diagnostics, 418–419
   pathophysiology, 416–417
   therapeutics, 419
Hydromorphone *see* **Opioids**

Iodine, 101–104
   pathophysiology, 102
Ionophores, 173–177
   diagnostics, 175
   lasalocid, 173, 174, 175
   monensin, 173, 174, 175
   pathophysiology, 173–174
   salinomycin, 173, 174, 175
   therapeutics, 176
Iron, 197–201
   antidote, 200
   chelating agents, 24, 200
   diagnostics, 199–200
   pathophysiology, 197–198
   therapeutics, 200
Isocoma pluriflora see **Rayless goldenrod (*Isocoma pluriflora*)**

Jimsonweed (*Datura stramonium*), 300–305, 301f
   diagnostics, 303
   pathophysiology, 300–302
   therapeutics, 304
Juglans nigra see **Black walnut (*Juglans nigra*)**

Kalmia spp. *see* **Cardiotoxic plants**
Kleingrass (*Panicum coloratum*), 306–309
   diagnostics, 308
   pathophysiology, 306–307
   therapeutics, 308–309

Lantana (*Lantana camara*), 310–314, 311f
   diagnostics, 313
   pathophysiology, 310–312
   therapeutics, 313–314
Latrodectus spp. *see* **Spiders (brown recluse and black widow)**
Lead, 202–206
   antidotes, 205
   chelating agents, 23, 24, 205
   diagnostics, 204
   pathophysiology, 202

therapeutics, 204–205
Levothyroxine, 121–124
   diagnostics, 122–123
   pathophysiology, 121–122
   therapeutics, 123
LGD-4033 see Selective androgen receptor modulators (SARMs)
Lily of the valley (*Convallaria majalis*) see Cardiotoxic plants
Locoweed (*Astragalus* and *Oxytropis*), 315–321, 316t, 317f
   diagnostics, 319
   pathophysiology, 315–318
   swainsonine, 315, 316
   therapeutics, 320
Lolitems, 238
   see also Tremorgenic mycotoxins
Loxosceles spp. see Spiders (brown recluse and black widow)

Malva parviflora see Cardiotoxic plants
Marijuana, 53–57, 54f
   pathophysiology, 53–54
   therapeutics, 56
   see also Synthetic cannabinoids
Medroxyprogesterone acetate (MPA), 106–109
   diagnostics, 107–108
   pathophysiology, 106–107
   therapeutics, 108
Methadone see Opioids
Methamphetamine/Amphetamine, 58–60
   diagnostics, 59
   pathophysiology, 58–59
   therapeutics, 59–60
Methylxanthine, 110–114
   caffeine, 110, 112–113
   diagnostics, 113
   pathophysiology, 110–112
   theobromine, 110, 112
   theophylline, 110, 112
   therapeutics, 113–114
Midazolam see Benzodiazepines
Milkweed see Cardiotoxic plants; Narrowleaf milkweed (*Asclepias fascicularis*)
Morphine see Opioids
MPA see Medroxyprogesterone acetate (MPA)

Mycotoxins see Aflatoxins; Fusaria; Slaframine; Tremorgenic mycotoxins

Nalbuphine see Opioids
Narrowleaf milkweed (*Asclepias fascicularis*), 322–325
   diagnostics, 324
   pathophysiology, 322–323
   therapeutics, 324
Nerium oleander, 330, 331f
   see also Oleander (*Nerium oleander* and *Cascabela thevetia*)
Nightshades (*Solanum* spp.), 326–328
   diagnostics, 327–328
   pathophysiology, 326–327
   therapeutics, 328
Nonsteroidal anti-inflammatory drugs (NSAIDs), 116–119
   diagnostics, 118
   pathophysiology, 116–117
   therapeutics, 118–119

Oak (*Quercus* spp.), 442–445
   diagnostics, 443–444
   pathophysiology, 442–443
   therapeutics, 444–445
Oleander (*Nerium oleander* and *Cascabela thevetia*), 330–335, 331f, 332f
   diagnostics, 333–334
   pathophysiology, 330–332
   therapeutics, 334–335
Opioids, 62–66
   antidotes, 65
   interactions, 65–66
   pathophysiology, 63
   receptors, 63
   therapeutics, 65–66
Organophosphate pesticides, 142–146, 493t
   antidote, 145
   diagnostics, 144
   pathophysiology, 142–143
   therapeutics, 145
Osphos (clodronate) see Bisphosphonates
Oxytropis see Locoweed (*Astragalus* and *Oxytropis*)

Pamidronate see Bisphosphonates
Panicum coloratum see Kleingrass (*Panicum coloratum*)

Paraquat, 151–154, 156–160
diagnostics, 158
pathophysiology, 156–157
therapeutics, 159
see also **Herbicides**
Paspalitrems, 238
see also **Tremorgenic mycotoxins**
Pentachlorophenol (PCP), 161–164
diagnostics, 162–163
pathophysiology, 161–162
therapeutics, 163
Persea spp. see **Cardiotoxic plants**
Pethidine see **Opioids**
Phosphides, 398–402
diagnostics, 400
pathophysiology, 398–399
therapeutics, 400–402
Pieris japonica see **Cardiotoxic plants**
Pit vipers see **Crotalids (Pit vipers)**
Poison hemlock (*Conium maculatum*) see Hemlock
Pyrethrins and pyrethroid insecticides, 165–170
diagnostics, 168
pathophysiology, 165–166
therapeutics, 168–169
Pyrota spp. see **Blister beetles (*Epicauta* spp. and *Pyrota* spp.)**
Pyrrolizidine alkaloids, 336–342
diagnostics, 340–341
pathophysiology, 336–339
plants associated with poisoning, 337t, 338f
therapeutics, 341–342

Quercus see **Oak (*Quercus* spp.)**

Ractopamine, 178–181
diagnostics, 180
pathophysiology, 178–179
therapeutics, 180–181
Raloxifene see **Selective estrogen receptor modulators (SERMs)**
Rattlesnakes, 460, 461f, 462f
see also **Crotalids (Pit vipers)**
Rayless goldenrod (*Isocoma pluriflora*), 344–348
diagnostics, 346–347
pathophysiology, 344–345
therapeutics, 347–348
tremetol, 344, 345
Red maple (*Acer rubrum*), 446–450
diagnostics, 448
pathophysiology, 446–447
therapeutics, 449
Remifentanil see **Opioids**
Reserpine, 78–82
pathophysiology, 79–80
therapeutics, 81–82
Rhizoctonia leguminicola, 235
see also **Slaframine**
***Rhododendron* spp.**, 350–354, 351f
diagnostics, 353
grayanotoxins, 352
pathophysiology, 350–352
therapeutics, 353–354
Robinia pseudoacacia see **Black locust (*Robinia pseudoacacia*)**
Russian knapweed (*Acroptilon repens*), 369–372, 370f
diagnostics, 371–372
equine nigropallidal encephalomalacia, 369
pathophysiology, 369–371
therapeutics, 372
Ryegrass toxicosis, 238
see also **Tremorgenic mycotoxins**

Salt see **Sodium chloride**
Selective androgen receptor (SARMs) and estrogen receptor (SERMs) modulators, 67–71
diagnostics, 70
interactions, 70
pathophysiology, 67–69
therapeutics, 70
Selenium, 207–211
Alkali disease, 209
diagnostics, 209–210
pathophysiology, 207–208
therapeutics, 210–211
Senecio jacobaea see **Tansy ragwort (*Senecio jacobaea*)**
Slaframine, 235–237
antidote, 237
diagnostics, 236

pathophysiology, 235
therapeutics, 236–237
Smoke, 421–426
   antidotes, 425
   diagnostics, 423–424
   pathophysiology, 421–422
   therapeutics, 424–425
Sodium chloride, 254–257
   diagnostics, 256
   hypernatremia forms, 255
   pathophysiology, 254–255
   therapeutics, 256–257
Sodium fluoroacetate (Compound 1080), 403–407
   diagnostics, 405–406
   pathophysiology, 403–404
   therapeutics, 406
Solanum spp. *see* **Nightshades (*Solanum* spp.)**
Spiders (brown recluse and black widow), 474–481, 475f
   antivenin, 23, 479
   diagnostics, 478–479
   pathophysiology, 474–476
   therapeutics, 479–480
Strychnine, 408–412
   diagnostics, 410
   pathophysiology, 408–409
   therapeutics, 410–411
Sudangrass (*Sorghum* spp.), 355–358
   diagnostics, 356–357
   pathophysiology, 355–356
   therapeutics, 357
Summer pheasants eye (*Adonis aestivalis*) *see* **Cardiotoxic plants**
Synthetic cannabinoids, 72–75
   diagnostics, 74
   pathophysiology, 72–73
   therapeutics, 74–75

Tamoxifen *see* **Selective estrogen receptor modulators (SERMs)**
Tansy ragwort (*Senecio jacobaea*), 359–363
   diagnostics, 361
   jacobine, 359
   pathophysiology, 359–360
   therapeutics, 361–362

Taxus spp. *see* **Yew (*Taxus* spp.)**
Testolone *see* **Selective androgen receptor modulators (SARMs)**
Theobromine, 110, 112
   see also **Methylxanthine**
Theophylline, 110, 112
   see also **Methylxanthine**
Tildren (tiludronate disodium) *see* **Bisphosphonates**
Toremifene *see* **Selective estrogen receptor modulators (SERMs)**
Tramadol *see* **Opioids**
Tremorgenic mycotoxins, 238–242
   diagnostics, 240
   lolitrems, 238
   paspalitrems, 238
   pathophysiology, 238
   therapeutics, 240–241
Trichothecenes, 231, 232
   see also **Fusaria**
Trifolium hybridum see **Alsike clover (*Trifolium hybridum*)**

Vitamin D (Calciferol), 125–127
   diagnostics, 126–127
   pathophysiology, 125–126
   therapeutics, 127

Water hemlock (*Cicuta* spp.) *see* Hemlock
White snakeroot (*Ageratina altissima*), 364–368
   diagnostics, 366–367
   pathophysiology, 364–365
   therapeutics, 367–368
   tremetol, 364, 365

Yellow star thistle (*Centaurea solstitialis*), 369–372, 370f
   diagnostics, 371–372
   equine nigropallidal encephalomalacia, 369
   pathophysiology, 369–371
   therapeutics, 372
Yew (*Taxus* spp.), 374–379, 375f
   diagnostics, 377
   pathophysiology, 374–376
   taxines, 374–376
   therapeutics, 377–378

Zearalenone, 231, 232
　see also **Fusaria**
Zigadenus spp. *see* **Death camas (*Zigadenus* spp.)**
Zilpaterol, 182–185
　diagnostics, 184
　pathophysiology, 182–183
　therapeutics, 184–185
Zoledronate *see* **Bisphosphonates**

This index is intended to assist clinicians with differential diagnoses of the specific toxins and toxicants documented in this book by providing a quick review of associated clinical signs or physiological conditions.

Abdominal pain
  Arsenic
  Cardiotoxic plants
  Fertilizers
  Methamphetamine/Amphetamine
  Oak (*Quercus* spp.)
  Oleander
  Paraquat and Diquat
  Rhododendron spp.
  Zilpaterol

Abortion
  Anticoagulants
  Fertilizers
  Fescue
  Hoary alyssum (*Berteroa incana*)
  Red maple (*Acer rubrum*)
  Tansy ragwort (*Senecio jacobaea*)

Acidosis
  Amitraz
  Boxelder (*Acer negundo*)
  Iron
  Oak (*Quercus* spp.)
  Phosphides
  Pyrethrins and pyrethroid insecticides
  Rhododendron spp.
  Smoke
  Sodium chloride
  Sodium fluoroacetate (Compound 1080)
  Strychnine

Acute kidney injury
  Beta$_2$ agonists
  NSAIDs
  Phosphides
  Rayless goldenrod (*Isocoma pluriflora*)
  Smoke
  Synthetic cannabinoids
  see also Azotemia; Nephrotoxicity; Renal failure

Agalactia
  Fescue

Aggression
  Locoweeds
  Methamphetamine/Amphetamine
  Methylxanthines
  SARMs/SERMs

Agitation
  Antipsychotic agents
  Benzodiazepines
  Beta$_2$ agonists
  Cobalt
  Cocaine
  Jimsonweed (*Datura stramonium*)
  Lead
  Methamphetamine/Amphetamine
  Ractopamine
  Sodium fluoroacetate (Compound 1080)
  Spiders
  Synthetic cannabinoids
  Yew (*Taxus* spp.)
  Zilpaterol

Alopecia
  Iodine
  Pentachlorophenol (PCP)
  Selenium

Blackwell's Five-Minute Veterinary Consult Clinical Companion: Equine Toxicology, First Edition. Edited by Lynn R. Hovda, Dionne Benson, and Robert H. Poppenga.
© 2022 John Wiley & Sons, Inc. Published 2022 by John Wiley & Sons, Inc.
Companion website: www.wiley.com/go/hovda/equine

Anaphylactic shock
 Medroxyprogesterone acetate (MPA)
Anemia
 Aflatoxins
 Anticoagulants
 Crotalid snakes (pit vipers)
 Hoary alyssum (*Berteroa incana*)
 Lead
 Locoweeds
 NSAIDs
 Pentachlorophenol (PCP)
 Red maple (*Acer rubrum*)
 Spiders
Anorexia
 Aflatoxins
 Anticoagulants
 Blister beetles
 Blue-green algae
 Cardiotoxic plants
 Ionophores
 Iron
 Kleingrass (*Panicum coloratum*)
 Lantana (*Lantana camara*)
 Lead
 Methylxanthines
 Nightshades (*Solanum*)
 Oleander
 Pentachlorophenol (PCP)
 Phosphides
 Pyrrolizidine alkaloids
 Selenium
 Slaframine
 Sodium chloride
Antinociception
 Dermorphin
Anxiety
 Benzodiazepine
 Carbamate pesticides
 Cobalt
 Cocaine
 Locoweeds
 Narrowleaf milkweed (*Asclepias fascicularis*)
 Organophosphate pesticides
Apathy
 Nightshades (*Solanum*)
Aphagia
 Paraquat and Diquat

Arrhythmias
 Anticoagulants
 Black locust (*Robinia pseudoacacia*)
 Cardiotoxic plants
 Cholecalciferol
 Cobalt
 Cocaine
 Crotalid snakes (pit vipers)
 Cyanide
 Hydrogen sulfide
 Levothyroxine
 Methylxanthines
 Narrowleaf milkweed (*Asclepias fascicularis*)
 Nightshades (*Solanum* spp.)
 Oleander
 Rayless goldenrod (*Isocoma pluriflora*)
 Rhododendron spp.
 Sodium fluoroacetate (Compound 1080)
 White snakeroot (*Ageratina altissima*)
 Yew (*Taxus* spp.)
 Zilpaterol
 see also Bradycardia; Tachycardia
Ascites
 Pyrrolizidine alkaloids
 Sodium fluoroacetate (Compound 1080)
 Tansy ragwort (*Senecio jacobaea*)
Asphyxia
 Hemlock
Aspiration pneumonia
 Botulism neurotoxin
 Crotalid snakes (pit vipers)
 Lead
 Rhododendron spp.
Ataxia
 Aflatoxins
 Amitraz
 Arsenic
 Benzodiazepines
 Beta$_2$ agonists
 Bromethalin
 Carbon monoxide
 Cobalt
 Cocaine
 Crotalid snakes (pit vipers)
 Cyanide
 Death camas (*Zigadenus* spp.)
 Elapids (coral snakes)

Fertilizers
Fumonisins
Gabapentin
Hydrogen sulfide
Ionophores
Iron
Jimsonweed (*Datura stramonium*)
Lead
Marijuana
Methamphetamine/Amphetamine
Narrowleaf milkweed (*Asclepias fascicularis*)
NSAIDs
Phosphides
Pyrrolizidine alkaloids
Russian knapweed (*Acroptilon repens*)
Smoke
Sodium chloride
Sodium fluoroacetate (Compound 1080)
Spiders
Sudan grass (*Sorghum* spp.)
Synthetic cannabinoids
Tansy ragwort (*Senecio jacobaea*)
Yellow star thistle (*Centaurea solstitialis*)

Azotemia
Arsenic
Blister beetles
Paraquat and Diquat
Phosphides
Zilpaterol
see also Acute kidney injury; Nephrotoxicity; Renal failure

Blindness
Carbon monoxide
Herbicides
Pyrrolizidine alkaloids
Sodium fluoroacetate (Compound 1080)

Bradycardia
Amitraz
Antipsychotic agents
Carbamate pesticides
Cardiotoxic plants
Death camas (*Zigadenus* spp.)
Fumonisins
Oleander
Opioids
Organophosphate pesticides
Rhododendron spp.
Synthetic cannabinoids
Yew (*Taxus* spp.)
see also Arrhythmias

Bronchoconstriction
Carbamate pesticides
Organophosphate pesticides

Bruxism
Alsike clover (*Trifolium hybridum*)
Blister beetles
Death camas (*Zigadenus* spp.)
Hemlock
Sodium fluoroacetate (Compound 1080)

Cachexia
Iodine
Levothyroxine

Calcification of soft tissues
Day blooming jessamine (*Cestrum diurnum*)
Vitamin D

Cardiac arrest
Methylxanthines
Yew (*Taxus* spp.)

Cardiac failure
Ionophores
Rayless goldenrod (*Isocoma pluriflora*)
Selenium
Smoke
White snakeroot (*Ageratina altissima*)

Cardiogenic shock
Paraquat and Diquat
Yew (*Taxus* spp.)

Cardiomegaly
Growth hormone

Cardiomyopathy
$Beta_2$ agonists
Cardiotoxic plants
Rayless goldenrod (*Isocoma pluriflora*)
White snakeroot (*Ageratina altissima*)

Catalepsy
Dermorphin

Cerebral edema
Aflatoxins
Bromethalin
Paraquat and Diquat

Circling
  Antipsychotic agents
  Fumonisins
  Methamphetamine/Amphetamine
Circulatory shock
  Arsenic
  Iron
CNS depression
  Benzodiazepines
  Bromethalin
  Carbamate pesticides
  Elapids (coral snakes)
  Herbicides
  Nightshades (*Solanum*)
  Opioids
  Organophosphate pesticides
Coagulopathy
  Aflatoxins
  Anticoagulants
  Iron
  Spiders
Colic
  Amitraz
  Anticoagulants
  Antipsychotic agents
  Beta$_2$ agonists
  Bisphosphonates
  Black locust (*Robinia pseudoacacia*)
  Black walnut (*Juglans nigra*)
  Blister beetles
  Blue-green algae
  Boxelder (*Acer negundo*)
  Carbamate pesticides
  Cardiotoxic plants
  Cobalt
  Death camas (*Zigadenus* spp.)
  Dermorphin
  Fertilizers
  Hemlock
  Herbicides
  Ionophores
  Iron
  Jimsonweed (*Datura stramonium*)
  Kleingrass (*Panicum coloratum*)
  Lead
  Marijuana
  Narrowleaf milkweed (*Asclepias ascicularis*)
  Nightshades (*Solanum*)
  NSAIDs
  Oak (*Quercus* spp.)
  Oleander
  Organophosphate pesticides
  Paraquat and Diquat
  Pentachlorophenol (PCP)
  Ractopamine
  Red maple (*Acer rubrum*)
  Rhododendron spp.
  Selenium
  Slaframine
  Sodium fluoroacetate (Compound 1080)
  Spiders
  Synthetic cannabinoids
  Tansy ragwort (*Senecio jacobaea*)
  Yew (*Taxus* spp.)
  Zilpaterol
Collapse
  Ionophores
  Medroxyprogesterone acetate (MPA)
  Pentachlorophenol (PCP)
  Tremorgenic mycotoxins
  Yew (*Taxus* spp.)
Coma
  Alsike clover (*Trifolium hybridum*)
  Benzodiazepines
  Blue-green algae
  Death camas (*Zigadenus* spp.)
  Hemlock
  Iron
  Nightshades (*Solanum*)
  Oleander
  Opioids
  Smoke
  Sodium chloride
  Sodium fluoroacetate (Compound 1080)
Conjunctivitis
  Alsike clover (*Trifolium hybridum*)
  Ammonia
  Pentachlorophenol (PCP)
Constipation
  Black locust (*Robinia pseudoaccacia*)
  Lantana (*Lantana camara*)
  Oak (*Quercus* spp.)
  Opioids
Convulsions *see* **Seizures**
Corneal effects

Herbicides
   SERMs
Cough
   Aflatoxins
   Ammonia
   Carbamate pesticides
   Hydrogen sulfide
   Organophosphate pesticides
   Paraquat and Diquat
   Smoke
   Synthetic cannabinoids
Cramps
   Bisphosphonates
   Spiders
Cyanosis
   Blue-green algae
   Red maple (*Acer rubrum*)
   Smoke
Cystitis
   Blister beetles
   Sudangrass (*Sorghum* spp.)

Death
   Alsike clover (*Trifolium hybridum*)
   Amitraz
   Anticoagulants
   Beta agonists
   Blister beetles
   Blue-green algae
   Bromethalin
   Cardiotoxic plants
   Crotalid snakes (pit vipers)
   Cyanide
   Fertilizers
   Fluoride
   Fumonisins
   Fusaria
   Hemlock
   Hydrogen sulfide
   Ionophores
   Jimsonweed (*Datura stramonium*)
   Lantana (*Lantana camara*)
   Lead
   Levothyroxine
   Medroxyprogesterone acetate (MPA)
   Methamphetamine/Amphetamine
   Methylxanthines
   Narrowleaf milkweed (*Asclepias fascicularis*)

   Oleander
   Opioids
   Paraquat
   Rayless goldenrod (*Isocoma pluriflora*)
   Red maple (*Acer rubrum*)
   Selenium
   Slaframine
   Sodium chloride
   Sodium fluoroacetate (Compound 1080)
   White snakeroot (*Ageratina altissima*)
   Yew (*Taxus* spp.)
Dehydration
   Amitraz
   Cardiotoxic plants
   Hoary alyssum (*Berteroa incana*)
   NSAIDs
   Pyrethrins and pyrethroid insecticides
   Red maple (*Acer rubrum*)
   Russian knapweed (*Acroptilon repens*)
   Slaframine
   Smoke
   Yellow star thistle (*Centaurea solstitialis*)
Dental lesions
   Fluoride
Depression
   Aflatoxins
   Alsike clover (*Trifolium hybridum*)
   Amitraz
   Anticoagulants
   Arsenic
   Bisphosphonates
   Black locust (*Robinia pseudoacacia*)
   Black walnut (*Juglans nigra*)
   Blister beetles
   Blue-green algae
   Cardiotoxic plants
   Cholecalciferol
   Death camas (*Zigadenus* spp.)
   Fluoride
   Fumonisins
   Hemlock
   Lead
   Locoweeds
   Marijuana
   Narrowleaf milkweed (*Asclepias fascicularis*)
   Oak (*Quercus* spp.)
   Oleander
   Pyrrolizidine alkaloids

Depression (*continued*)
  Rayless goldenrod (*Isocoma pluriflora*)
  Red maple (*Acer rubrum*)
  Russian knapweed (*Acroptilon repens*)
  SARMs/SERMs
  Slaframine
  Smoke
  Sodium chloride
  White snakeroot (*Ageratina altissima*)
  Yellow star thistle (*Centaurea solstitialis*)
  see also CNS depression; Respiratory depression
Dermal irritation
  Fusaria
Dermatitis
  Paraquat and Diquat
  Pentachlorophenol (PCP)
  Pyrrolizidine alkaloids
Diarrhea
  Aflatoxins
  Antipsychotic agents
  Arsenic
  Black locust (*Robinia pseudoacacia*)
  Blister beetles
  Blue-green algae
  Carbamate pesticides
  Cardiotoxic plants
  Fluoride
  Hemlock
  Herbicides
  Hoary alyssum (*Berteroa incana*)
  Ionophores
  Iron
  Methamphetamine/Amphetamine
  Nightshades (*Solanum*)
  NSAIDs
  Oak (*Quercus* spp.)
  Oleander
  Organophosphate pesticides
  Paraquat and Diquat
  Pyrrolizidine alkaloids
  Selenium
  Slaframine
  Sodium chloride
  Tansy ragwort (*Senecio jacobaea*)
  Yew (*Taxus* spp.)
Drowsiness
  Amitraz
  Nightshades (*Solanum*)
  Pyrrolizidine alkaloids
  Russian knapweed (*Acroptilon repens*)
  Synthetic cannabinoids
  Yellow star thistle (*Centaurea solstitialis*)
Dysgalactia
  Fescue
Dysmetria
  Tremorgenic mycotoxins
Dysphagia
  Botulism neurotoxin
  Boxelder (*Acer negundo*)
  Fumonisins
  Lead
  Rayless goldenrod (*Isocoma pluriflora*)
  White snakeroot (*Ageratina altissima*)
Dyspnea
  Black locust (*Robinia pseudoacacia*)
  Boxelder (*Acer negundo*)
  Carbamate pesticides
  Cardiotoxic plants
  Cyanide
  Fertilizers
  Herbicides
  Narrowleaf milkweed (*Asclepias fascicularis*)
  Organophosphate pesticides
  Paraquat and Diquat
  Phosphides
  Pyrrolizidine alkaloids
  Selenium
  Smoke
  Spiders
  Yew (*Taxus* spp.)
Dystocia
  Fescue
Dysuria
  Blister beetles
  Boxelder (*Acer negundo*)

Ecchymoses
  Aflatoxins
  Fumonisins
  Hoary alyssum (*Berteroa incana*)
  Red maple (*Acer rubrum*)
Edema
  Amitraz
  Arsenic
  Black walnut (*Juglans nigra*)

Cardiotoxic plants
Crotalid snakes (pit vipers)
Fusaria
Hoary alyssum (*Berteroa incana*)
Iron
NSAIDs
Oak (*Quercus* spp.)
Paraquat and Diquat
Pentachlorophenol (PCP)
Pyrrolizidine alkaloids
Spiders
White snakeroot (*Ageratina altissima*)
see also Cerebral edema; Macular edema; Pulmonary edema

Emesis
Carbamate pesticides
Organophosphate pesticides

Emphysema
Smoke

Epistaxis
Aflatoxins
Anticoagulants

Esophageal obstruction
Boxelder (*Acer negundo*)
Lead
Rayless goldenrod (*Isocoma pluriflora*)
White snakeroot (*Ageratina altissima*)

Excitation
Alsike clover (*Trifolium hybridum*)
Beta₂ agonists
Black locust (*Robinia pseudoacacia*)
Cocaine
Fluoride
Fumonisins
Opioids
Paraquat and Diquat
Ractopamine

Exercise intolerance
Anticoagulants
Ionophores
Tansy ragwort (*Senecio jacobaea*)
Vitamin D

Facial paralysis
Crotalid snakes (pit vipers)
Fumonisins

Falling
Fumonisins
Methylxanthines

Narrowleaf milkweed (*Asclepias fascicularis*)

Feed refusal
Aflatoxins
Fusaria
Herbicides

Fetal death
Locoweeds

Fetal malformations
Sudangrass (*Sorghum* spp.)

Fever
Blister beetles
Jimsonweed (*Datura stramonium*)
Phosphides
Spiders

Gastrointestinal hemorrhage
Aflatoxins
Anticoagulants
Arsenic
Herbicides
Iron
Nightshades (*Solanum* spp.)
Selenium

Gastrointestinal irritation
Fertilizers
Fusaria
Herbicides
Marijuana
Nightshades (*Solanum* spp.)
Paraquat and Diquat

Gastrointestinal ulcers
Blister beetles
Iron
Nightshades (*Solanum* spp.)
NSAIDs
Phosphides

Gestation, prolonged
Fescue

Goiter
Iodine

Hair abnormalities
Aflatoxins
Alsike clover (*Trifolium hybridum*)
Iodine
Lead
Locoweeds
Pyrethrins and pyrethroid insecticides
Selenium

Head movements
  Antipsychotic agents
  Bisphosphonates
  Dermorphin
  Tremorgenic mycotoxins
Head pressing
  Aflatoxins
  Alsike clover (*Trifolium hybridum*)
  Bromethalin
  Fertilizers
  Fumonisins
  Iron
  Kleingrass (*Panicum coloratum*)
  Pyrrolizidine alkaloids
  Russian knapweed (*Acroptilon repens*)
  Tansy ragwort (*Senecio jacobaea*)
  Yellow star thistle (*Centaurea solstitialis*)
Hematuria
  Anticoagulants
  Arsenic
  Blister beetles
  Cobalt
  Hoary alyssum (*Berteroa incana*)
  Oak (*Quercus* spp.)
  Paraquat and Diquat
  Pentachlorophenol (PCP)
  Red maple (*Acer rubrum*)
Hemoconcentration
  Amitraz
  Arsenic
  Blister beetles
  Paraquat and Diquat
  Pyrethrins and pyrethroid insecticides
Hemorrhage
  Anticoagulants
  see also Gastrointestinal hemorrhage;
    Pulmonary hemorrhage
Hemothorax
  Anticoagulants
Hepatopathy
  Aflatoxins
  Alsike clover (*Trifolium hybridum*)
  Blue-green algae
  Fumonisins
  Iron
  Kleingrass (*Panicum coloratum*)
  Lantana (*Lantana camara*)
  NSAIDs
  Phosphides
  Pyrrolizidine alkaloids
  SARMs
  Tansy ragwort (*Senecio jacobaea*)
  White snakeroot (*Ageratina altissima*)
Hyperactivity
  Carbamate pesticides
  Jimsonweed (*Datura stramonium*)
  Levothyroxine
  Methamphetamine/Amphetamine
  Organophosphate pesticides
  Ractopamine
Hyperammonemia
  Black locust (*Robinia pseudoacacia*)
  Blue-green algae
  Pyrrolizidine alkaloids
  Tansy ragwort (*Senecio jacobaea*)
Hyperbilirubinemia
  Aflatoxins
  Alsike clover (*Trifolium hybridum*)
  Arsenic
  Blue-green algae
  Lantana (*Lantana camara*)
  Paraquat and Diquat
  Pyrrolizidine alkaloids
Hypercalcemia
  Cholecalciferol
  Day blooming jessamine (*Cestrum diurnum*)
  Vitamin D
Hyperemia
  Arsenic
  Blister beetles
  Selenium
Hyperesthesia
  Lead
  Strychnine
Hyperexcitability *see* **Excitation**
Hyperglycemia
  Amitraz
  Arsenic
  Beta$_2$ agonists
  Blister beetles
  Boxelder (*Acer negundo*)
  Growth hormone
  Sodium fluoroacetate (Compound 1080)
  Zilpaterol
Hyperkalemia
  Blue-green algae

Cardiotoxic plants
Oleander
Hypermetria
Antipsychotic agents
Phosphides
Hyperphosphatemia
Day-blooming jessamine (*Cestrum diurnum*)
Vitamin D
Hypersalivation *see* **Salivation, excessive**
Hypertension
Cocaine
Growth hormone
Methamphetamine/Amphetamine
Ractopamine
Synthetic cannabinoids
Hyperthermia
Aflatoxins
Cocaine
Fescue
Methamphetamine/Amphetamine
Pentachlorophenol (PCP)
Phosphides
Pyrethrins and pyrethroid insecticides
Sodium chloride
Strychnine
Synthetic cannabinoids
Hypoalbuminemia
Anticoagulants
NSAIDs
Pyrrolizidine alkaloids
Tansy ragwort (*Senecio jacobaea*)
Hypocalcemia
Bisphosphonates
Black locust (*Robinia pseudoacacia*)
Blister beetles
Cobalt
Oak (*Quercus* spp.)
Sodium fluoroacetate (Compound 1080)
Hypochloremia
Arsenic
Beta$_2$ agonists
Ractopamine
Zilpaterol
Hypoglycemia
Blue-green algae
Growth hormone
Opioids
Hypokalemia

Arsenic
Blister beetles
Dermorphin
Medroxyprogesterone acetate (MPA)
Oleander
Synthetic cannabinoids
Hypomagnesemia
Blister beetles
Oak (*Quercus* spp.)
Hyponatremia
Arsenic
Beta$_2$ agonists
Dermorphin
Ractopamine
Zilpaterol
Hypoproteinemia
Anticoagulants
NSAIDs
Oak (*Quercus* spp.)
Pyrrolizidine alkaloids
Hyposthenuria
Blister beetles
Cholecalciferol
Oak (*Quercus* spp.)
Hypotension
Amitraz
Anticoagulants
Carbon monoxide
Cyanide
Death camas (*Zigadenus* spp.)
Elapids (coral snakes)
Growth Hormone
Hydrogen sulfide
Oleander
Opioids
Rhododendron spp.
Spiders
Hypothermia
Amitraz
Death camas (*Zigadenus* spp.)
Opioids
Hypovolemia
Blister beetles
Blue-green algae
Herbicides
Hoary alyssum (*Berteroa incana*)
Iron

Hypoxemia
  Smoke

Icterus
  Aflatoxins
  Alsike clover (*Trifolium hybridum*)
  Fumonisins
  Iron
  Kleingrass (*Panicum coloratum*)
  Lantana (*Lantana camara*)
  Oak (*Quercus* spp.)
  Pyrrolizidine alkaloids
  Tansy ragwort (*Senecio jacobaea*)

Ileus
  Jimsonweed (*Datura stramonium*)
  Phosphides

Impaction, intestinal
  Amitraz
  Lead
  Opioids
  Pyrrolizidine alkaloids
  Tansy ragwort (*Senecio jacobaea*)

Inappetence
  Blister beetles
  Bromethalin
  Cholecalciferol
  Jimsonweed (*Datura stramonium*)
  Lantana (*Lantana camara*)
  Oak (*Quercus* spp.)
  Rayless goldenrod (*Isocoma pluriflora*)
  Tansy ragwort (*Senecio jacobaea*)
  White snakeroot (*Ageratina altissima*)
  Zilpaterol

Incoordination
  Alsike clover (*Trifolium hybridum*)
  Fertilizers
  Fescue
  Hemlock
  Methylxanthine
  Sudangrass (*Sorghum* spp.)
  Yew (*Taxus* spp.)

Irritability
  Nightshades (*Solanum* spp.)
  Paraquat and Diquat
  Smoke
  Synthetic cannabinoids

Jaundice
  Lantana (*Lantana camara*)
  Pyrrolizidine alkaloids

Joint swelling
  Lead

Keratitis
  Alsike clover (*Trifolium hybridum*)

Kyphosis
  Day blooming jessamine (*Cestrum diurnum*)
  Vitamin D

Lacrimation, excessive
  Alsike clover (*Trifolium hybridum*)
  Blue-green algae
  Carbamate pesticides
  Hemlock
  Herbicides
  Hydrogen sulfide
  Iodine
  Organophosphate pesticides
  Slaframine

Lameness
  Anticoagulants
  Crotalid snakes (pit vipers)
  Day blooming jessamine (*Cestrum diurnum*)
  Fluoride
  Lead
  Selenium

Laminitis
  Beta$_2$ agonists
  Black locust (*Robinia pseudoacacia*)
  Black walnut (*Juglans nigra*)
  Blister beetles
  Fescue
  Hoary alyssum (*Berteroa incana*)
  Red maple (*Acer rubrum*)
  Zilpaterol

Laryngeal hemiplegia
  Lead
  Tansy ragwort (*Senecio jacobaea*)

Lethargy
  Anticoagulants
  Bisphosphonates
  Blister beetles
  Blue-green algae
  Boxelder (*Acer negundo*)

Ionophores
Iron
Lantana (*Lantana camara*)
NSAIDs
Pyrrolizidine alkaloids
Red maple (*Acer rubrum*)
Russian knapweed (*Acroptilon repens*)
Selenium
Slaframine
Sodium chloride
Yellow star thistle (*Centaurea solstitialis*)
Liver damage *see* **Hepatopathy**

Mania
Pyrrolizidine alkaloids
Tansy ragwort (*Senecio jacobaea*)
Melena
Anticoagulants
Iron
Methemoglobinemia
Iron
Phosphides
Red maple (*Acer rubrum*)
Smoke
Miosis
Antipsychotic agents
Carbamate pesticides
Organophosphate pesticides
Synthetic cannabinoids
Muscle atrophy
Ionophores
Locoweeds
Muscle fasciculations
Antipsychotic agents
Benzodiazepines
Beta$_2$ agonists
Cobalt
Lead
Phosphides
Tremorgenic mycotoxins
Muscle twitching
Carbamate pesticides
Organophosphate pesticides
Muscle weakness
Aflatoxins
Alsike clover (*Trifolium hybridum*)
Amitraz

Benzodiazepines
Black locust (*Robinia pseudoacacia*)
Blue-green algae
Botulism neurotoxin
Boxelder (*Acer negundo*)
Cardiotoxic plants
Cyanide
Death camas (*Zigadenus* spp.)
Fluoride
Hemlock
Ionophores
Lead
Narrowleaf milkweed (*Asclepias fascicularis*)
Nightshades (*Solanum*)
NSAIDs
Oak (*Quercus* spp.)
Oleander
Pentachlorophenol (PCP)
Pyrrolizidine alkaloids
Rayless goldenrod (*Isocoma pluriflora*)
Red maple (*Acer rubrum*)
Rhododendron spp.
Selenium
Sodium chloride
Sodium fluoroacetate (Compound 1080)
White snakeroot (*Ageratina altissima*)
Yew (*Taxus* spp.)
Mydriasis
Amitraz
Carbamate pesticides
Cocaine
Hemlock
Jimsonweed (*Datura stramonium*)
Narrowleaf milkweed (*Asclepias fascicularis*)
Nightshades (*Solanum*)
Organophosphate pesticides
Synthetic cannabinoids
Myoglobinuria
Boxelder (*Acer negundo*)
Rayless goldenrod (*Isocoma pluriflora*)
Strychnine
White snakeroot (*Ageratina altissima*)

Nasal discharge
Ammonia
Carbamate pesticides
Iodine

Nasal discharge (*continued*)
  Organophosphate pesticides
  Rhododendron spp.
  Smoke
Nausea
  Hemlock
  Hydrogen sulfide
  Nightshades (*Solanum*)
Necrosis
  Arsenic
  Crotalid snakes (pit vipers)
  Fusaria
  Paraquat and Diquat
  Spiders
Nephrotoxicity
  Gabapentin
  Paraquat and Diquat
  Pyrethrins and pyrethroid insecticides
  see also Acute kidney injury; Azotemia; Renal failure
Nystagmus
  Anticoagulants
  Bisphosphonates
  Bromethalin
  Synthetic cannabinoids

Oliguria
  Arsenic
  Paraquat and Diquat
Opportunistic infections
  Pentachlorophenol (PCP)
Oral ulcers
  Herbicides
  NSAIDs
  Paraquat and Diquat

Paralysis
  Blue-green algae
  Botulism neurotoxin
  Bromethalin
  Carbamate pesticides
  Fumonisins
  Hemlock
  Nightshades (*Solanum*)
  Organophosphate pesticides
  Spiders
Paspalum staggers
  Tremorgenic mycotoxins

Peripheral neuropathy
  Lead
Petechiae
  Aflatoxins
  Fumonisins
  Hoary alyssum (*Berteroa incana*)
  Red maple (*Acer rubrum*)
Photosensitization
  Alsike clover (*Trifolium hybridum*)
  Blue-green algae
  Hydrogen sulfide
  Jimsonweed (*Datura stramonium*)
  Kleingrass (*Panicum coloratum*)
  Pyrrolizidine alkaloids
  Tansy ragwort (*Senecio jacobaea*)
Pneumothorax
  Smoke
Polydipsia
  Herbicides
  Oak (*Quercus* spp.)
Polyuria
  Bisphosphonates
  Blister beetles
  Cholecalciferol
  Day blooming jessamine (*Cestrum diurnum*)
  Herbicides
  Oak (*Quercus* spp.)
  Slaframine
Pregnancy abnormalities
  Fescue
Priapism
  Antipsychotic agents
Proteinuria
  Anticoagulants
  Arsenic
  Ionophores
  Lead
  Oak (*Quercus* spp.)
  Paraquat and Diquat
  Pyrethrins and pyrethroid insecticides
  Red maple (*Acer rubrum*)
  Zilpaterol
Pruritus
  Alsike clover (*Trifolium hybridum*)
  Spiders
Ptyalism *see* Salivation, excessive
Pulmonary edema
  Arsenic

Carbamate pesticides
Death camas (Zigadenus spp.)
Hydrogen sulfide
Oleander
Paraquat
Phosphides
Pyrrolizidine alkaloids
Selenium
Smoke
Tansy ragwort (Senecio jacobaea)
Yew (Taxus spp.)

Pulmonary hemorrhage
Anticoagulants
Cocaine
Death camas (Zigadenus spp.)
Levothyroxine
Paraquat and Diquat
Pyrrolizidine alkaloids
Tansy ragwort (Senecio jacobaea)

Pyrexia
Beta$_2$ agonists
Black walnut (Juglans nigra)
Red maple (Acer rubrum)

Recumbency
Arsenic
Benzodiazepines
Botulism neurotoxin
Boxelder (Acer negundo)
Hemlock
Narrowleaf milkweed (Asclepias fascicularis)
Nightshades (Solanum)
Rayless goldenrod (Isocoma pluriflora)
Sodium fluoroacetate (Compound 1080)
Sudangrass (Sorghum spp.)
White snakeroot (Ageratina altissima)

Red bag presentation
Fescue

Renal failure
Bisphosphonates
Cholecalciferol
Spiders
See also Acute kidney injury; Nephrotoxicity; Azotemia

Renal tubular necrosis
Aflatoxins
Arsenic
Blue-green algae

Herbicides
NSAIDs
Pentachlorophenol (PCP)
Rayless goldenrod (Isocoma pluriflora)
White snakeroot (Ageratina altissima)

Respiratory depression
Benzodiazepines
Bromethalin
Elapids (coral snakes)
Opioids
Rhododendron spp.

Respiratory distress
Antipsychotic agents
Crotalid snakes (pit vipers)
Cyanide
Fertilizers
Smoke
Strychnine

Respiratory paralysis
Hydrogen sulfide
Strychnine

Restlessness
Anticoagulants
Beta$_2$ agonists
Carbamate pesticides
Organophosphate pesticides
Pentachlorophenol (PCP)
Zilpaterol

Retained fetal membranes
Fescue

Retching
Death camas (Zigadenus spp.)
Synthetic cannabinoids

Rhabdomyolysis
Beta$_2$ agonists
Blister beetles
Boxelder (Acer negundo)
Cocaine
Crotalid snakes (pit vipers)
Gabapentin
Rayless goldenrod (Isocoma pluriflora)
Synthetic cannabinoids
White snakeroot (Ageratina altissima)

Ryegrass staggers
Tremorgenic mycotoxins

Salivation, excessive
  Arsenic
  Blister beetles
  Blue-green algae
  Carbamate pesticides
  Cardiotoxic plants
  Death camas (*Zigadenus* spp.)
  Fluoride
  Hemlock
  Herbicides
  Nightshades (*Solanum*)
  Organophosphate pesticides
  Pyrethrins and pyrethroid insecticides
  Rhododendron spp.
  Slaframine
  Strychnine
Sedation
  Amitraz
  Benzodiazepines
  Dermorphin
  Gabapentin
Seizures
  Aflatoxins
  Amitraz
  Bromethalin
  Carbamate pesticides
  Carbon monoxide
  Cardiotoxic plants
  Cocaine
  Cyanide
  Fertilizers
  Fluoride
  Fumonisins
  Hemlock
  Hydrogen sulfide
  Jimsonweed (*Datura stramonium*)
  Lead
  Narrowleaf milkweed (*Asclepias fascicularis*)
  Oleander
  Opioids
  Organophosphate pesticides
  Pentachlorophenol (PCP)
  Phosphides
  Pyrethrins and pyrethroid insecticides
  Smoke
  Sodium chloride
  Spiders
  Strychnine
  Synthetic cannabinoids
  Yew (*Taxus* spp.)
Somnolence
  Aflatoxins
  Amitraz
  Fumonisins
  Tansy ragwort (*Senecio jacobaea*)
Stiffness
  Blister beetles
  Boxelder (*Acer negundo*)
  Carbamate pesticides
  Cholecalciferol
  Day blooming jessamine (*Cestrum diurnum*)
  Fluoride
  Lead
  Organophosphate pesticides
  Pentachlorophenol (PCP)
  Ractopamine
  Rayless goldenrod (*Isocoma pluriflora*)
  Slaframine
  Strychnine
  Tremorgenic mycotoxins
  Vitamin D
  White snakeroot (*Ageratina altissima*)
Stillbirth
  Fescue
Sweating
  Amitraz
  Antipsychotic agents
  Beta$_2$ agonists
  Boxelder (*Acer negundo*)
  Carbamate pesticides
  Cardiotoxic plants
  Dermorphin
  Ionophores
  Methylxanthines
  Narrowleaf milkweed (*Asclepias fascicularis*)
  Organophosphate pesticides
  Phosphides
  Ractopamine
  Rayless goldenrod (*Isocoma pluriflora*)
  Sodium fluoroacetate (Compound 1080)
  White snakeroot (*Ageratina altissima*)
  Zilpaterol
Swelling *see* **Edema**

Tachycardia
  Amitraz

Anticoagulants
Beta$_2$ agonists
Black walnut (*Juglans nigra*)
Blister beetles
Boxelder (*Acer negundo*)
Carbamate pesticides
Carbon monoxide
Cardiotoxic plants
Cholecalciferol
Cobalt
Cocaine
Fertilizers
Hemlock
Hoary alyssum (*Berteroa incana*)
Iodine
Jimsonweed (*Datura stramonium*)
Levothyroxine
Methamphetamine/Amphetamine
Oak (*Quercus* spp.)
Oleander
Organophosphate pesticides
Phosphides
Ractopamine
Rayless goldenrod (*Isocoma pluriflora*)
Red maple (*Acer rubrum*)
Rhododendron spp.
Selenium
Smoke
Sodium chloride
Sodium fluoroacetate (Compound 1080)
Synthetic cannabinoids
Vitamin D
White snakeroot (*Ageratina altissima*)
Zilpaterol
see also Arrhythmias

Tachypnea
Amitraz
Ammonia
Black walnut (*Juglans nigra*)
Boxelder (*Acer negundo*)
Carbamate pesticides
Carbon monoxide
Cardiotoxic plants
Dermorphin
Hemlock
Hoary alyssum (*Berteroa incana*)
Hydrogen sulfide
Iodine

Jimsonweed (*Datura stramonium*)
Levothyroxine
Medroxyprogesterone acetate (MPA)
Methamphetamine/Amphetamine
Organophosphate pesticides
Paraquat and Diquat
Pentachlorophenol (PCP)
Phosphides
Smoke

Teratogenicity
Locoweeds

Thrombocytopenia
Anticoagulants
Crotalid snakes (pit vipers)
Iron
Pentachlorophenol (PCP)
Spiders

Tongue weakness
Botulism neurotoxin

Trembling
Death camas (*Zigadenus* spp.)
Narrowleaf milkweed (*Asclepias fascicularis*)
Nightshades (*Solanum*)
Yew (*Taxus* spp.)

Tremors
Aflatoxins
Anticoagulants
Arsenic
Beta$_2$ agonists
Blister beetles
Blue-green algae
Boxelder (*Acer negundo*)
Bromethalin
Cardiotoxic plants
Cobalt
Cyanide
Fertilizers
Fumonisins
Hemlock
Hydrogen sulfide
Ionophores
Jimsonweed (*Datura stramonium*)
Locoweeds
Methamphetamine/Amphetamine
Methylxanthines
Oleander
Phosphides
Pyrethrins and pyrethroid insecticides

Tremors (*continued*)
    Ractopamine
    Rayless goldenrod (*Isocoma pluriflora*)
    Sodium chloride
    Spiders
    Synthetic cannabinoids
    Tremorgenic mycotoxins
    White snakeroot (*Ageratina altissima*)
    Zilpaterol

Ulcers
    Spiders
    see also Gastrointestinal ulcers; Oral ulcers

Urination, excessive
    Blue-green algae
    Carbamate pesticides
    Herbicides
    Organophosphate pesticides

Vomiting
    Fluoride
    Hemlock

Weakness *see* **Muscle weakness**

Weight loss
    Aflatoxins
    Anticoagulants
    Cholecalciferol
    Day blooming jessamine (*Cestrum diurnum*)
    Hydrogen sulfide
    Iodine
    Kleingrass (*Panicum coloratum*)
    Lead
    Levothyroxine
    Locoweeds
    Pentachlorophenol (PCP)
    Pyrrolizidine alkaloids
    Tansy ragwort (*Senecio jacobaea*)
    Vitamin D

Yawning
    Alsike clover (*Trifolium hybridum*)
    Pyrrolizidine alkaloids
    Tansy ragwort (*Senecio jacobaea*)